ACP | MKSAP® 18

Medical Knowledge Self-Assessment Program®

Rheumatology

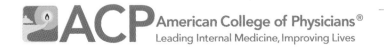
American College of Physicians®
Leading Internal Medicine, Improving Lives

Welcome to the Rheumatology Section of MKSAP 18!

In these pages, you will find updated information on approaches to the patient with rheumatologic disease, principles of therapeutics, rheumatoid arthritis, osteoarthritis, systemic lupus erythematosus, infectious arthritis, inflammatory myopathies, systemic sclerosis, systemic vasculitis, autoinflammatory diseases, genetic diseases of connective tissue, and other clinical challenges. All of these topics are uniquely focused on the needs of generalists and subspecialists *outside* of rheumatology.

The core content of MKSAP 18 has been developed as in previous editions—all essential information that is newly researched and written in 11 topic areas of internal medicine—created by dozens of leading generalists and subspecialists and guided by certification and recertification requirements, emerging knowledge in the field, and user feedback. MKSAP 18 also contains 1200 all-new peer-reviewed, psychometrically validated, multiple-choice questions (MCQs) for self-assessment and study, including **96** in Rheumatology. MKSAP 18 continues to include *High Value Care* (HVC) recommendations, based on the concept of balancing clinical benefit with costs and harms, with associated MCQs illustrating these principles and HVC Key Points called out in the text. Internists practicing in the hospital setting can easily find comprehensive *Hospitalist*-focused content and MCQs, specially designated in blue and with the ⊞ symbol.

If you purchased MKSAP 18 Complete, you also have access to MKSAP 18 Digital, with additional tools allowing you to customize your learning experience. MKSAP Digital includes regular text updates with new, practice-changing information, 200 new self-assessment questions, and enhanced custom-quiz options. MKSAP Complete also includes more than 1200 electronic, adaptive learning–enhanced flashcards for quick review of important concepts, as well as an updated and enhanced version of Virtual Dx, MKSAP's image-based self-assessment tool. As before, MKSAP 18 Digital is optimized for use on your mobile devices, with iOS- and Android-based apps allowing you to sync between your apps and online account and submit for CME credits and MOC points online.

Please visit us at the MKSAP Resource Site (mksap.acponline.org) to find out how we can help you study, earn CME credit and MOC points, and stay up to date.

On behalf of the many internists who have offered their time and expertise to create the content for MKSAP 18 and the editorial staff who work to bring this material to you in the best possible way, we are honored that you have chosen to use MKSAP 18 and appreciate any feedback about the program you may have. Please feel free to send any comments to mksap_editors@acponline.org.

Sincerely,

Patrick Alguire

Patrick C. Alguire, MD, FACP
Editor-in-Chief
Senior Vice President Emeritus
Medical Education Division
American College of Physicians

Rheumatology

Committee

Michael Pillinger, MD, FACP, Section Editor[2]
Professor of Medicine
Biochemistry and Molecular Pharmacology
Director of Rheumatology Training
New York University School of Medicine/NYU Langone
    Health
Section Chief, Rheumatology
New York Harbor Health Care System, New York Campus
United States Department of Veterans Affairs
New York, New York

Aryeh M. Abeles, MD[2]
Associate Clinical Professor of Medicine
Division of Rheumatology
University of Connecticut Health Center
Farmington, Connecticut

Gregory C. Gardner, MD, FACP[1]
Gilliland-Henderson Professor of Medicine
Fellowship Program Director
Division of Rheumatology
University of Washington
Seattle, Washington

Sharon L. Kolasinski, MD, FACP[1]
Professor of Clinical Medicine
Division of Rheumatology
University of Pennsylvania Perelman School of Medicine
Director, Rheumatology, Penn Musculoskeletal Center
Philadelphia, Pennsylvania

Svetlana Krasnokutsky Samuels, MD, MSci[2]
Assistant Professor of Medicine
Division of Rheumatology
New York University School of Medicine/NYU Langone
    Health
New York, New York

Bonita S. Libman, MD, FACP[2]
Professor of Medicine
Division Chief and Fellowship Program Director
Division of Rheumatology and Clinical Immunology
The Robert Larner MD College of Medicine at the University
    of Vermont Medical Center
Burlington, Vermont

Vikas Majithia, MD, MPH, FACP[2]
Professor of Internal Medicine
Division Chief and Fellowship Program Director
Division of Rheumatology, Department of Medicine
University of Mississippi Medical Center
Jackson, Mississippi

Editor-in-Chief

Patrick C. Alguire, MD, FACP[2]
Senior Vice President Emeritus, Medical Education
American College of Physicians
Philadelphia, Pennsylvania

Deputy Editor

Robert L. Trowbridge, Jr., MD, FACP[2]
Associate Professor of Medicine
Tufts University School of Medicine
Maine Medical Center
Portland, Maine

Rheumatology Reviewers

Grant W. Cannon, MD, MACP[2]
Ana M. Cilursu, MD, FACP[1]
Gautam A. Deshpande, MD, FACP[2]
LTC Jess D. Edison, MD, FACP[1]
Amr F. Edrees, MD, FACP[1]
Nkechinyere Emejuaiwe, MD, FACP[1]
Luis R. Espinoza, MD, MACP[1]
Steven Eyanson, MD, FACP[1]
Mitchell D. Forman, DO, MACP[1]
James G. Freeman, MD, FACP[1]

Hospital Medicine Rheumatology Reviewers

Nihar N. Shah, MD, FACP[1]
Maria E. Tudor, DO, FACP[1]

Rheumatology ACP Editorial Staff

Megan Zborowski, Senior Staff Editor, Self-Assessment and Educational Programs

Margaret Wells, Director, Self-Assessment and Educational Programs

Becky Krumm, Managing Editor, Self-Assessment and Educational Programs

ACP Principal Staff

Davoren Chick, MD, FACP[2]
Senior Vice President, Medical Education

Patrick C. Alguire, MD, FACP[2]
Senior Vice President Emeritus, Medical Education

Sean McKinney[1]
Vice President, Medical Education

Margaret Wells[1]
Director, Self-Assessment and Educational Programs

Becky Krumm[1]
Managing Editor

Valerie Dangovetsky[1]
Administrator

Ellen McDonald, PhD[1]
Senior Staff Editor

Megan Zborowski[1]
Senior Staff Editor

Randy Hendrickson[1]
Production Administrator/Editor

Julia Nawrocki[1]
Digital Content Associate/Editor

Linnea Donnarumma[1]
Staff Editor

Chuck Emig[1]
Staff Editor

Jackie Twomey[1]
Staff Editor

Joysa Winter[1]
Staff Editor

Kimberly Kerns[1]
Administrative Coordinator

Disclosure of relationships with any entity producing, marketing, reselling, or distributing health care goods or services consumed by, or used on, patients.

Aryeh M. Abeles, MD
Consultantship
Celgene
Speakers Bureau
AbbVie

Patrick C. Alguire, MD, FACP
Royalties
UpToDate

Grant W. Cannon, MD, MACP
Research Grants/Contracts
Amgen

Davoren Chick, MD, FACP
Royalties
Wolters Kluwer Publishing
Consultantship
EBSCO Health's DynaMed Plus
Other
Owner and sole proprietor of Coding 101 LLC; research consultant (spouse) for Vedanta Biosciences Inc.

Gautam A. Deshpande, MD, FACP
Honoraria
Astellas Pharma US Inc., Daiichi Sankyo Inc.

Svetlana Krasnokutsky Samuels, MD, MSci
Consultantship
Crealta Holdings LLC/Horizon Pharma plc, Ironwood Pharmaceuticals Inc.

Bonita S. Libman, MD, FACP
Research Grants/Contracts
Human Genome Sciences/GlaxoSmithKline plc, Novartis, Pfizer Inc.

Vikas Majithia, MD, MPH, FACP
Research Grants
Human Genome Sciences, GlaxoSmithKline plc

Michael Pillinger, MD, FACP
Research Grants/Contracts
Takeda Inc.
Consultantship/Speakers Bureau
AstraZeneca, Crealta Holdings LLC/Horizon Pharma plc, Ironwood Pharmaceuticals Inc., SOBI

Robert L. Trowbridge, Jr., MD, FACP
Consultantship
American Board of Internal Medicine

Acknowledgments

The American College of Physicians (ACP) gratefully acknowledges the special contributions to the development and production of the 18th edition of the Medical Knowledge Self-Assessment Program® (MKSAP® 18) made by the following people:

Graphic Design: Barry Moshinski (Director, Graphic Services), Michael Ripca (Graphics Technical Administrator), and Jennifer Gropper (Graphic Designer).

Production/Systems: Dan Hoffmann (Director, Information Technology), Scott Hurd (Manager, Content Systems), Neil Kohl (Senior Architect), and Chris Patterson (Senior Architect).

MKSAP 18 Digital: Under the direction of Steven Spadt (Senior Vice President, Technology), the digital version of MKSAP 18 was developed within the ACP's Digital Products and Services Department, led by Brian Sweigard (Director, Digital Products and Services). Other members of the team included Dan Barron (Senior Web Application Developer/Architect), Chris Forrest (Senior Software Developer/Design Lead), Kathleen Hoover (Senior Web Developer), Kara Regis (Manager, User Interface Design and Development), Brad Lord (Senior Web Application Developer), and John McKnight (Senior Web Developer).

The College also wishes to acknowledge that many other persons, too numerous to mention, have contributed to the production of this program. Without their dedicated efforts, this program would not have been possible.

MKSAP Resource Site (mksap.acponline.org)

The MKSAP Resource Site (mksap.acponline.org) is a continually updated site that provides links to MKSAP 18 online answer sheets for print subscribers; access to MKSAP 18 Digital; Board Basics® e-book access instructions; information on Continuing Medical Education (CME), Maintenance of Certification (MOC), and international Continuing Professional Development (CPD) and MOC; errata; and other new information.

International MOC/CPD

For information and instructions on submission of international MOC/CPD, please go to the MKSAP Resource Site (mksap.acponline.org).

Continuing Medical Education

The American College of Physicians is accredited by the Accreditation Council for Continuing Medical Education (ACCME) to provide continuing medical education for physicians.

The American College of Physicians designates this enduring material, MKSAP 18, for a maximum of 275 *AMA PRA Category 1 Credits*™. Physicians should claim only the credit commensurate with the extent of their participation in the activity.

Up to 22 *AMA PRA Category 1 Credits*™ are available from July 31, 2018, to July 31, 2021, for the MKSAP 18 Rheumatology section.

Learning Objectives

The learning objectives of MKSAP 18 are to:

- Close gaps between actual care in your practice and preferred standards of care, based on best evidence
- Diagnose disease states that are less common and sometimes overlooked and confusing
- Improve management of comorbid conditions that can complicate patient care
- Determine when to refer patients for surgery or care by subspecialists
- Pass the ABIM Certification Examination
- Pass the ABIM Maintenance of Certification Examination

Target Audience

- General internists and primary care physicians
- Subspecialists who need to remain up to date in internal medicine
- Residents preparing for the certifying examination in internal medicine
- Physicians preparing for maintenance of certification in internal medicine (recertification)

ABIM Maintenance of Certification

Check the MKSAP Resource Site (mksap.acponline.org) for the latest information on how MKSAP tests can be used to apply to the American Board of Internal Medicine (ABIM) for Maintenance of Certification (MOC) points following completion of the CME activity.

Successful completion of the CME activity, which includes participation in the evaluation component, enables the participant to earn up to 275 medical knowledge MOC points in the ABIM's MOC program. It is the CME activity provider's responsibility to submit participant completion information to ACCME for the purpose of granting MOC credit.

Earn Instantaneous CME Credits or MOC Points Online

Print subscribers can enter their answers online to earn instantaneous CME credits or MOC points. You can submit your answers using online answer sheets that are provided at mksap.acponline.org, where a record of your MKSAP 18 credits will be available. To earn CME credits or to apply for MOC points, you need to answer all of the questions in a test and earn a score of at least 50% correct (number of correct answers divided by the total number of questions). Please note that if you are applying for MOC points, you must also enter your birth date and ABIM candidate number.

Take either of the following approaches:

1. Use the printed answer sheet at the back of this book to record your answers. Go to mksap.acponline.org, access the appropriate online answer sheet, transcribe your answers, and submit your test for instantaneous CME credits or MOC points. There is no additional fee for this service.
2. Go to mksap.acponline.org, access the appropriate online answer sheet, directly enter your answers, and submit your test for instantaneous CME credits or MOC points. There is no additional fee for this service.

Earn CME Credits or MOC Points by Mail or Fax

Pay a $20 processing fee per answer sheet and submit the printed answer sheet at the back of this book by mail or fax, as instructed on the answer sheet. Make sure you calculate your score and enter your birth date and ABIM candidate number, and fax the answer sheet to 215-351-2799 or mail the answer sheet to Member and Customer Service, American College of Physicians, 190 N. Independence Mall West, Philadelphia, PA 19106-1572, using the courtesy envelope provided in your MKSAP 18 slipcase. You will need your 10-digit order number and 8-digit ACP ID number, which are printed on your packing slip. Please allow 4 to 6 weeks for your score report to be emailed back to you. Be sure to include your email address for a response.

If you do not have a 10-digit order number and 8-digit ACP ID number, or if you need help creating a username and password to access the MKSAP 18 online answer sheets, go to mksap.acponline.org or email custserv@acponline.org.

Disclosure Policy

It is the policy of the American College of Physicians (ACP) to ensure balance, independence, objectivity, and scientific rigor in all of its educational activities. To this end, and consistent with the policies of the ACP and the Accreditation Council for Continuing Medical Education (ACCME), contributors to all ACP continuing medical education activities are required to disclose all relevant financial relationships with any entity producing, marketing, re-selling, or distributing health care goods or services consumed by, or used on, patients. Contributors are required to use generic names in the discussion of therapeutic options and are required to identify any unapproved, off-label, or investigative use of commercial products or devices. Where a trade name is used, all available trade names for the same product type are also included. If trade-name products manufactured by companies with whom contributors have relationships are discussed, contributors are asked to provide evidence-based citations in support of the discussion. The information is reviewed by the committee responsible for producing this text. If necessary, adjustments to topics or contributors' roles in content development are made to balance the discussion. Further, all readers of this text are asked to evaluate the content for evidence of commercial bias and send any relevant comments to mksap_editors@acponline.org so that future decisions about content and contributors can be made in light of this information.

Resolution of Conflicts

To resolve all conflicts of interest and influences of vested interests, ACP's content planners used best evidence and updated clinical care guidelines in developing content, when such evidence and guidelines were available. All content underwent review by peer reviewers not on the committee to ensure that the material was balanced and unbiased. Contributors' disclosure information can be found with the list of contributors' names and those of ACP principal staff listed in the beginning of this book.

Hospital-Based Medicine

For the convenience of subscribers who provide care in hospital settings, content that is specific to the hospital setting has been highlighted in blue. Hospital icons (⬛) highlight where the hospital-only content begins, continues over more than one page, and ends.

High Value Care Key Points

Key Points in the text that relate to High Value Care concepts (that is, concepts that discuss balancing clinical benefit with costs and harms) are designated by the HVC icon [**HVC**].

Educational Disclaimer

The editors and publisher of MKSAP 18 recognize that the development of new material offers many opportunities for error. Despite our best efforts, some errors may persist in print. Drug dosage schedules are, we believe, accurate and in accordance with current standards. Readers are advised, however, to ensure that the recommended dosages in MKSAP 18 concur with the information provided in the product information material. This is especially important in cases of new, infrequently used, or highly toxic drugs. Application of the information in MKSAP 18 remains the professional responsibility of the practitioner.

The primary purpose of MKSAP 18 is educational. Information presented, as well as publications, technologies, products, and/or services discussed, is intended to inform subscribers about the knowledge, techniques, and experiences of the contributors. A diversity of professional opinion exists, and the views of the contributors are their own and not those of the ACP. Inclusion of any material in the program does not constitute endorsement or recommendation by the ACP. The ACP does not warrant the safety, reliability, accuracy, completeness, or usefulness of and disclaims any and all liability for damages and claims that may result from the use of information, publications, technologies, products, and/or services discussed in this program.

Publisher's Information

Disclaimer Regarding Direct Purchases from Online Retailers

CME and/or MOC for MKSAP 18 is available only if you purchase the program directly from ACP. CME credits and MOC points cannot be awarded to those purchasers who have purchased the program from non-authorized sellers such as Amazon, eBay, or any other such online retailer.

Unauthorized Use of This Book Is Against the Law

MKSAP 18 ISBN: 978-1-938245-47-3
Rheumatology ISBN: 978-1-938245-53-4

Printed in the United States of America.

For order information in the U.S. or Canada call 800-ACP-1915. All other countries call 215-351-2600 (Monday to Friday, 9 AM – 5 PM ET). Fax inquiries to 215-351-2799 or email to custserv@acponline.org.

Errata

Errata for MKSAP 18 will be available through the MKSAP Resource Site at mksap.acponline.org as new information becomes known to the editors.

Table of Contents

Rheumatology High Value Care Recommendations

The American College of Physicians, in collaboration with multiple other organizations, is engaged in a worldwide initiative to promote the practice of High Value Care (HVC). The goals of the HVC initiative are to improve health care outcomes by providing care of proven benefit and reducing costs by avoiding unnecessary and even harmful interventions. The initiative comprises several programs that integrate the important concept of health care value (balancing clinical benefit with costs and harms) for a given intervention into a broad range of educational materials to address the needs of trainees, practicing physicians, and patients.

HVC content has been integrated into MKSAP 18 in several important ways. MKSAP 18 includes HVC-identified key points in the text, HVC-focused multiple choice questions, and, for subscribers to MKSAP Digital, an HVC custom quiz. From the text and questions, we have generated the following list of HVC recommendations that meet the definition below of high value care and bring us closer to our goal of improving patient outcomes while conserving finite resources.

High Value Care Recommendation: A recommendation to choose diagnostic and management strategies for patients in specific clinical situations that balance clinical benefit with cost and harms with the goal of improving patient outcomes.

Below are the High Value Care Recommendations for the Rheumatology section of MKSAP 18.

- An accurate history and a thorough musculoskeletal examination can avoid unnecessary testing.
- Do not obtain antinuclear antibody testing for patients with nonspecific symptoms and a normal clinical examination.
- Do not obtain antinuclear antibody subserology testing without a strong clinical suspicion of an underlying connective tissue disease.
- Plain radiography is usually the first-line imaging test performed in the evaluation of rheumatologic diseases.
- Ultrasonography is an inexpensive means to assess soft-tissue abnormalities, assess disease activity, and assist with tendon or joint injections.
- Acetaminophen is not beneficial for osteoarthritis and lower back pain, even at high doses.
- Topical NSAIDs are beneficial for patients at high risk for toxicity from oral NSAIDs (see Item 20).
- The most useful laboratory studies to aid in the diagnosis of rheumatoid arthritis are rheumatoid factor and anti-cyclic citrullinated peptide antibodies.
- Weight loss can lower the risk for developing osteoarthritis (see Item 78).
- Laboratory testing is usually not necessary to diagnose osteoarthritis.
- A muscle strengthening program is part of the management plan for knee osteoarthritis (see Item 73).
- Arthroscopic surgery is generally not indicated for knee osteoarthritis unless there is a mechanical disorder.
- Nonpharmacologic therapy (education, exercise, psychosocial support) remains a cornerstone of treatment for fibromyalgia.
- Plain radiography of the sacroiliac joints is the first imaging test in patients with suspected ankylosing spondylitis (see Item 94).
- HLA-B27 cannot independently confirm or exclude a diagnosis of spondylitis.
- Antibiotics are not usually effective in treating reactive arthritis.
- Löfgren syndrome (a triad of bilateral hilar lymphadenopathy, erythema nodosum, and migratory polyarthralgia) is highly specific for sarcoidosis, obviating the need for tissue biopsy.
- Plain radiography is the initial radiographic study of choice for osteonecrosis, and MRI is indicated when plain radiographs are normal (see Item 81).

Rheumatology

Approach to the Patient with Rheumatologic Disease

Inflammatory Versus Noninflammatory Pain

The differentiation between inflammatory and noninflammatory signs and symptoms is central to the evaluation of patients with musculoskeletal pain. Autoimmune conditions typically present with inflammation, whereas mechanical or degenerative disorders are characteristically noninflammatory. The cardinal signs of inflammation are pain, erythema, swelling, and warmth; with the exception of pain, noninflammatory conditions usually lack these features. Importantly, patients may simultaneously experience more than one type of pain. **Table 1** compares the features of inflammatory and noninflammatory pain.

The Musculoskeletal Examination

An accurate history and a thorough musculoskeletal physical examination are essential to diagnose and differentiate inflammatory and noninflammatory symptoms and can help to avoid unnecessary testing. Musculoskeletal pain may be articular, periarticular, or referred. Pain with passive range of motion suggests an articular condition, whereas pain with active range of motion suggests a periarticular condition.

See MKSAP 18 General Internal Medicine for more information.

Arthritis

Monoarthritis

Monoarthritis involves a single joint and is classified as acute or chronic. Acute monoarthritis can be noninflammatory (for example, trauma, hemarthrosis, or internal derangement) or inflammatory (for example, crystal induced or infectious). Evaluation for infectious arthritis should be guided by the clinical presentation and examination, but suspicion should always be high. Joint aspiration is usually the most effective means of diagnosing the underlying cause.

Chronic inflammatory monoarthritis (>26 weeks) can be caused by chronic infection (for example, mycobacterial, fungal, or *Borrelia burgdorferi*) or by autoimmune rheumatologic disease. Synovial fluid analysis will confirm inflammation but may be inadequate for diagnosis; assessment for systemic disease (serologies and other laboratory studies) and, in some cases, synovial biopsy may be required.

Chronic noninflammatory monoarthritis is usually caused by osteoarthritis.

TABLE 1. Features of Inflammatory Versus Noninflammatory Pain

Feature	Inflammatory Pain	Noninflammatory Pain
Physical examination findings	Erythema; warmth; soft-tissue swelling; joint effusions; reduced ROM is frequent	Minimal or no warmth; no soft-tissue swelling; bony enlargement and joint effusions may occur in osteoarthritis; reduced ROM may occur
Morning stiffness	>60 min; worsens with immobility	<30 min
Constitutional symptoms	Fever; fatigue; malaise	Generally absent
Synovial fluid	Leukocyte count >2000/μL (2.0 × 10^9/L), predominantly neutrophils in acute inflammation and monocytes in chronic inflammation	Leukocyte count between 200-2000/μL (0.2-2.0 × 10^9/L), predominantly monocytes
Other laboratory findings	Elevated inflammatory markers (ESR, CRP); anemia of chronic disease	Inflammatory markers usually normal or minimally elevated

CRP = C-reactive protein; ESR = erythrocyte sedimentation rate; ROM = range of motion.

Oligoarthritis

Oligoarthritis involves two to four joints, typically in an asymmetric pattern. Acute inflammatory oligoarthritis may be caused by gonorrhea or rheumatic fever. Chronic inflammatory oligoarthritis can be caused by autoimmune conditions such as spondyloarthritis.

Chronic noninflammatory oligoarthritis is usually caused by osteoarthritis.

Polyarthritis

Polyarthritis involves five or more joints. In many cases, it involves the small joints of the hands and/or feet. Acute polyarthritis (<6 weeks in duration) can be caused by viral infections (for example, parvovirus B19, HIV, hepatitis B virus, or rubella) or may be an early manifestation of a chronic inflammatory polyarthritis (>6 weeks in duration) such as rheumatoid arthritis, systemic lupus erythematosus, or psoriatic arthritis.

Soft-Tissue Abnormalities

Common nonarticular sources of musculoskeletal symptoms are the soft tissues (tendons, ligaments, and bursae) around or away from the joints. Isolated tendon and/or ligament involvement is usually suggestive of noninflammatory disorders such as mechanical injury/irritation, overuse, or degeneration (for example, rotator cuff disorders or tennis elbow). Disorders of widespread musculoskeletal pain (such as fibromyalgia) also have symptoms localizing to these structures.

The enthesis is a complex structure at the site of the insertion of a tendon or ligament onto the bone. Inflammation of the enthesis (enthesitis) is highly suggestive of spondyloarthritis. When enthesitis is particularly severe, the inflammation may extend along the associated tendon and local ligaments, resulting in dactylitis ("sausage digits").

See MKSAP 18 General Internal Medicine for more information.

KEY POINTS

HVC
- Joint aspiration is usually the most effective means of diagnosing the underlying cause of acute monoarthritis.
- Chronic inflammatory arthritis can be caused by autoimmune diseases, whereas chronic noninflammatory arthritis is usually caused by osteoarthritis.
- Isolated tendon and/or ligament involvement is usually suggestive of noninflammatory disorders such as mechanical injury/irritation, overuse, or degeneration.
- Inflammation of the enthesis (enthesitis) is highly suggestive of spondyloarthritis.

Extra-Articular Manifestations of Rheumatologic Disease

Constitutional Symptoms

Fever, morning stiffness, and fatigue occur in numerous rheumatologic conditions. Fever is usually low grade but may be high and spiking in some conditions (for example, adult-onset Still disease and autoinflammatory diseases). Morning stiffness lasting more than 60 minutes is most commonly described in rheumatoid arthritis but also occurs in other forms of inflammatory arthritis. Significant and even disabling fatigue is a prominent feature of fibromyalgia and chronic fatigue syndrome.

Skin Involvement

Skin involvement is common in rheumatologic conditions and may go unnoticed by the patient (**Table 2**). Skin involvement may also occur as an adverse effect of medications used to treat rheumatologic conditions, including skin infections secondary to immunosuppressive therapy.

Eye Involvement

Eye involvement in different rheumatologic diseases usually follows fairly distinct patterns, and the location and type of involvement can help narrow the differential diagnosis (**Table 3**). If not quickly recognized and treated, certain forms of eye involvement can have devastating consequences, including permanent loss of vision.

Internal Organ Involvement

Rheumatologic diseases frequently affect internal organs, with different diseases tending to follow characteristic patterns (**Table 4**).

KEY POINT

- Rheumatologic disease can cause constitutional symptoms and extra-articular manifestations affecting the skin, eyes, and internal organs.

Laboratory Studies

Laboratory studies are useful for diagnosing rheumatologic diseases, identifying the extent/severity of involvement, evaluating disease activity, and monitoring therapeutic responses. Because of limited specificity, these tests should always be interpreted in the context of the clinical history and physical examination and should be used with great caution, if at all, in the setting of low pretest probability.

Tests That Measure Inflammation

Erythrocyte Sedimentation Rate

The erythrocyte sedimentation rate (ESR) measures the fall of erythrocytes (mm/h) through anticoagulated plasma. Erythrocytes tend to be negatively charged on their surfaces, leading to repulsion and a prolonged ESR. Fibrinogen and other acute phase reactants neutralize the erythrocytes' surface charges, promoting their ability to settle at a faster rate. Elevated fibrinogen levels and high ESRs are seen in many rheumatologic diseases, as well as in nonrheumatologic inflammatory conditions such as chronic infections and malignancies. The normal ESR increases with age and is usually higher in women. A well-accepted rule of thumb is to

TABLE 2. Dermatologic Manifestations of Rheumatologic Disease

Rheumatologic Disease	Dermatologic Manifestations
Systemic lupus erythematosus	Butterfly (malar) rash; photosensitive rash; discoid lupus erythematosus; subacute cutaneous lupus erythematosus; oral ulcerations (on the tongue/hard palate; usually painless); alopecia; lupus panniculitis (painful, indurated subcutaneous swelling with overlying erythema of the skin)
Dermatomyositis	Gottron papules (erythematous plaques on extensor surfaces of MCP and PIP joints); photodistributed poikiloderma, including shawl sign (over the back and shoulders) and V sign (over the posterior neck/back or neck/upper chest); heliotrope rash (violaceous rash on the upper eyelids); mechanic's hands (hyperkeratotic, fissured skin on the palmar and lateral aspects of fingers); nailfold capillary abnormalities; holster sign (poikilodermic rash along lateral thigh); can occur in the absence of myositis (amyopathic dermatomyositis)
Systemic sclerosis	Skin thickening and hardening; nailfold capillary changes
Vasculitis	Palpable purpura; cutaneous nodules; ulcers; necrosis
Behçet syndrome	Painful oral and genital ulcers; erythema nodosum; acne/folliculitis; pathergy (skin inflammation/ulceration from minor trauma)
Sarcoidosis	Erythema nodosum; infiltrated plaques; maculopapular and papular lesions; nodules; soft infiltrates of the nose (lupus pernio); on blanching with a glass slide, sarcoid skin lesions reveal "apple jelly" discoloration
Psoriatic arthritis	Plaque psoriasis typically on extensor surfaces, umbilicus, gluteal fold, scalp, and behind ears; pustular psoriasis on palms and soles; nail pitting; onychodystrophy
Reactive arthritis	Keratoderma blennorrhagicum (psoriasiform rash on soles, toes, palms); circinate balanitis (psoriasiform rash on penis)
Adult-onset Still disease	Evanescent, salmon-colored rash on trunk and proximal extremities
Rheumatic fever (secondary to streptococcal infection)	Erythema marginatum (annular pink to red nonpruritic rash with central clearing)
Lyme disease	Erythema chronicum migrans (slowly expanding, often annual lesion with central clearing)

MCP = metacarpophalangeal; PIP = proximal interphalangeal.

TABLE 3. Ocular Manifestations of Systemic Inflammatory Disease

Systemic Inflammatory Disease	Ocular Manifestations
Ankylosing spondylitis, reactive arthritis, and inflammatory bowel disease (anterior chamber); sarcoidosis and Behçet syndrome (anterior and/or posterior chamber); granulomatosis with polyangiitis (posterior chamber)	Uveitis (inflammation of the anterior and/or posterior chamber and/or retina)
Rheumatoid arthritis; spondyloarthritis; systemic vasculitis	Episcleritis
Rheumatoid arthritis; relapsing polychondritis; inflammatory bowel disease; systemic vasculitis	Scleritis
Systemic vasculitis; antiphospholipid syndrome	Retinal ischemia
Sjögren syndrome	Dryness of the eyes (keratoconjunctivitis sicca)
Giant cell arteritis	Anterior/posterior ischemic optic neuropathy; central retinal artery occlusion; loss of vision
Sarcoidosis; granulomatosis with polyangiitis	Exophthalmos/retrobulbar inflammatory infiltrate
Reactive arthritis	Conjunctivitis

adjust the upper limit of normal as age in years divided by 2 for men and (age in years + 10)/2 for women.

In addition to inflammatory conditions, elevated ESRs can be seen in pregnancy, diabetes mellitus, and end-stage kidney disease. Due to rheostatic properties, anemia and macrocytosis are also associated with an increased ESR. An excessively low ESR can occur in low fibrinogen states such as liver or heart failure and in conditions promoting rouleaux formation (for example, polycythemia vera). Sickle cell disease and microcytosis (including spherocytosis) may also lower ESR.

A markedly elevated ESR (>100 mm/h) should alert physicians to conditions such as giant cell arteritis, multiple myeloma, metastatic cancer, or other overwhelming inflammatory states (infection or autoimmune disease).

TABLE 4. Internal Organ Involvement in Rheumatologic Disease

Organ	Disease	Type of Involvement
Heart		
	Kawasaki disease	Coronary artery vasculitis
	Systemic sclerosis	Arrhythmia; myocardial fibrosis
	SLE	Pericarditis; valvular disease; myocarditis
	RA	Pericarditis; myocarditis
	Rheumatic fever; antiphospholipid syndrome	Valvular disease
	GCA	Aortic aneurysm/dissection; aortitis; large-vessel obstruction
Lung		
	RA	Serositis; ILD; rheumatoid nodules
	SLE; CTDs; Henoch-Schönlein purpura	Serositis; pneumonitis; pulmonary hemorrhage from vasculitis
	AAV	Pulmonary hemorrhage; cavitary nodules
	Diffuse cutaneous systemic sclerosis	ILD; pulmonary hypertension
	Limited cutaneous systemic sclerosis	Pulmonary hypertension
	Antiphospholipid syndrome	Pulmonary embolism
	Sarcoidosis	Hilar lymphadenopathy; ILD
	Goodpasture syndrome	Pulmonary hemorrhage
Kidney		
	SLE; CTDs; AAV; systemic vasculitis (except PAN)	Glomerulonephritis
	PAN	Renal artery vasculitis; pseudoaneurysms
	Antiphospholipid syndrome	Renal infarct; renal vein thrombosis
	Sjögren syndrome	Acute interstitial nephritis/renal tubular acidosis
	Goodpasture syndrome	Glomerulonephritis
Gastrointestinal System		
	PAN	Mesenteric vasculitis
	Henoch-Schönlein purpura	Intestinal vasculitis and ulcerations
	Diffuse and limited cutaneous systemic sclerosis	Esophageal and small bowel hypomotility
	Behçet syndrome	Mucosal ulcerations
	Familial Mediterranean fever	Peritonitis
Nervous System		
	SLE; CTDs; AAV; systemic vasculitis	Mononeuritis multiplex; peripheral neuropathy
	PACNS	CNS vasculitis

AAV = ANCA-associated vasculitis; CNS = central nervous system; CTD = connective tissue disease; GCA = giant cell arteritis; ILD = interstitial lung disease; PACNS = primary angiitis of the central nervous system; PAN = polyarteritis nodosa; RA = rheumatoid arthritis; SLE = systemic lupus erythematosus.

C-Reactive Protein

C-reactive protein (CRP) is produced by the liver mainly in response to interleukin-6 generated by leukocytes during the inflammatory state. CRP levels and ESR usually follow a common pattern, but CRP is often more rapidly responsive to changes in inflammation. In rheumatologic conditions, CRP is typically elevated 2 to 10 times the normal level; a higher level (especially >10 mg/dL [100 mg/L]) should prompt consideration of an alternative diagnosis such as infection. CRP is thought to be a better marker than ESR in measuring inflammation in spondyloarthritis. In contrast, in some patients with systemic lupus erythematosus (SLE), the CRP may remain normal despite active disease. CRP can be elevated in obesity, and a low CRP can occur with the use of certain antibiotics and interleukin-6 blockers.

Complement

The complement system is an essential part of the immune response, promoting vasodilation, attracting leukocytes, and assisting in the lysis of opsonized bacteria during humoral immunity.

Complement components are acute phase reactants and rise in many inflammatory states. However, in response to immune complex formation diseases (SLE and cryoglobulinemic and urticarial vasculitis) and certain other states, complement cascades are activated, and complement levels fall due to excessive consumption. Paradoxically, genetic deficiency of early complement components may increase the risk for lupus-like autoimmune diseases.

C3 and C4 are the commonly measured complement components. The CH50 assay should not be performed routinely due to cost and limited utility.

Autoantibody Tests

Rheumatologic diseases are commonly associated with autoantibodies, but their presence does not equate with the diagnosis of an underlying condition because they lack specificity and may be seen in other conditions and healthy persons. In commercial laboratories, autoantibody testing has been automated using enzyme-linked immunosorbent assay in a sequential algorithm, which may simplify physician assessment but tends to have reduced sensitivity and specificity.

Rheumatoid factor is an IgM antibody directed against the Fc portion of IgG immunoglobulin. Although characteristically associated with rheumatoid arthritis (RA), rheumatoid factor is present in fewer than 70% of patients with RA and is common in several other diseases. Anti–cyclic citrullinated peptide antibodies are more specific for RA but less sensitive. The presence of both autoantibodies together increases the likelihood of RA.

Antinuclear antibodies (ANA) are directed against nuclear antigens and are traditionally associated with SLE. About one third of the healthy population has a low-titer (1:40) ANA, and 3% to 5% have a titer of 1:160 or more. ANA can also be seen in other autoimmune conditions, infection, and malignancy, and it may be drug induced. An isolated positive ANA with nonspecific symptoms and normal clinical examination does not establish the diagnosis of a connective tissue disease.

A higher titer of ANA is more often associated with an underlying rheumatologic disease, although not always SLE. However, almost all patients with SLE (>95%) have a positive ANA. ANA titer does not correlate with disease activity and should not be used for activity assessment.

ANA specificity or subserology testing (that is, testing for antibodies to specific nuclear components such as DNA or centromeres) should be reserved for patients with a positive ANA and a clinical syndrome suggestive of an underlying connective tissue disease. ANA subserology testing should not be routinely performed, even in the setting of a positive ANA, without a strong clinical suspicion of underlying connective tissue disease.

Table 5 provides details on these and other autoantibodies and their associations with specific conditions.

Imaging Studies
Radiography

Plain radiography is an essential modality in the evaluation of many rheumatologic diseases and can assess and differentiate inflammatory arthritis, osteoarthritis, and crystal arthropathies (**Table 6**). Plain radiography has limitations because it gives a two-dimensional picture of three-dimensional structures, is limited in its ability to visualize soft tissues, and may not detect early or small erosive changes. Despite these limitations, plain radiography is usually the first imaging test ordered in the evaluation of rheumatologic diseases because it is readily available, is inexpensive, exposes patients to only a low level of ionizing radiation, and is useful in monitoring arthritis progression.

CT

CT provides multiple views and orientations from a single study but is more useful for bony abnormalities than for soft-tissue inflammation or fluid collections. CT is more sensitive for detecting bone erosions than plain radiographs or MRI. However, CT is more expensive than plain radiography and exposes the patient to more radiation.

MRI

MRI is the most sensitive routine radiologic technique for detecting soft-tissue abnormalities, inflammation, and fluid collections but is less effective than CT in demonstrating bony abnormalities or erosions. MRI is sensitive for detecting early spine and sacroiliac joint inflammation and may be indicated for the evaluation of suspected spondyloarthritis if plain radiographs are negative. MRI does not expose patients to radiation but is associated with high cost, limited availability, and possible patient intolerance due to claustrophobia or body habitus. The American College of Rheumatology Choosing Wisely list recommends against routine MRI of the peripheral joints to monitor RA due to inadequate data supporting its use.

Ultrasonography

The use of ultrasonography to evaluate patients with rheumatologic diseases has expanded dramatically in the past 10 years.

TABLE 5. Autoantibodies in Rheumatologic Disease

Autoantibody	Rheumatologic Disease	Sensitivity/Specificity	Comments
ANA	SLE; also SSc, Sjögren, MCTD	SLE: >95% sensitivity, poor specificity; indirect IFA is the most appropriate methodology	Does not correlate with disease activity
Anti–double-stranded DNA	SLE	SLE: 50%-60% sensitivity, >95% specificity; *Crithidia* IFA or Farr assays more specific than ELISA	Found in more severe disease, especially kidney disease; antibody levels commonly follow disease activity and are useful to monitor
Anti-Smith	SLE	SLE: 30% sensitivity, 99% specificity	Most specific test for SLE; does not correlate with disease activity
Anti-U1-RNP	MCTD; SLE	High sensitivity for MCTD	High titer seen in MCTD (>1:10,000); does not correlate with disease activity
Anti-Ro/SSA; anti-La/SSB	Sjögren; SLE; RA; SSc	Sjögren: 70% sensitivity; SLE: 20% sensitivity	Sicca symptoms; in SLE, associated with photosensitive rash; offspring of mothers who are positive for anti-Ro/SSA or anti-La/SSB are at increased risk for neonatal lupus erythematosus (rash and congenital heart block)
Antiribosomal P	SLE	15% sensitivity	Associated with CNS lupus and lupus hepatitis
Anti-Scl-70 (antitopoisomerase-1)	DcSSc	10%-30% sensitivity	Seen more often in patients with DcSSc who have pulmonary fibrosis
Anticentromere	LcSSc (CREST)	10%-30% sensitivity	Patients with LcSSc with this antibody are more likely to develop pulmonary arterial hypertension
c-ANCA (antiproteinase-3)	GPA	90% sensitivity when disease is active; high specificity in classic presentations	Correlation with disease activity is unclear
p-ANCA (antimyeloperoxidase)	MPA; EGPA	MPA: 80% sensitivity; EGPA: 60% sensitivity; less specific than c-ANCA	Atypical p-ANCA (antimyeloperoxidase negative) can be seen in inflammatory bowel disease and with positive ANA
Anti–Jo-1	Polymyositis	20%-30% sensitivity	Associated with antisynthetase syndrome, including lung inflammation
Rheumatoid factor	RA; Sjögren; cryoglobulinemia	RA: 70% sensitivity; limited specificity, especially in patients without a classic disease presentation	RF is common in multiple other diseases (e.g., hepatitis C, endocarditis, SLE); 30% with RA are RF negative but may become positive later in RA course
Anti-cyclic citrullinated peptide	RA	RA: 70% sensitivity; 95% specificity	Can be positive in RF-negative RA patients; often present before RF becomes positive; associated with erosions; predicts disease progression in undifferentiated arthritis
Antihistone	DILE	95% sensitivity; poor specificity	Also seen in primary SLE
Cryoglobulins	Vasculitis; hepatitis C; myeloma; SLE; RA	Type II or III cryoglobulins seen in cryoglobulinemic vasculitis	May be present in connective tissue diseases in the absence of vasculitis

ANA = antinuclear antibodies; CNS = central nervous system; CREST = calcinosis, Raynaud phenomenon, esophageal dysmotility, sclerodactyly, and telangiectasia; DcSSc = diffuse cutaneous systemic sclerosis; DILE = drug-induced lupus erythematosus; EGPA = eosinophilic granulomatosis with polyangiitis; ELISA = enzyme-linked immunosorbent assay; GPA = granulomatosis with polyangiitis; IFA = immunofluorescence assay; LcSSc = limited cutaneous systemic sclerosis; MCTD = mixed connective tissue disease; MPA = microscopic polyangiitis; RA = rheumatoid arthritis; RF = rheumatoid factor; RNP = ribonucleoprotein; SLE = systemic lupus erythematosus; SSc = systemic sclerosis.

Ultrasonography is relatively inexpensive, can scan across three-dimensional structures, and can provide real-time data in the clinic without exposure to ionizing radiation. It can assess soft-tissue abnormalities, including synovitis, tendonitis, bursitis, and effusions; assess disease activity using Doppler; and assist with tendon or joint injections. However, it is operator dependent, and training/practice is needed to achieve competence.

KEY POINTS

- Plain radiography is usually the first imaging test ordered in the evaluation of rheumatologic diseases because it is readily available, is inexpensive, exposes patients to only a low level of ionizing radiation, and is useful in monitoring arthritis progression.

HVC

(Continued)

TABLE 6. Radiographic Findings of Common Rheumatologic Diseases	
Rheumatologic Disease	**Radiographic Findings**
Rheumatoid arthritis	Bony erosions; periarticular osteopenia; subluxations; soft-tissue swelling; MCP, PIP, and wrist involvement
Osteoarthritis	Asymmetric joint-space narrowing; osteophytes; subchondral sclerosis and cystic changes; degenerative disk disease with collapse of disks; degenerative joint disease with facet joint osteophytes; spondylolisthesis (anterior/posterior misalignment of the spine); kyphosis
Diffuse idiopathic skeletal hyperostosis	Calcification of the anterior longitudinal ligament; bridging horizontal syndesmophytes; usually seen in the thoracic spine and more prominent on the right side of the spine
Ankylosing spondylitis	Sacroiliitis; squaring of the vertebral bodies; bridging vertical syndesmophytes; shiny corners; ankylosis does not skip vertebrae
Psoriatic arthritis	Destructive arthritis with erosions and osteophytes; DIP involvement is common; pencil-in-cup deformity on hand radiograph; arthritis mutilans; syndesmophytes
Gout	Punched-out erosions with sclerotic borders and overhanging edges; periarticular soft-tissue swelling with calcifications in tophaceous deposits
Calcium pyrophosphate deposition	Chondrocalcinosis, most commonly of the knees, shoulders, wrists, pubic symphysis; osteoarthritis, including in locations atypical for primary osteoarthritis (MCPs, wrists, shoulders)

DIP = distal interphalangeal; MCP = metacarpophalangeal; PIP = proximal interphalangeal.

KEY POINTS *(continued)*

HVC
- CT is more sensitive for detecting bony abnormalities or erosions than plain radiographs or MRI, whereas MRI is the most sensitive routine radiologic technique for detecting soft-tissue abnormalities, inflammation, and fluid collections.

HVC
- Ultrasonography is an inexpensive means to assess soft-tissue abnormalities, assess disease activity, and assist with tendon or joint injections, but it is operator dependent.

Joint Aspiration

Joint aspiration and synovial fluid analysis are essential for discriminating between inflammatory and noninflammatory effusions or for distinguishing between infectious arthritis and acute crystal arthropathies. In the evaluation of any monoarthritis or when infection is being considered, joint aspiration should be performed to diagnose the underlying cause. Aspirated synovial fluid should be sent for leukocyte count, Gram stain, and cultures, as well as evaluation for crystals under polarized light. See **Table 7** for more information.

There is no absolute cutoff of synovial fluid leukocyte counts for ruling out infectious arthritis; however, counts greater than 50,000/µL (50×10^9/L) with polymorphonuclear cell predominance have a high likelihood of infection. Counts less than 2000/µL (2.0×10^9/L) are usually associated with noninflammatory etiologies. Notably, crystals can coexist with infection, and their presence does not rule out infection if suspicion is high.

Tissue Biopsy

When appropriate, tissue biopsy of involved organs can be helpful in diagnosing numerous rheumatologic conditions such as vasculitis (lung, kidney, or temporal artery biopsy) and SLE (skin biopsy). Tissue biopsy may also help assess disease

TABLE 7. Synovial Fluid Analysis						
	Normal	**Noninflammatory**	**Inflammatory**	**Crystal Induced**	**Infectious**	**Hemorrhagic**
Appearance	Clear/yellow/ transparent	Clear/yellow/ transparent	Yellow/white/ translucent/ opaque	Yellow/white/ translucent/ opaque	Yellow/white/ opaque	Red/opaque
Leukocyte count	<200/µL (0.2×10^9/L)	200-2000/µL (0.2-2.0×10^9/L)	2000-20,000/µL (2.0-20×10^9/L) (may be higher)	10,000-50,000/µL (10-50×10^9/L) (may be higher)	>50,000/µL (50×10^9/L) (may be lower)	—
Other studies	Negative Gram stain; negative culture	Negative Gram stain; negative culture	Negative Gram stain; negative culture	Negative Gram stain; positive crystals[a]	Positive Gram stain[b]; positive culture[c]	Negative Gram stain; negative culture

[a]Crystal description: Urate crystals are needle shaped and bright. Viewed under polarized light, they are negatively birefringent; they appear yellow when parallel to the axis of the polarized field and blue when perpendicular to the axis. Calcium pyrophosphate crystals are rhomboid, pale, and weakly (not as vividly) positively birefringent; they appear blue when parallel to the axis and yellow when perpendicular.

[b]Gram stain sensitivity for infection is approximately 30% to 50%.

[c]Nearly all cultures are positive except for infection caused by *Neisseria gonorrhoeae*, which may be positive in 50% or fewer cases.

activity (for example, kidney biopsy in SLE). The benefits should be appropriately balanced with possible risks of the procedure.

KEY POINTS

- Synovial fluid leukocyte counts greater than 50,000/μL (50×10^9/L) with polymorphonuclear cell predominance have a high likelihood of infection; counts less than 2000/μL (2.0×10^9/L) are usually associated with noninflammatory etiologies.
- Tissue biopsy of involved organs can be helpful in diagnosing numerous rheumatologic conditions and in assessing disease activity in some conditions.

Principles of Therapeutics

Overview

This section reviews the indications for use, mechanisms of action, major toxicities, and monitoring requirements of medications used in rheumatologic disease. Drug applications in specific disease states are elaborated upon in their respective sections.

Anti-Inflammatory Agents

Glucocorticoids

Glucocorticoids are effective in many rheumatologic diseases, including rheumatoid arthritis (RA), acute crystal arthropathy, systemic vasculitis, polymyalgia rheumatica, systemic lupus erythematosus (SLE), inflammatory myopathies, and autoinflammatory diseases. Advantages include rapid onset of action, ease of use, low cost, and universal availability; in many disease states, they are disease modifying and sometimes lifesaving.

Glucocorticoids have numerous adverse effects, which are more likely to occur with higher doses and longer treatment. These include osteoporosis, immunosuppression, skin fragility, glaucoma, cataracts, weight gain, diabetes mellitus, hypertension, psychomotor agitation, osteonecrosis, and hypothalamic-pituitary-adrenal axis suppression.

Patients anticipated to be taking ≥2.5-mg prednisone for ≥3 months should be risk-assessed for glucocorticoid-induced osteoporosis and appropriately managed. Those who are at moderate or high risk for osteoporotic fractures and placed on chronic glucocorticoid therapy should begin oral bisphosphonates.

NSAIDs

NSAIDs prevent prostaglandin production by inhibiting the two isoforms of cyclooxygenase (COX), COX-1 and COX-2. COX-2 is an inducible enzyme typically expressed in inflammatory milieus, whereas COX-1 is constitutively expressed and helps maintain organismal homeostasis. Nearly all available COX inhibitors are nonselective (inhibit both isoenzymes), down-regulating prostaglandin production in inflammatory states and interfering with housekeeping functions of prostanoids (for example, renal blood flow and gut mucosal integrity maintenance) (**Table 8**). Nonselective COX inhibitors also inhibit thromboxane A_2, inhibiting platelet function and promoting bleeding.

Although they alleviate symptoms, COX inhibitors are not disease modifying, with the apparent exception of ankylosing spondylitis. Major concerns surrounding all COX inhibitors include increased risk for gastrointestinal bleeding (particularly in those already at risk) and adverse cardiovascular events; therefore, they should be prescribed at the lowest dose for the shortest time possible. COX inhibitors should generally be avoided in patients on concomitant anticoagulation.

Selective COX-2 inhibitors were developed to spare COX-1 and reduce gastrointestinal risk; although effective for this purpose, the most selective COX-2 inhibitors were found to increase the risk of cardiovascular events and were removed from the market.

NSAIDs vary with regard to kinetics, COX-1/2 selectivity, and other features, and carry somewhat different degrees of risk; having experience with several different NSAIDs is potentially beneficial in clinical practice.

Topical NSAIDs such as diclofenac are available by prescription for arthritis and pose a lower risk for systemic side effects than oral NSAIDs. They may be preferred for patients at high risk for toxicity from oral NSAIDs and/or for those ≥75 years of age. However, they are often expensive.

TABLE 8.	Potential Toxicities of NSAID Use
Category	**Toxicity**
Cardiovascular	Myocardial infarction; exacerbation of heart failure
Hemostatic	Platelet dysfunction
Gastrointestinal	Dyspepsia; reflux; peptic ulcer disease; gastrointestinal bleeding
Obstetric/Gynecologic	Bleeding; delayed labor; premature ductus arteriosus closure
Pulmonary	Asthma exacerbation
Renal	Hypertension; decreased glomerular filtration; increased salt and water retention; increased renin production; uncommonly, allergic interstitial nephritis or acute tubular necrosis

Colchicine

Colchicine inhibits microtubules and impairs neutrophil function. It is most commonly employed for gout and acute calcium pyrophosphate crystal arthritis (pseudogout). It is also used to treat hypersensitivity vasculitis and familial Mediterranean fever.

Gastrointestinal side effects (particularly diarrhea) are common. With overdose, severe (even fatal) myelosuppression can occur. Dosing must be adjusted for kidney disease. When given chronically, colchicine can rarely cause neuromuscular toxicity, particularly if coadministered with statin drugs. Concomitant administration of strong CYP3A4 inhibitors (for example, clarithromycin) that reduce the hepatic catabolism of colchicine should be avoided.

KEY POINTS

- Although effective inflammatory agents in many rheumatologic diseases, glucocorticoids have numerous adverse side effects, including osteoporosis, immunosuppression, skin fragility, glaucoma, cataracts, weight gain, diabetes mellitus, hypertension, psychomotor agitation, osteonecrosis, and hypothalamic-pituitary-adrenal axis suppression.

- Because of the increased risk for gastrointestinal bleeding and adverse cardiovascular events, cyclooxygenase inhibitors should be prescribed at the lowest dose for the shortest time possible.

Analgesics and Pain Pathway Modulators

Acetaminophen

The efficacy of acetaminophen for osteoarthritis and lower back pain is increasingly questioned, with recent controlled trials and meta-analyses demonstrating no benefit from the drug, even at high doses (3000-4000 mg/d).

Tramadol

Tramadol is a mixed opioid analgesic and weak serotonin-norepinephrine reuptake inhibitor; potential for addiction is lower than for traditional opioids, which are generally avoided in rheumatologic treatment.

Duloxetine

Duloxetine is a serotonin-norepinephrine reuptake inhibitor that is FDA approved for the management of chronic musculoskeletal pain and fibromyalgia. Duloxetine provides modest pain relief for knee osteoarthritis, chronic lower back pain, and fibromyalgia. Patients must be slowly weaned off the drug when discontinuing to avoid withdrawal symptoms.

Gabapentinoids

Gabapentinoids (gabapentin and pregabalin) inhibit voltage-gated calcium channels, reducing pain signaling. Pregabalin is FDA approved for fibromyalgia. Common side effects (dizziness, disequilibrium, somnolence, weight gain, peripheral edema, cognitive difficulties) may limit its utility, and discontinuation is sometimes warranted. Gabapentin also modestly improves fibromyalgia symptoms, with a similar side-effect profile.

KEY POINT

- The efficacy of acetaminophen for osteoarthritis and **HVC** lower back pain is increasingly questioned, with recent controlled trials and meta-analyses demonstrating no benefit from the drug, even at high doses.

Disease-Modifying Antirheumatic Drugs

Nonbiologic Disease-Modifying Antirheumatic Drugs

Table 9 summarizes the mechanisms of action, indications, and common monitoring parameters of various nonbiologic disease-modifying antirheumatic drugs (DMARDs). See Medications and Pregnancy for information on these drugs in pregnancy.

Methotrexate

Methotrexate is a first-line medication for treating RA and other autoimmune diseases. Once-weekly dosing is generally between 10 to 25 mg and can be given orally or subcutaneously. At doses above 15 mg, parenteral administration is more reliable but much more expensive.

Potential side effects include headaches, fatigue, and nausea (particularly around the time of weekly dosing). Hepatotoxicity and cytopenias can occur (especially macrocytic anemia), and dose adjustment is required with kidney disease. Methotrexate should be avoided in patients with significant hepatic or kidney disease. Folic acid supplements minimize toxicity while preserving efficacy. Limiting alcohol intake is recommended.

Hydroxychloroquine

Hydroxychloroquine is an immunomodulator that is widely used in SLE, in which it decreases mortality and the likelihood of developing nephritis. It is rarely sufficient as single-drug therapy for RA but is useful as an adjunctive therapy.

Sulfasalazine

Sulfasalazine is used to treat RA and nonaxial psoriatic arthritis, but use has decreased because of the relative effectiveness of methotrexate and leflunomide. It is now most frequently used as part of combination DMARD therapy for RA and in women considering pregnancy. Serious side effects include blood dyscrasias, hepatitis, and hypersensitivity reactions. Because of its benefit for inflammatory bowel disease (IBD), it may constitute a useful strategy for patients with IBD-associated arthritis.

TABLE 9. Nonbiologic Disease-Modifying Antirheumatic Drugs

Agent	Mechanism	Indications	Common Monitoring Parameters
Methotrexate	Low dose: anti-inflammatory agent via up-regulation of adenosine A_{2A} signaling High dose: antimetabolite/folate antagonist used in neoplastic disease	RA; psoriasis; psoriatic arthritis; IBD; SLE (arthritis only); reactive arthritis; DM; PM; vasculitis	Baseline: chest radiography, hepatitis screening, CBC, LCTs, serum creatinine Thereafter: CBC, LCTs, serum creatinine after the first month, then approximately every 2-3 months[a]
Hydroxychloroquine	Uncertain; appears to involve stabilization of lysosomal vacuoles, leading to inhibition of antigen processing and/or inhibition of Toll-like receptor activation	SLE; RA	Baseline: CBC, LCTs, serum creatinine Retinal examinations at baseline and annual examination after 5 years of therapy to evaluate for retinopathy
Sulfasalazine	Unknown; the prodrug is broken down into 5-amino salicylic acid (active metabolite in the gastrointestinal tract) and sulfapyridine (exerts systemic action)	RA; SpA; IBD	Baseline: CBC, LCTs, serum creatinine Thereafter: CBC, LCTs, serum creatinine every 3-6 months
Leflunomide	Inhibits the mitochondrial enzyme dihydroorotate dehydrogenase to block pyrimidine synthesis (decreasing lymphocyte production); antiproliferative	RA	Baseline: hepatitis screening, CBC, LCTs, serum creatinine Thereafter: CBC, LCTs, serum creatinine after 4 weeks, then every 3 months
Azathioprine	A prodrug of 6-mercaptopurine; purine analogue; inhibits DNA synthesis essential for proliferating T- and B-lymphocytes	SLE; DM; PM; vasculitis; IBD	Baseline: CBC, LCTs, serum creatinine Thereafter: CBC, LCTs, serum creatinine every 3 months[a]
Cyclophosphamide	Alkylating agent; blocks DNA synthesis and causes cell death, especially of T cells	Severe and life-threatening disease in SLE, DM, PM, and vasculitis; may be used when other agents fail	Close monitoring clinically and measuring CBC, chemistries, LCTs, urinalysis every 4-8 weeks
Mycophenolate mofetil	Active metabolite (mycophenolic acid) inhibits purine synthesis; preferentially inhibits T- and B-lymphocytes	SLE (especially lupus nephritis); vasculitis (maintenance therapy); DM; PM; SSc	Baseline: CBC, LCTs, serum creatinine Thereafter: CBC, LCTs, serum creatinine after 4 weeks and then every 3 months[a]
Cyclosporine	Inhibits calcineurin (a transcription activating factor); preferentially targets T cells	SLE; psoriasis; RA	Baseline: CBC, LCTs, serum creatinine Thereafter: CBC, LCTs, serum creatinine every 2-3 months[a]
Tofacitinib	Janus kinase inhibitor	RA	Baseline: CBC, LCTs, creatinine, lipid panel Thereafter: CBC, LCTs, creatinine every 8 weeks, lipids after 8 weeks and then every 6 months
Apremilast	Inhibits phosphodiesterase 4	Psoriasis; psoriatic arthritis	Baseline: weight Thereafter: weight, neuropsychiatric effects

CBC = complete blood count; DM = dermatomyositis; IBD = inflammatory bowel disease; LCTs = liver chemistry tests; PM = polymyositis; RA = rheumatoid arthritis; SLE = systemic lupus erythematosus; SpA = spondyloarthritis; SSc = systemic sclerosis.

[a]Recommended monitoring interval is for a stable dose but may be shorter after initiation or in the case of abnormal results and must be individualized to the patient's risk of toxicity.

Leflunomide

Leflunomide is FDA approved for rheumatoid and psoriatic arthritis, with comparable efficacy to methotrexate. Patients must be monitored for hepatotoxicity and myelosuppression. Other common side effects include nausea, headaches, rash, diarrhea, and transaminitis. An uncommon side effect is peripheral neuropathy, but it is usually self-limited if the drug is discontinued. The active metabolite of leflunomide (teriflunomide) has a half-life of nearly 3 weeks; therefore, when the drug needs to be eliminated quickly, an 11-day cholestyramine washout is necessary.

Azathioprine

Azathioprine is an immunosuppressant used in various inflammatory diseases. Concomitant use with xanthine oxidase inhibitors (allopurinol, febuxostat) is contraindicated. Azathioprine's primary toxicity is myelosuppression. Thiopurine methyltransferase enzyme testing allows for identification of patients with decreased or absent enzyme activity at high myelosuppression risk.

Cyclophosphamide

Cyclophosphamide is a powerful immunosuppressant with a rapid onset of action (days to weeks). It treats vasculitis,

CONT.

life-threatening complications of SLE, and interstitial lung disease. Cyclophosphamide has largely been displaced by newer and safer drugs for first-line treatment of ANCA-associated vasculitis and lupus nephritis (rituximab and mycophenolate mofetil, respectively) but is still used in severe cases or when these agents fail. Serious potential side effects include severe immunosuppression, leukopenia, hemorrhagic cystitis, and ovarian failure, as well as long-term risk for bladder cancer, leukemia, and lymphoma. ⊞

Mycophenolate Mofetil

Mycophenolate mofetil is currently the first-line agent for lupus nephritis and may be effective for systemic sclerosis and associated interstitial lung disease. Gastrointestinal side effects are common, particularly diarrhea. Myelosuppression may occur.

Calcineurin Inhibitors

Calcineurin inhibitors include cyclosporine and tacrolimus. Although cyclosporine is now rarely used in rheumatology, one of its most common side effects is hyperuricemia, and cyclosporine-induced gout is an important consideration in patients taking the drug who present with acute monoarthritis. There is currently renewed interest in tacrolimus as a possible alternative therapy for lupus nephritis.

Tofacitinib

Tofacitinib is an oral agent that inhibits Janus kinase (JAK) signaling. Tofacitinib is FDA approved for RA and has efficacy equal to biologic DMARDs. Risks include hyperlipidemia, hepatotoxicity, and leukopenia.

Apremilast

Apremilast is modestly effective for psoriasis and psoriatic arthritis. It does not cause immunosuppression or myelosuppression. However, apremilast is less efficacious than biologic DMARDs and has a slow onset of action, and its effect on progression of erosive damage is unknown. Adverse events include gastrointestinal side effects (mainly nausea and diarrhea) and weight loss. It should be used with caution in patients with a history of depression.

KEY POINTS

- Methotrexate is a first-line medication for treating rheumatoid arthritis and other autoimmune diseases.

- Hydroxychloroquine is widely used in systemic lupus erythematosus, in which it decreases mortality and the likelihood of developing nephritis.

- Cyclophosphamide has been largely displaced by newer drugs for first-line treatment of ANCA-associated vasculitis and lupus nephritis but is still used in severe cases or when other agents fail.

- The oral agent tofacitinib is FDA approved for rheumatoid arthritis and has efficacy equal to biologic agents.

Biologic Disease-Modifying Antirheumatic Drugs

Biologic DMARDs are highly specific, parenterally administered, protein-based agents with extracellular targets (specific proinflammatory cytokines, cytokine receptors, or clusters of differentiation cell surface molecules on immune cells; **Figure 1**). The end of the generic name of a biologic agent indicates what type of molecule it is: -*mab* indicates monoclonal antibody; -*kin* indicates an interleukin-type substance; -*ra* is for a receptor antagonist; and -*cept* is for receptor molecules.

Table 10 and **Table 11** summarize the structures, targets, indications, and common monitoring parameters of various biologic DMARDs. See Medications and Pregnancy for information on these drugs in pregnancy. Biologic DMARDs increase the risk for infection to variable degrees. Targeted screening is therefore necessary before initiation (see Vaccination and Screening in Immunosuppression).

The cost of biologic agents is significant and may be a barrier to access.

Tumor Necrosis Factor α Inhibitors

Tumor necrosis factor (TNF)-α inhibitors are large protein-based molecules that require parenteral administration (see Table 10). They are widely used for treating RA, psoriasis, psoriatic arthritis, and ankylosing spondylitis, and are also approved for several nonrheumatologic diseases.

TNF-α inhibitors are generally well tolerated, with increased risk for infection the primary safety concern. They pose a particularly high risk for reactivation of tuberculosis, so all patients being considered for TNF-α inhibitor therapy need to be screened and receive appropriate prophylaxis. TNF-α inhibitors do not appear to increase the risk of new cancers, aside from nonmelanoma and possibly melanoma skin cancer; the risk for malignant recurrence is unclear. These agents may also exacerbate heart failure and rarely provoke a demyelinating condition. Over time, TNF-α inhibitors may often lose efficacy owing to formation of anti-drug antibodies.

Other Biologic Disease-Modifying Antirheumatic Drugs

Multiple biologic DMARDs with additional extracellular and cell-surface targets have been approved by the FDA in the past decade. Most of these agents are started after one or two TNF-α inhibitors have failed. See Table 11 for more information. ⊞

Biosimilars

Biosimilar agents are "copycat" versions of brand-name biologic medications. The drugs are not exact replicas (hence the term "biosimilar" rather than "generic"); therefore, they must go through phase III testing to garner regulatory approval. In 2016, the FDA approved three biosimilar anti-TNF agents.

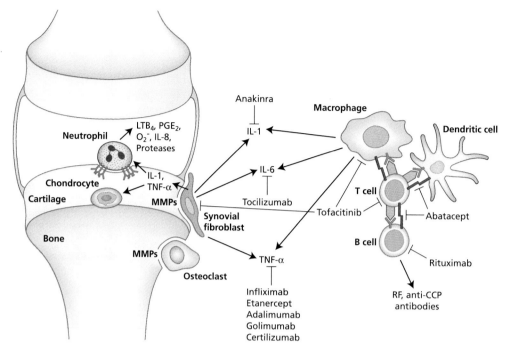

FIGURE 1. The inflammatory cascade in rheumatoid arthritis (RA). Dendritic cells, macrophages, and B cells present inciting antigens to T cells. Macrophages secrete multiple cytokines, including ILs and TNF-α, which are also secreted by activated synovial fibroblasts. The activated fibroblasts secrete matrix metalloproteinases (MMPs) and other enzymes that contribute to the degradation of articular cartilage and activate neutrophils, which mediate joint damage through proteases and other enzymes. Activated osteoclasts additionally secrete MMPs that contribute to marginal erosions of bone. ILs, TNF-α, T cells, and B cells may all be targeted for inhibition by the various disease-modifying antirheumatic drugs useful in RA. CCP = cyclic citrullinated peptide; IL = interleukin; LTB$_4$ = leukotriene B$_4$; MMP = matrix metalloproteinase; O$_2$ = oxygen; PGE$_2$ = prostaglandin E$_2$; RF = rheumatoid factor; TNF = tumor necrosis factor.

TABLE 10. Tumor Necrosis Factor α Inhibitors[a]

Agent	Agent Structure	Indications
Adalimumab	Humanized monoclonal antibody	RA; psoriatic arthritis; ankylosing spondylitis; IBD
Etanercept	Fusion protein made of two p75 TNF-α receptors linked to IgG Fc segment	RA; psoriatic arthritis; ankylosing spondylitis
Certolizumab pegol	Fab' segment of humanized monoclonal antibody attached to polyethylene glycol strands	RA; psoriatic arthritis; ankylosing spondylitis
Golimumab	Humanized monoclonal antibody	RA; psoriatic arthritis; ankylosing spondylitis
Infliximab	Chimeric (mouse-human) monoclonal antibody	RA; psoriatic arthritis; ankylosing spondylitis; IBD

IBD = inflammatory bowel disease; RA = rheumatoid arthritis; TNF = tumor necrosis factor.

[a]Common monitoring parameters for TNF-α inhibitors include tuberculosis, fungal, and other infections as well as complete blood count, serum creatinine, and liver chemistry tests at baseline and thereafter every 3 to 6 months.

KEY POINTS

- All biologic agents increase the risk for infection; therefore, targeted screening is necessary before initiation.

- Tumor necrosis factor α inhibitors are widely used for treating rheumatoid arthritis, psoriasis, psoriatic arthritis, and ankylosing spondylitis; they are also approved for treating some nonrheumatologic diseases.

HVC
- Non–tumor necrosis factor (TNF)-α biologic agents are usually started after one or two TNF-α inhibitors have failed.

Urate-Lowering Therapy
Allopurinol

Allopurinol is the most commonly used urate-lowering agent. It competitively inhibits the enzyme xanthine oxidase, blocking the conversion of hypoxanthine (a breakdown product of purines) to uric acid. Allopurinol is metabolized to oxypurinol, which also inhibits xanthine oxidase. Allopurinol is FDA approved for doses up to 800 mg/d. According to the American College of Rheumatology, allopurinol should be initiated at 100 mg/d and titrated in 100-mg increments as needed, and

TABLE 11. Other Biologic Disease-Modifying Antirheumatic Drugs[a]

Agent	Agent Structure	Target	Indications	Comments
Abatacept	Soluble CTLA4 receptor/IgG Fc segment chimera	CD80/CD86; blocks T-cell costimulation	RA	Preferred for those with history of severe infection; relatively contraindicated in COPD
Rituximab	Chimeric (mouse-human) monoclonal antibody	CD20[+] B cells	RA; ANCA-associated vasculitis; occasionally for SLE (off-label); hyper-IgG4 syndrome	Given as an intravenous infusion over several hours; has a higher risk of infusion reactions than other biologic DMARDs; can cause hypogammaglobulinemia
Tocilizumab	Humanized monoclonal antibody	IL-6 receptor	RA; JIA; Castleman disease; GCA	Can cause transaminitis, hyperlipidemia, leukopenia, thrombocytopenia; avoid in those with history of diverticulitis because of an attendant risk of bowel perforation
Belimumab	Human monoclonal antibody	BLyS/BAFF	SLE	Phase III trials showed a small but statistically significant improvement versus standard therapy alone, with a glucocorticoid-sparing effect
Ustekinumab	Human monoclonal antibody	IL-12/IL-23	Psoriasis; psoriatic arthritis	Injectable; less robust effect than other biologic DMARDs
Secukinumab	Human monoclonal antibody	IL-17a	Psoriatic arthritis; ankylosing spondylitis	Phase III trials suggest equal efficacy to TNF-α inhibitors; can cause flares of IBD
Anakinra	Recombinant receptor antagonist	IL-1β receptor	RA; CAPS[b]; AOSD (off-label); acute gouty arthritis (off-label)	Rarely used in RA because efficacy is inferior to other biologic DMARDs; reversible neutropenia can develop
Canakinumab	Human monoclonal antibody	IL-1β	CAPS[b]	Newer, more expensive IL-1 inhibitor
Rilonacept	Dual IL-1β receptors chimerically attached to IgG Fc segment	IL-1	CAPS[b]; refractory gout	Newer, more expensive IL-1 inhibitor

AOSD = adult-onset Still disease; BAFF = B-cell-activating factor; BLyS = B-lymphocyte stimulator; CAPS = cryopyrin-associated periodic syndromes; DMARD = disease-modifying antirheumatic drug; GCA = giant cell arteritis; IBD = inflammatory bowel disease; IL = interleukin; JIA = juvenile idiopathic arthritis; RA = rheumatoid arthritis; SLE = systemic lupus erythematosus; TNF = tumor necrosis factor.

[a]Prior to initiating any biologic, tuberculosis screening must be performed. Complete blood counts should be performed every 3 to 6 months for all biologics, and aspartate aminotransferase/alanine aminotransferase and a lipid panel should be checked every 2 to 3 months for tocilizumab.

[b]The cryopyrin-associated periodic syndromes (CAPS) include familial cold autoinflammatory syndrome, Muckle-Wells syndrome, and neonatal-onset multisystem inflammatory disease (chronic infantile neurologic, cutaneous, articular syndrome).

for those with stage 4 or 5 chronic kidney disease, allopurinol should be initiated at 50 mg/d and titrated in 50-mg increments as needed.

The biggest risk the drug poses is DRESS (drug reaction with eosinophilia and systemic symptoms) syndrome, a rare reaction that usually occurs in the presence of chronic kidney disease and diuretic use and has a high mortality rate (see MKSAP 18 Dermatology). A recently discovered DRESS risk factor is the HLA-B*5801 allele, which is more common in persons of Han Chinese, Thai, and Korean descent. Screening for HLA-B*5801 in high-risk populations is recommended before initiating therapy. Xanthine oxidase inhibitors cannot be coadministered with purine analogues (such as azathioprine). H

Febuxostat

Febuxostat is a noncompetitive xanthine oxidase inhibitor. As with allopurinol, transaminitis rarely occurs, and liver enzymes should be monitored. Concomitant use with purine analogues is contraindicated. Incidence of DRESS syndrome is rare.

Uricosuric Agents

Probenecid is an organic acid transport inhibitor that decreases renal reuptake of uric acid. Probenecid is uncommonly used because of limited efficacy, as well as inconvenience and limitations on use.

Lesinurad is a recently approved, highly potent inhibitor of renal uric acid reuptake targeting the urate transporter URAT1. It is approved only for combination use with febuxostat or allopurinol. Lesinurad can rarely cause renal toxicity and should not be given to those with an estimated creatinine clearance less than 45 mL/min.

Pegloticase

Unlike most other mammals, humans lack a functioning uricase to break down uric acid. Pegloticase is a recombinant, nonhuman, infusible pegylated uricase that is highly effective at lowering serum urate. Pegloticase is reserved for severe and/or refractory gout. Because of its extreme potency, mobilization flares of gout are common, and prophylaxis against acute gouty attacks is required. Pegloticase is administered intravenously every 2 weeks; if the pre-infusion serum urate increases to more than 6.0 mg/dL (0.35 mmol/L) on two occasions, it is likely that antibodies have formed, and the drug should be discontinued to prevent infusion reactions.

KEY POINTS

- Allopurinol is the most commonly used urate-lowering agent; the biggest risk the drug poses is DRESS (drug reaction with eosinophilia and systemic symptoms) syndrome, which has a high mortality rate.
- Concomitant use of xanthine oxidase inhibitors (allopurinol or febuxostat) with purine analogues is contraindicated.

Medications and Pregnancy

Some rheumatologic medications can have adverse effects on pregnancy. See **Table 12** for a discussion of these agents and their relative risks.

KEY POINTS

- Methotrexate is highly teratogenic and abortifacient; it must be discontinued at least 3 months before pregnancy.
- Hydroxychloroquine is relatively safe in pregnancy and should not be discontinued if it is needed.
- Leflunomide is extremely teratogenic and must not be used before or during pregnancy; upon discontinuation, cholestyramine administration is required to remove the drug from the body in all women of childbearing potential and specifically in those wishing to become pregnant.

Vaccination and Screening in Immunosuppression

Patients should be updated with vaccinations before initiating biologic DMARD regimens. Vaccine response may be diminished once on treatment, and patients on some immunosuppressants (including all biologic DMARDs and tofacitinib) should not receive live attenuated vaccines (such as for herpes zoster, live attenuated influenza, and yellow fever) because of risk for viral activity in an immunocompromised host. Despite diminished efficacy, patients already on a biologic DMARD should receive any non-live vaccines that are indicated as per standard of care. Patients receiving traditional oral DMARDs (for example, hydroxychloroquine, methotrexate, and sulfasalazine) may receive any and all vaccines as needed.

Before initiating immunosuppressive therapy, the following screening is recommended:

- Tuberculosis screening with tuberculin skin testing or interferon-γ release assay, particularly for patients initiating biologic DMARDs

- Hepatitis B and C serologies (for biologic DMARDs and drugs that can cause hepatotoxicity)
- HIV screening

Patients with latent or active tuberculosis, active hepatitis B, or untreated HIV infection require initiation of appropriate therapy before initiating immunosuppression. Repeat screening for tuberculosis should be performed annually if there are risk factors for ongoing tuberculosis exposure.

KEY POINTS

- Vaccinations should be updated before initiating biologic disease-modifying antirheumatic drug regimens.
- Screening (and therapy if needed) for tuberculosis, hepatitis B and C serologies, and HIV is appropriate before initiating immunosuppressive therapy.

Nonpharmacologic and Nontraditional Management

Because rheumatologic diseases frequently affect the musculoskeletal system, nonpharmacologic measures are often employed to address pain not eliminated by medications. These measures include physical therapy, occupational therapy, surgery, weight reduction, psychosocial support, and self-management programs. Many patients turn to complementary and alternative medicine as adjuncts to traditional medical interventions.

Physical and Occupational Therapy

The physical therapist can aid the primary care provider in assessing a patient's aerobic fitness and conditioning as well as the patient's ability to carry out activities of daily living. Pain and functional limitation can be addressed through manual therapy, assistive devices, joint protection techniques, and thermal treatments. A targeted exercise program can be initiated, and adapting the program for home use is critical. Tendinitis, bursitis, many forms of arthritis, and chronic soft tissue pain due to overuse, injury, and chronic pain syndromes (such as fibromyalgia) are among the diagnoses appropriate for physical therapy referral.

Occupational therapists assess upper extremity functioning, including the ability to perform self-care and job-related tasks. Braces and splints may be provided for painful or unstable joints. An ergonomic evaluation of the workstation may accompany instruction in improved body mechanics and avoidance of repetitive trauma.

Complementary and Alternative Medicine

Nontraditional options for symptom management are employed by about one third of patients overall and up to 90% of patients with chronic pain, including arthritis and rheumatologic diseases. Commonly used over-the-counter supplements include fish oil, vitamins, glucosamine, and chondroitin. Providers should ask about supplement use because

TABLE 12. Rheumatologic Medications and Pregnancy[a]

Medication/Class	Comments
Anti-Inflammatory Agents	
NSAIDs	May impede implantation and may be associated with a small increased risk of miscarriage when used before 20 weeks' gestation. Use of NSAIDs after 30 weeks' gestation can lead to premature closure of the ductus arteriosus.
Glucocorticoids	When taken in the first trimester, can increase the risk of fetal cleft palate, and can raise the risk of maternal gestational diabetes throughout the pregnancy.
	Useful in the management of active autoimmune disease in pregnancy. Non-fluorinated glucocorticoids (e.g., prednisone, prednisolone, methylprednisolone) have limited ability to cross the placenta and are preferred, except when treating the fetus (e.g., neonatal lupus erythematosus).
Colchicine	Should be used only if the potential benefit justifies the potential risk to the fetus.
Analgesics	
Acetaminophen	Generally considered safe at standard dosing, but does cross the placenta.
Opiates	Some opiates/opioids cross the placenta; may cause fetal opioid withdrawal at birth.
Tramadol	Should be used only if the potential benefit justifies the potential risk to the fetus; postmarketing reports suggest the possibility of neonatal seizures, withdrawal syndrome, and stillbirth.
Topical agents	Topical use may limit serum levels; individual agents should be reviewed for pregnancy impact prior to use.
Nonbiologic DMARDs	
Methotrexate	Highly teratogenic and abortifacient; must be discontinued at least 3 months before pregnancy.
Hydroxychloroquine	Relatively safe in pregnancy and should not be discontinued if needed.
Sulfasalazine	Relatively safe during pregnancy.
Leflunomide	Extremely teratogenic; must not be used before/during pregnancy; upon discontinuation, cholestyramine administration is required to remove the drug from the body in all women of childbearing potential and specifically in those wishing to become pregnant; should be followed up with measurement of leflunomide and its metabolite levels to ensure removal of the drug.
Azathioprine	Routine use in pregnancy is not recommended; however, azathioprine may be safer than some other DMARDs and may be used if an immunosuppressive agent is imperative.
Cyclophosphamide	Not used in pregnancy unless absolutely necessary.
Mycophenolate mofetil	Teratogenic; should not be used in pregnancy; discontinue for 3 months before attempting pregnancy.
Cyclosporine	May be used in pregnancy only if benefits outweigh the risks.
Tofacitinib	May be teratogenic at high doses.
Biologic DMARDs	
TNF-α inhibitors	Accumulating retrospective data suggest low risk in pregnancy, but evidence is limited; can be continued if absolutely needed; different agents may have different considerations regarding crossing the placenta.
Ustekinumab; anakinra; secukinumab	Should be used only if the potential benefit justifies the undefined risk to the fetus.
Abatacept; belimumab; canakinumab; rilonacept; rituximab; tocilizumab	Should be used only if the potential benefit justifies the potential risk to the fetus.
Urate-Lowering Therapy (rarely needed in premenopausal women)	
Allopurinol	Should be used only if the potential benefit justifies the potential risk to the fetus.
Febuxostat	Should be used only if the potential benefit justifies the potential risk to the fetus.
Probenecid	No current evidence for adverse impact on pregnancy.
Pegloticase	Should be used only if the potential benefit justifies the potential risk to the fetus.

DMARD = disease-modifying antirheumatic drug; TNF = tumor necrosis factor.

[a]See MKSAP 18 General Internal Medicine for information on the FDA pregnancy categories.

patients rarely volunteer this information. Significant drug interactions may occur; for example, some herbal preparations can interact with anticoagulants.

Mind-body interventions such as tai chi, meditation, and yoga can improve psychological well-being, strength, balance, and pain level. Chiropractic and osteopathic manipulation as well as massage remain popular. Randomized controlled trials support the use of tai chi for arthritis; smaller trials suggest benefit from meditation techniques, yoga, massage, and manipulative medicine for various musculoskeletal problems.

Role of Surgery

Surgical procedures such as carpal tunnel release or rotator cuff tendon repair can address conditions that arise from repetitive trauma, injury, and degenerative changes in the soft tissue. Synovectomy of inflammatory pannus is occasionally employed when a single or limited number of joints in patients with RA do not respond to medications. Total joint arthroplasty, particularly of the knee or hip, can reduce or eliminate pain and restore function in patients with an inadequate response to medication and physical or occupational therapy.

KEY POINT

- Nonpharmacologic measures used in rheumatologic diseases include physical or occupational therapy, surgery, weight reduction, psychosocial support, and self-management programs.

Rheumatoid Arthritis
Pathophysiology and Risk Factors

Rheumatoid arthritis (RA) is a systemic autoimmune disease characterized by a chronic inflammatory polyarthritis affecting large and small joints with a predilection for the small joints of the hands and feet. RA has a prevalence of 0.5% to 1% in the general population, with some specific populations having rates as high as 7%.

Genetic Factors

Genes provide 60% of the risk for RA. Among some 100 genetic loci currently recognized as associated with RA risk, the most important is the class II HLA group, especially HLA-D alleles. These risk alleles code for the shared epitope, a five amino acid sequence that binds and presents citrullinated peptide antigens important in the pathophysiology of RA. Because citrulline is an amino acid that does not normally occur in humans, citrullinated proteins are immunogenic, especially in people who also have the shared epitope.

Citrulline is formed by the action of the enzyme peptidyl-arginine deiminase (PADI), which is found at sites of inflammation and serves to deiminate arginine to form citrullinated peptides. Many of the genes associated with RA modify

immune responses to provide a milieu for the development of autoantibodies.

Environmental Factors

Environmental factors provide 40% of the risk for RA. One of the most provocative environmental factors is smoking. Smoking can lead to lung inflammation, which activates enzymes such as PADI, and may promote citrullination. Patients who smoke and are at risk for RA because of family history must be counseled about smoking cessation.

Infectious Agents

A potential risk factor for the development of RA is periodontal disease. *Porphyromonas gingivalis*, a bacterium associated with periodontitis, produces PADI enzymes and provides a potential link to citrullinated peptide formation. Other infectious agents implicated include mycoplasma, Epstein-Barr virus, and parvovirus B19. However, a direct infectious cause of RA has not been identified. There is also interest in the role of the intestinal microbiome in RA. Gut dysbiosis has been postulated to promote early RA, possibly by activating proinflammatory lymphocytes.

Hormones

Women are two to three times as likely as men to develop RA. The role of estrogen and other gender-specific factors is incompletely understood but appears to promote a proinflammatory and/or proautoimmune milieu. Estrogen receptors are present on synovial fibroblasts and may lead to the production of cartilage-damaging metalloproteases. Stimulation of estrogen receptors on macrophages can increase tumor necrosis factor α production, a key RA inflammatory cytokine.

KEY POINT

- Potential risk factors for rheumatoid arthritis include genetic and environmental factors, infectious agents, and hormones; genes provide 60% of the risk.

Diagnosis

The 2010 American College of Rheumatology (ACR) and the European League Against Rheumatism (EULAR) classification criteria for RA are more sensitive but less specific than the prior 1987 criteria and emphasize early diagnosis and treatment to prevent the permanent consequences of chronic inflammation (**Table 13**).

Clinical Manifestations

RA is a chronic disorder, and onset of symptoms is usually gradual. Patients with RA typically report joint pain and inflammatory symptoms, including swelling and morning stiffness often lasting several hours. Stiffness is generally worse with rest but alleviated by ongoing activity. Joint swelling (softness or bogginess of the affected joint) is palpable on joint examination.

TABLE 13. The 2010 American College of Rheumatology/European League Against Rheumatism Classification Criteria for Rheumatoid Arthritis	
Criteria	Score[a]
Joint Involvement[b]	
1 large joint (shoulders, elbows, hips, knees, ankles)	0
2-10 large joints	1
1-3 small joints (MCPs, PIPs, wrists, 2-5 MTPs)	2
4-10 small joints	3
More than 10 small joints	5
Serology	
Negative RF or anti-CCP antibodies	0
Low-positive RF or anti-CCP antibodies (under 3 times the upper limit of normal)	2
High-level RF or anti-CCP antibodies (above 3 times the upper limit of normal)	3
Acute Phase Reactants	
Normal CRP or ESR	0
Abnormal CRP or ESR	1
Duration	
Less than 6 weeks	0
More than 6 weeks	1

CCP = cyclic citrullinated peptide; CRP = C-reactive protein; ESR = erythrocyte sedimentation rate; MCP = metacarpophalangeal; MTP = metatarsophalangeal; PIP = proximal interphalangeal; RF = rheumatoid factor.

[a]Six points needed for classification as rheumatoid arthritis.

[b]At least one joint with definite clinical synovitis that is not better explained by another disease.

From Aletaha D, Neogi T, Silman AJ, Funovits J, Felson DT, Bingham CO 3rd, et al. 2010 Rheumatoid arthritis classification criteria: an American College of Rheumatology/European League Against Rheumatism collaborative initiative. Arthritis Rheum. 2010 Sep;62(9):2569-81. doi: 10.1002/art.27584. [PMID: 20872595] Copyright 2010, American College of Rheumatology. Adapted with permission from John Wiley & Sons, Inc.

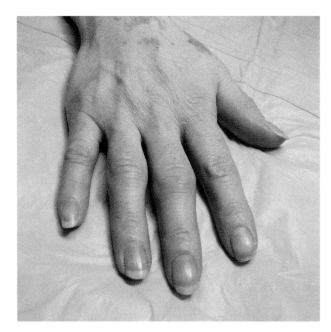

FIGURE 2. Early rheumatoid arthritis of the hands, with swelling in the third and fourth proximal interphalangeal joints.

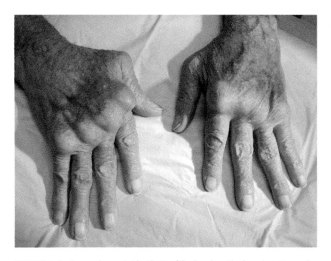

FIGURE 3. Severe rheumatoid arthritis of the hands, with ulnar deviation and subluxation at the metacarpophalangeal joints on both sides.

The pattern of joint involvement is useful for diagnosing RA. RA characteristically affects the metacarpophalangeal joints, metatarsophalangeal joints, and proximal interphalangeal joints of the hands and feet but spares the distal interphalangeal joints of both the upper and lower extremities (**Figure 2** and **Figure 3**). Wrists, elbows, shoulders, hips, knees, and ankles also can be involved. RA affects joints symmetrically (that is, joints on both sides of the body are generally involved), but severity may be asymmetric. RA may occasionally present as persistent involvement in a single joint. RA spares the thoracic and lumbar spine but affects the cervical spine, especially the C1-C2 (atlantoaxial) articulation. See **Table 14** for more information.

Laboratory Studies

The most useful laboratory studies to aid in the diagnosis of RA are rheumatoid factor and anti–cyclic citrullinated peptide (CCP) antibodies. Rheumatoid factor is found in approximately 70% of patients with RA and may be present at the time of disease onset. Because other diseases can be associated with rheumatoid factor, its specificity for RA is somewhat limited. Anti-CCP antibodies are also present in 70% of patients with RA but have a specificity of 95%. Anti-CCP antibodies are also more predictive than rheumatoid factor for erosive disease.

Approximately 10% to 20% of patients diagnosed with RA are seronegative (that is, neither rheumatoid factor nor anti-CCP antibodies is positive). Although categorized as having RA, these patients have somewhat different genetics and risk factors and generally have a better prognosis than those with seropositive RA.

TABLE 14. Consequences of Persistent Inflammation on Joints and Supporting Structures

Joint Area	Implications
C1-C2 articulation and transverse ligament	Laxity of the transverse ligament results in increased posterior motion of the dens on C2; with neck flexion, the dens can impact the midbrain and other vital neurologic structures
Shoulder and rotator cuff tendons	Restricted range of motion of the glenohumeral joint and rotator cuff tears
Elbow joint	Elbow contractures and difficulty with hand pronation and supination
Wrist carpal joints and finger tendons	Restricted range of motion of wrist; carpal tunnel syndrome; rupture of finger extensor tendons, especially the fourth and fifth
MCPs and surrounding structures	Ulnar deviation and subluxation of MCPs
PIPs and surrounding structures	Swan neck or boutonniere deformity due to inflammatory disruption of periarticular support structures
Hip joint	Axial migration of the femoral head in the acetabulum (protrusio acetabuli)
Knee joint	Tricompartmental joint-space narrowing
Ankle and mid-foot joints and tendons	Restricted range of motion of ankle; progressive pronated flat foot deformity
MTPs and surrounding structures	Fibular deviation of MTPs; cock-up deformities; skin ulceration underneath subluxed MTP heads

MCP = metacarpophalangeal; MTP = metatarsophalangeal; PIP = proximal interphalangeal.

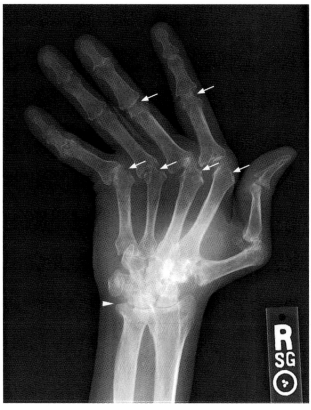

FIGURE 4. Radiograph showing advanced rheumatoid arthritis in the hand. There is ulnar deviation at the metacarpophalangeal joints; marginal erosions most prominently at the second through fourth metacarpophalangeal joints and the second and third proximal interphalangeal joints (*arrows*); and joint-space narrowing at the wrist, metacarpophalangeal, and proximal interphalangeal joints, which also represents erosive disease. Note the loss of the ulnar styloid (*arrowhead*), another common sign of bony erosion in rheumatoid arthritis.

Erythrocyte sedimentation rate and C-reactive protein are elevated in 75% of patients with RA and can be used to monitor treatment response. The systemic inflammation inherent to RA is commonly reflected by an anemia of inflammation and modest thrombocytosis.

Imaging Studies

Plain radiography of the hands and/or feet is a standard imaging study for RA and can aid in diagnosis and assessing progression, although early radiographs may be normal. Radiographic changes include periarticular osteopenia, marginal erosions, and joint-space narrowing (**Figure 4** and **Figure 5**). Radiography of the cervical spine with flexion/extension views is appropriate if C1-C2 subluxation is suspected.

MRI and ultrasonography are more sensitive than plain radiography and may have utility in following disease, assessing risk of progression, and determining response to therapy. Ultrasonography is becoming a standard tool for detecting joint fluid, synovial tissue thickening, early erosions, and increased vascularity. MRI is used for measuring bone marrow edema, synovitis, and erosions; it is also specifically indicated if atlantoaxial involvement is suspected.

KEY POINTS

- Clinical manifestations of classic rheumatoid arthritis typically include pain, swelling, and prolonged morning stiffness in symmetric small joints.

- The most useful laboratory studies to aid in the diagnosis of rheumatoid arthritis (RA) are rheumatoid factor and anti–cyclic citrullinated peptide (CCP) antibodies; anti-CCP antibodies have a specificity of 95% for RA. **HVC**

- Plain radiography of the hands and/or feet is a standard imaging study for rheumatoid arthritis; radiographic changes include periarticular osteopenia, marginal erosions, and joint-space narrowing, although early radiographs may be normal. **HVC**

Complications and Extra-Articular Manifestations

Joints

RA joint damage is a consequence of the development of synovitis within the joint. The synovial lining, normally only a few

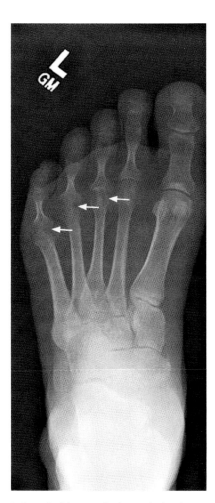

FIGURE 5. Radiograph of rheumatoid arthritis in the foot showing marginal erosions and joint-space narrowing at the third, fourth, and fifth metatarsophalangeal joints (*arrows*). Erosion at the fifth metatarsophalangeal joint is often the first radiographic sign of rheumatoid arthritis foot involvement.

cells thick, becomes significantly expanded and produces cartilage-damaging metalloproteases. Receptor activator of nuclear factor kappa B ligand (RANKL), produced by inflammatory cells, activates osteoclasts to erode bone. The metalloproteases and activated osteoclasts result in various irreversible changes to the joints (see Table 14).

Skin

The most common RA skin changes are rheumatoid nodules, present in up to 30% of patients. Nodules typically occur in the olecranon region and can be confused with gouty tophi, but can also occur over the hand and feet joints and even in the lungs. Nodulosis can rarely be induced by certain drugs (for example, methotrexate and leflunomide) but may respond to others (for example, hydroxychloroquine and colchicine). Patients with RA are also at an increased risk for neutrophilic dermatoses such as pyoderma gangrenosum or Sweet syndrome. Palpable purpura may result from small-vessel cutaneous vasculitis.

Eyes

The most common eye manifestation in RA is dry eye (keratoconjunctivitis sicca). It occurs in 10% to 15% of patients and can be severe. Most of these patients also have dry mouth and are classified as having secondary Sjögren syndrome. Less common (1%) are episcleritis (inflammation of the superficial scleral vessels) and scleritis (inflammation of deep scleral vessels). RA is one of the most common diseases associated with scleritis, which can be vision-threatening and lead to thinning of the sclera and perforation. Keratitis (corneal inflammation) can occur, which is ulcerative and occurs at the periphery of the cornea; severe keratitis is known as corneal melt. Both scleritis and keratitis require immediate referral to an ophthalmologist.

Lungs

Air trapping reflecting small airway disease occurs in up to 50% of patients with RA. Pleural disease occurs in up to 5%; pleural effusions are exudative and can be large. RA pleural effusions are characterized by low glucose and pH (mimicking bacterial or tubercular infection and malignancy) and low complement levels, as well as elevated levels of total protein, rheumatoid factor, and lactate dehydrogenase. Inflammatory cells in the RA effusion are characteristically mononuclear; a neutrophil-predominant effusion suggests infection. Interstitial lung disease contributes to excess mortality in RA and may develop in 50% of patients, but clinically significant disease is seen in 10%. Bronchiectasis and bronchiolitis occur, and the bronchiolitis can be obliterative/constrictive. Upper airway involvement from cricoarytenoid arthritis occurs rarely; symptoms include hoarseness, sore throat, dysphagia, and stridor. Cricoarytenoid arthritis can pose problems for endotracheal intubation.

Heart

Atherosclerotic heart disease remains the major cause of excess death in patients with RA, although recent data suggest that cardiovascular disease risk may be decreasing toward that of the general population. Nonetheless, patients with RA should be considered at high cardiovascular risk for purposes of perioperative evaluation, and cardiovascular disease risk factors such as dyslipidemia and hypertension should be addressed. Clinically significant pericarditis is rare. Granulomatous myocarditis, valvular disease (mainly mitral), conduction block, and aortitis are reported to occur in RA but are very rare.

Hematologic

Anemia of inflammation is the most common RA hematologic abnormality. Felty syndrome consists of neutropenia and splenomegaly and occurs in patients with long-standing, severe, seropositive RA. These patients are at risk for serious bacterial infection, lower extremity ulceration, lymphoma, and vasculitis. With current treatment, Felty syndrome has become rare.

CONT.

Patients with RA can also have a large granular lymphocyte syndrome that can progress to large granular lymphocyte leukemia. Findings overlap with Felty syndrome and include neutropenia, anemia, thrombocytopenia, splenomegaly, and recurrent infections. Patients with RA are at increased risk for lymphomas (particularly large B-cell lymphomas), and risk is correlated with disease activity.

Blood Vessels

A small-vessel cutaneous vasculitis occurs in a small percentage of patients with RA, leading to palpable purpura or periungual infarcts. A very rare, larger-vessel vasculitis similar to polyarteritis nodosa can affect multiple organ systems; prior to current therapy, it had a 5-year mortality of 30% to 50%.

KEY POINT

- Extra-articular manifestations and complications of rheumatoid arthritis include rheumatoid nodules, rheumatoid vasculitis, dry eye, small airway disease, interstitial lung disease, pleural effusions, and anemia of inflammation.

Management

See Principles of Therapeutics for details on the uses, mechanisms of action, major toxicities, and/or monitoring requirements of the medications used in RA.

General Considerations

The 2015 ACR RA treatment guidelines (https://www.rheumatology.org/Practice-Quality/Clinical-Support/Clinical-Practice-Guidelines/Rheumatoid-Arthritis) advocate for early diagnosis and aggressive early therapy of RA to prevent irreversible cartilage and bone damage. The 2010 ACR RA classification criteria emphasize sensitivity to permit early diagnosis and institution of disease-modifying therapy (see Table 13). A key treatment goal is to treat to target, with the target being achievement of remission or low disease activity. Disease activity assessment involves making a measured determination using combinations of numbers of tender and swollen joints (typically utilizing 28 joints that exclude the feet), patient and physician impressions of disease activity, and, in some activity scoring systems, measurement of the erythrocyte sedimentation rate or C-reactive protein. These parameters are combined into a composite score, thus assigning a disease activity ranging from remission, to low, moderate, or high. The Clinical Disease Activity Index (CDAI) and Disease Activity Score 28 (DAS28) are two commonly used instruments to assess disease activity and response to treatment. Treating to target in RA results in less radiographic damage, reduced cardiovascular risk, and increased work productivity compared with conventional care.

The 2015 ACR RA treatment guidelines can assist in making initial treatment decisions in early RA. Treatment is typically advanced at 12-week intervals with the goal of reaching remission or low disease activity as rapidly as possible. Patients who remain in remission or a low disease activity state for 6 months or longer may be able to reduce treatment intensity. Treatment decisions for established RA are more complex. An initial approach to the treatment of both early and established RA is outlined in **Figure 6**.

Disease-Modifying Antirheumatic Drugs
Nonbiologic Disease-Modifying Antirheumatic Drugs

Methotrexate is the anchor drug in RA, used in both monotherapy and combination therapy. It can be titrated to doses as high as 25 mg per week in partial responders; the treating physician should generally maximize methotrexate dosing before adding other agents. At doses greater than 15 mg weekly, methotrexate oral absorption approaches its effective limit; switching to subcutaneous administration allows for higher serum drug levels. Folic acid supplements minimize toxicity without diminishing efficacy. Of patients with RA taking methotrexate alone, 30% to 50% achieve remission or low disease activity.

Sulfasalazine, leflunomide, and hydroxychloroquine also can be used as monotherapy agents in RA. Leflunomide may

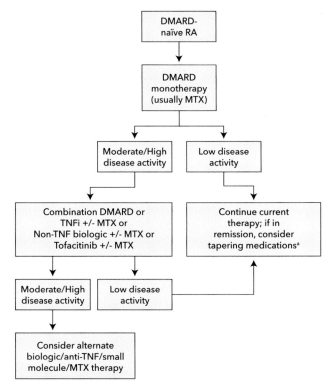

FIGURE 6. A simplified algorithm presenting an initial approach to the treatment of both early and established rheumatoid arthritis (RA). All patients with RA should receive a disease-modifying antirheumatic drug initially and be advanced to more aggressive and/or combination therapy as needed to control disease. Disease activity should be assessed, wherever possible, using a formal, validated, and consistent disease activity index. Refer to the American College of Rheumatology RA treatment guidelines for more complex algorithms accounting for differences between agents and patient-specific complexities. DMARD = disease-modifying antirheumatic drug; MTX = methotrexate; RA = rheumatoid arthritis; TNFi = tumor necrosis factor inhibitor.

ᵃDo not discontinue all RA treatments.

be useful in those who cannot tolerate methotrexate. Hydroxychloroquine is the least potent agent but can be used in very early disease when the disease activity score is low. It is also used as part of triple therapy (methotrexate, sulfasalazine, and hydroxychloroquine). Data suggest that triple therapy is comparable to methotrexate combined with a tumor necrosis factor α inhibitor, except in the area of radiographic progression.

Biologic Disease-Modifying Antirheumatic Drugs

Biologic DMARDs can be used as monotherapy but are typically added to methotrexate when moderate to high disease activity persists. Tumor necrosis factor (TNF)-α inhibitors are the most frequently used biologic DMARDs; these agents have a relatively rapid onset of action and demonstrate synergy with methotrexate. The combination of methotrexate and a TNF-α inhibitor has also been shown to have a "disconnect effect," meaning that even patients with continued clinical disease activity may demonstrate little to no damage to cartilage and bone. This effect also has been shown with rituximab or tocilizumab in combination with methotrexate. Other biologic DMARDs used in RA include abatacept (a selective T-cell costimulation modulator) and tofacitinib (a small-molecule Janus kinase inhibitor).

Until better data are available to guide therapeutic decisions, choice of a biologic DMARD remains empiric and based on patient characteristics, including what agents should be avoided due to patient comorbidity (for example, avoiding abatacept in a patient with COPD).

NSAIDs

NSAIDs were once the mainstay of therapy of RA. These agents are not disease modifying and do not prevent joint damage. They are used primarily to control symptoms while waiting for the full effect of DMARDs to be realized or in patients with postinflammatory osteoarthritis.

Glucocorticoids

Unlike NSAIDs, glucocorticoids may have a disease-modifying effect. A recent study tested 10 mg/d of prednisone versus placebo for 2 years in combination with methotrexate; the prednisone group had no more side effects than the placebo group but gained better control of disease activity, used less methotrexate, needed fewer additional medications, and had less radiographic damage. Low-dose prednisone (5-10 mg/d) can be used to rapidly improve RA symptoms while waiting for long-term medications to become effective, or they can be used short term for disease flares. Long-term therapy with glucocorticoids, however, may be associated with substantial adverse effects including osteoporosis, diabetes mellitus, and infection.

Surgery

Surgical therapy has become much less common in RA with current treatment strategies. However, some patients may require a synovectomy for a single persistently swollen joint, carpal tunnel release, repair of a ruptured tendon, total joint replacement (shoulder, metacarpophalangeal joints, hip, knee, or ankle), or joint fusion for a painful damaged joint (wrist or ankle). See MKSAP 18 General Internal Medicine for a discussion of perioperative RA medication management.

KEY POINTS

- In rheumatoid arthritis, treating to target of remission or low disease activity results in less radiographic damage, reduced cardiovascular risk, and increased work productivity compared with conventional care.

- Methotrexate is the anchor drug in rheumatoid arthritis; it is used as monotherapy and as a component of combination therapy.   **HVC**

- Tumor necrosis factor α inhibitors are the most frequently used biologics to treat rheumatoid arthritis; they have a relatively rapid onset of action and demonstrate synergy with methotrexate.

- In rheumatoid arthritis, NSAIDs are not disease modifying and do not prevent joint damage; they are used primarily to control symptoms while waiting for the full effect of disease-modifying antirheumatic drugs to be realized or in patients with postinflammatory osteoarthritis.   **HVC**

- Low-dose prednisone can be used in rheumatoid arthritis to rapidly improve symptoms until long-term medications become effective, or they can be used short term for disease flares.

Pregnancy

There is an increased risk for developing RA in the first year after a first pregnancy. Breastfeeding may decrease this risk. For women with established RA, two thirds will go into remission or low disease activity during pregnancy, and one third will not improve or will get worse. Medication management is a major issue, and pregnancy plans should be discussed with any woman of childbearing age who will be placed on therapy. A discussion of RA medications in pregnancy is located in Principles of Therapeutics.

KEY POINT

- There is an increased risk for developing rheumatoid arthritis (RA) in the first year after a first pregnancy; for women with established RA, two thirds will go into remission or achieve low disease activity during pregnancy, whereas one third will not improve or will get worse.

Osteoarthritis
Pathophysiology

Osteoarthritis (OA) is a chronic progressive multifactorial disorder of maladaptive cellular repair responses to joint stress.

Previously deemed a "wear and tear" disease and an inevitable consequence of aging, OA is now recognized as a disorder driven by a complex interplay of genetics, joint injury, cell stress, extracellular matrix degradation, and inflammation. It affects all the tissues of the joint and is characterized by cartilage and meniscal degradation, subchondral bone changes (bone marrow lesions, subchondral sclerosis), and osteophyte formation. Other findings include synovial inflammation with hypertrophy and effusion as well as weakening of the periarticular muscle. Morphologic changes in cartilage reflect collagen and proteoglycan alterations driven by imbalanced anabolic and catabolic repair processes. In addition, inflammatory cytokines such as interleukin-1β and tumor necrosis factor α are produced in the synovium and cartilage; they drive joint tissue destruction and stimulate synthesis of additional inflammatory mediators.

Epidemiology and Risk Factors

OA is the most common form of arthritis worldwide and a leading cause of pain and disability, affecting approximately 30 million U.S. adults. OA is the leading cause of lower extremity disability among older adults, with an estimated lifetime risk for knee OA approaching 50%. Prevalence is projected to more than double by the year 2030, largely due to increasing obesity rates and aging of the population. Incidence and prevalence rates vary by joint and depend upon whether a clinical or radiographic definition is being applied. Recent efforts examining whether patients with OA are at increased risk for cardiovascular morbidity and all-cause mortality have been inconclusive, with positive associations appearing to relate more to functional decline and disability than to OA-specific pathologic processes.

Epidemiological risk factors for OA include age greater than 55, race/ethnicity, female sex, obesity, genetics, and occupations that include repetitive motions or physical labor. Age and female sex are strong nonmodifiable risk factors for OA of different sites. Obesity is the most important modifiable risk factor, especially for knee OA. Increased body mass is also a risk factor for hand OA, perhaps underscoring the systemic nature of the disease and a role for metabolic and/or inflammatory mechanisms in its pathogenesis. Single inherited conditions rarely predispose to OA; however, mutations in proteins involved in bone or articular cartilage structure or metabolism are possible risk factors.

Risk factors involving the joint itself include abnormal loading, injury, malalignment, and intrinsic cartilage or bone tissue defects. Injury may be acute (for example, anterior cruciate ligament tear) or may be more minor and repetitive (for example, physical labor or overuse); regardless of cause, injuries have been linked with the future development of OA of various sites. Hip dislocation, congenital dysplasia, femoroacetabular impingement, knee malalignment, and shape of the knee joint are also associated with incident OA.

Given its multifactorial etiology, an individual patient may develop OA as a consequence of one or more risk factors; how the interaction of these risk factors culminates in OA is complex and not fully understood.

KEY POINTS

- Osteoarthritis is a chronic progressive disorder characterized by cartilage and meniscal degradation, subchondral bone changes, and osteophyte formation.
- Risk factors for osteoarthritis include epidemiological factors (age, race/ethnicity, female sex, genetics, obesity) and joint-specific factors (malalignment, cartilage defects, joint injury).

Classification

Primary Osteoarthritis

The most common type of OA is primary OA, in which no identifiable proximal cause is recognized. Although almost any joint may be affected by OA, primary OA typically involves specific joints, including the distal interphalangeal (DIP) and proximal interphalangeal (PIP) finger joints, the first carpometacarpal joint at the base of the thumb, the hip and knee joints, and the cervical and lumbar spine.

Erosive Osteoarthritis

Erosive (inflammatory) OA is a subset of primary hand OA. Clinically, erosive OA mostly affects the DIP and PIP joints, is more inflammatory and painful than typical hand OA (with erythema and swelling), and is more common in women. Radiographs reveal diagnosis-defining central erosions (in contrast to marginal erosions seen in rheumatoid arthritis) with a "seagull" or "gull-wing" appearance in the finger joints (**Figure 7**); joint ankylosis (bony fusion) may also occur. Whether erosive OA comprises a separate disease entity or is part of the continuum of OA remains controversial.

Secondary Osteoarthritis

Secondary OA is historically defined in the presence of a predisposing disorder; however, an increasing number of risk factors are being identified for primary OA, thus blurring the lines between the primary and secondary forms of the disease. Pathologic changes, clinical presentations, symptoms, and management are indistinguishable between primary and secondary OA. When OA is observed in a joint not typically affected by primary OA, however, secondary causes should be entertained. Commonly recognized causes of secondary OA include a history of frank damage such as trauma, joint infection, or surgical repair (such as anterior cruciate ligament repair or meniscectomy); congenitally abnormal joints (for example, hip dysplasia); systemic metabolic, endocrine, and neuropathic disorders, particularly those that affect cartilage; and underlying inflammatory arthritis with accompanying damage (for example, rheumatoid or psoriatic arthritis) (**Table 15**).

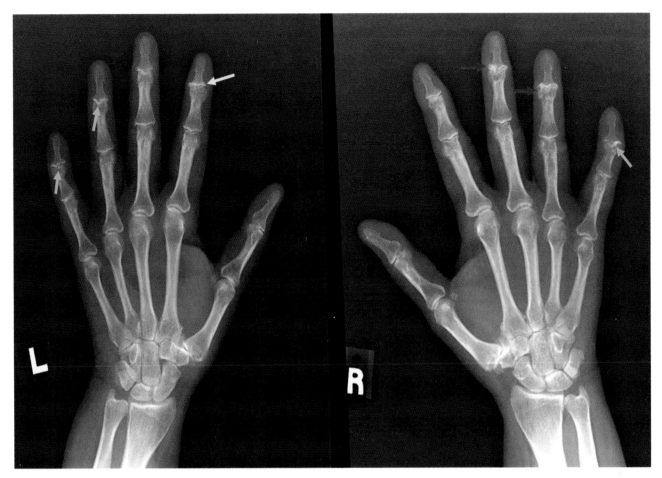

FIGURE 7. Plain radiographs showing erosive hand osteoarthritis (OA). Note the classic "gull-wing" appearance of the fourth and fifth distal interphalangeal (DIP) joints on the left and the fifth DIP joint on the right (*green arrows*), reflecting central erosion of cartilage on the proximal surface of the joint. Also seen is bony ankylosis, a feature of erosive OA, of the right fourth DIP joint and developing in the right third DIP joint (*red arrows*). Additionally, the left second DIP joint exhibits the findings of classic (nonerosive) hand OA (joint-space narrowing, subchondral sclerosis, and osteophytes without the "gull-wing" appearance) (*yellow arrow*).

TABLE 15.	Secondary Causes of Osteoarthritis
Secondary Cause	**Joint(s) Typically Involved**
Hemochromatosis	Second/third MCP joints
Calcium pyrophosphate deposition	MCP joints; wrists; knees; hips; shoulders; atlanto-axial joint
Alkaptonuria/ochronosis	Spine; hips; knees
Acromegaly	Knees; shoulders; spine
Hyperparathyroidism	Wrists; MCP joints
Joint injury	Knees

MCP = metacarpophalangeal.

Diffuse Idiopathic Skeletal Hyperostosis

Diffuse idiopathic skeletal hyperostosis (DISH) is a noninflammatory condition characterized by calcification and ossification of spinal ligaments (especially the anterior longitudinal ligament) and entheses (tendon and ligament attachments to bone). Unlike OA, DISH is more common in men. DISH usually presents as back pain and stiffness, with the thoracic spine most often involved. Although spinal ligamentous ossification is also seen in ankylosing spondylitis, the spinal calcifications in DISH are more "flowing," wider and less vertically oriented than those seen with ankylosing spondylitis. There is additionally no involvement of the sacroiliac joints in DISH.

Radiographic changes characteristic of DISH include confluent ossification of at least four contiguous vertebral levels, usually on the right side of the spine (**Figure 8**). Patients with DISH have less involvement of the left side of the thoracic spine, perhaps secondary to the aorta serving as a mechanical barrier to the production of bony hyperostosis.

KEY POINTS

- The most common type of osteoarthritis (OA) is primary OA, in which no identifiable proximal cause is recognized.

- Erosive osteoarthritis (OA) mostly affects the distal interphalangeal and proximal interphalangeal joints, is more inflammatory and painful than typical hand OA (with erythema and swelling), and is more common in women.

(Continued)

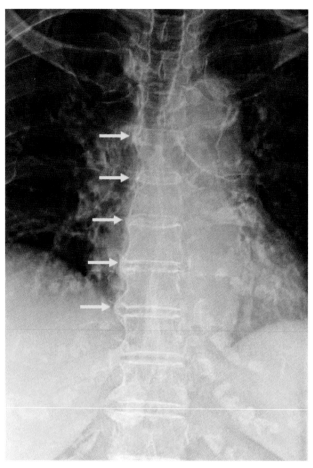

FIGURE 8. Plain lumbar radiograph of a patient with diffuse idiopathic skeletal hyperostosis (DISH). Note the calcification at sites of tendinous and ligamentous insertion of the spine, taking the form of flowing ossification of multiple contiguous vertebrae (*arrows*). Also seen here is the typical extensive involvement of the right side of the spine and relative sparing of the left (calcification of the anterior longitudinal ligament is also common, but not readily observed in this view).

Courtesy of Soterios Gyftopoulos, MD, MSc.

KEY POINTS *(continued)*

- Commonly recognized causes of secondary osteoarthritis include a history of frank damage; congenitally abnormal joints; systemic metabolic, endocrine, and neuropathic disorders; and underlying inflammatory arthritis.

- Diffuse idiopathic skeletal hyperostosis is a noninflammatory condition characterized by calcification and ossification of spinal ligaments and entheses; radiographs usually show confluent "flowing" ossification of at least four contiguous vertebral levels, usually on the right side of the spine.

Diagnosis

Clinical Manifestations

OA diagnosis is based on history and physical examination; radiography is confirmatory but may not be necessary. In early OA, clinical findings may not be accompanied by radiographic changes; conversely, some patients with prominent radiographic changes may have minimal or no symptoms. Patients with OA are typically over 50 years of age; diagnosis at an earlier age should prompt inquiry into a history of prior joint damage, endocrine or metabolic disorders, or a genetic proclivity for early disease.

Joints most commonly affected are the hands (DIPs and PIPs) (**Figure 9**), feet (first metatarsophalangeal joint and mid foot), knees, hips, and spine, but the distribution is variable. Localized OA, in which a single joint is affected, is more often a consequence of injury or joint asymmetry and often occurs in weight-bearing joints (hip or knee). Generalized OA, which affects multiple joint groups (for example, hands, spine, knees, and hips), is more likely the result of a combination of genetic and environmental factors and may be more symmetric in distribution.

Patients with OA usually describe an insidious onset of intermittent symptoms, which become more persistent and severe over time. The most common symptom is joint pain that is exacerbated by activity and alleviated with rest. Patients also describe morning stiffness usually lasting less than 30 minutes, in contrast to the prolonged morning stiffness of inflammatory arthritis. A single joint may initially be involved with eventual involvement of multiple joints.

On joint examination, crepitus, decreased range of motion, bony enlargement, and sometimes effusion may be present. Patients with long-standing hand OA may have Heberden and Bouchard nodes (bony enlargement of the DIP and PIP joints, respectively) and squaring of the first carpometacarpal joint. Hip involvement typically manifests as groin pain and decreased range of motion, especially internal rotation. Knee symptoms include pain on walking, especially on stairs, and difficulty transferring from a seated to standing position. Spondylosis, or OA affecting the spine, can affect the vertebral bodies, facet joints, and neural foramina, and may lead to spinal stenosis.

Patients with OA generally do not have systemic features. Pain and structural changes, however, ultimately result in functional impairment, pain, disability, psychosocial isolation, and reduced quality of life.

Laboratory and Imaging Studies

Laboratory testing is usually not necessary for diagnosis of OA but is helpful if other causes of arthritis are being considered, such as crystal arthropathy, rheumatoid arthritis, psoriatic arthritis, or hemochromatosis (all of which can coexist with OA). Acute phase reactants should be normal in OA. Routine laboratory testing (complete blood count, kidney and hepatic function) are not necessary for diagnosing OA but may be important when considering pharmacologic therapy, especially in the elderly and those with comorbidities.

If effusion is present, evaluation for concurrent crystal arthritis, infections, or other inflammatory causes should be

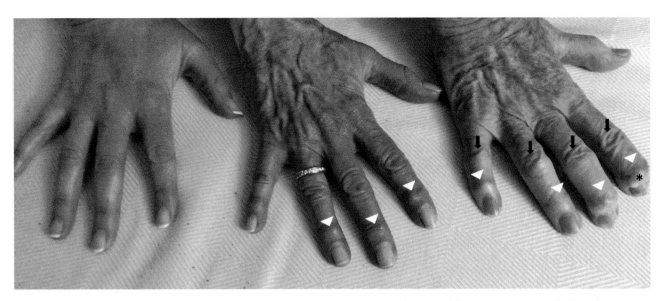

FIGURE 9. Progression of hand osteoarthritis (OA). This image illustrates the progression from normal hand joints (*left*), to distal interphalangeal (DIP) joint bony hypertrophy (Heberden nodes) of hand OA (*middle*), to extensive hand OA findings of Heberden nodes and proximal interphalangeal (PIP) joint bony hypertrophy (Bouchard nodes) (*right*). The hand on the right also displays a gouty nodule (tophus) overlying the Heberden node on the second DIP joint, underlining the potential coexistence of these two arthropathies. White arrowheads = Heberden nodes; black arrows = Bouchard nodes; black asterisk = tophus.

considered, ideally by synovial fluid analysis. OA synovial fluid is typically clear in appearance and noninflammatory, with a leukocyte count ≤2000/μL (2.0×10^9/L).

Although imaging is not necessary to make an OA diagnosis, it can be helpful to confirm the diagnosis, establish baseline severity, and exclude other diagnoses. Radiographic features of OA include asymmetric joint-space narrowing, subchondral sclerosis, osteophytes, and bone cysts; however, these changes may not be present in early disease. Even in established OA, symptoms may correlate poorly with imaging findings. Although MRI and ultrasonography can detect subtle OA changes at an earlier stage and are increasingly used in OA research, they are not needed for routine OA diagnosis. MRI may be indicated in the setting of symptoms suggestive of a concomitant mechanical disorder (joint catching, locking, instability), but incidental abnormalities such as meniscal tears are commonly seen on MRI in patients with OA and may prompt unnecessary surgical intervention.

Differential Diagnosis

Diagnosing OA may be problematic when OA is present in atypical joints, when an accurate history is difficult to obtain, or when a concurrent inflammatory arthropathy may be present. Calcium pyrophosphate deposition may occur in joints also typical for OA (hands or knees) but is associated with intermittent "flares," and radiographs show cartilage calcification (chondrocalcinosis). Gout and OA commonly co-associate, particularly in the DIP joints. Rheumatoid arthritis typically affects the hands, but unlike OA, the DIP joints are rarely affected, and signs and symptoms of chronic and persistent inflammation are seen. The presence of rheumatoid factor,

anti–cyclic citrullinated peptide antibodies, and elevated inflammatory markers favors the diagnosis of rheumatoid arthritis but does not eliminate the possibility of concurrent OA. Psoriatic arthritis can involve the DIP joints, but also commonly includes prolonged morning stiffness, joint swelling, dactylitis, and a history of psoriasis. Synovial fluid analysis can also be helpful in distinguishing between OA and these inflammatory disorders.

Other conditions to consider when evaluating a patient for OA include nonarticular sources of pain such as bursitis and tendinitis. Hip pain that is not in the anterior groin but instead around the lateral hip and buttock may indicate trochanteric bursitis or lumbosacral radiculopathy. Similarly, knee pain may be secondary to pes anserine bursitis or iliotibial band syndrome rather than intra-articular pathology. The pes anserine bursa is located along the proximal medial aspect of the tibia; thus, pes anserine bursitis should be considered when there is spontaneous pain along the inner (inferomedial) aspect of the knee joint. Patients with iliotibial band syndrome typically present with pain at the lateral aspect of the knee, usually exacerbated by physical activity, such as walking up or down stairs, running, or cycling.

KEY POINTS

- The most common symptom of osteoarthritis is joint pain that is exacerbated by activity and alleviated with rest; morning stiffness usually lasts less than 30 minutes.

- Laboratory testing is usually not necessary to diagnose osteoarthritis but is helpful if other causes of arthritis are being considered, such as crystal arthropathy, rheumatoid arthritis, psoriatic arthritis, and hemochromatosis. **HVC**

(Continued)

- Radiographic features of osteoarthritis (OA) include asymmetric joint-space narrowing, subchondral sclerosis, osteophytes, and bone cysts; however, these changes may not be present in early disease, and symptoms may correlate poorly with imaging findings, even in established OA.

Management

To date, no agents have been FDA approved to prevent, delay, or remit the structural progression of disease in OA. Instead, current treatment is directed to the management of pain and disability. Evidence-based guidelines for OA management are available from the American College of Rheumatology (ACR), the Osteoarthritis Research Society International (OARSI), the European League Against Rheumatism (EULAR), and others; however, there is poor consensus among these guidelines. Nevertheless, there is agreement that optimal OA management requires a combination of nonpharmacologic and pharmacologic modalities. Patients with OA should receive individualized multidisciplinary treatment that takes into account their expectations, functional and activity levels, occupational and vocational needs, joints affected, severity of disease, and any coexisting medical problems.

Nonpharmacologic Therapy

The nonpharmacologic approach to OA starts with assessment of physical status, activities of daily living, health education, motivation, beliefs, and other biopsychosocial factors. An individualized management plan includes education on OA and joint protection, an exercise regimen, weight loss, proper footwear, and assistive devices as appropriate. Physical activity includes graduated aerobic exercise and strength training, with attention paid to strengthening periarticular structures and minimizing injury. Tai chi has also been shown to be as beneficial as physical therapy for knee OA pain. A recent study reports that the combination of diet and exercise is more effective at decreasing OA-related knee pain and dysfunction than either diet or exercise alone. Furthermore, a 2015 Cochrane review, which included 54 knee OA studies, concluded that land-based therapeutic exercise provides short-term benefit in terms of reduced knee pain and improved physical function that is sustained for at least 2 to 6 months after cessation of formal treatment.

Pharmacologic Therapy

In the absence of disease-modifying OA drugs, pharmacologic treatment is considered when symptoms are present and bothersome to the patient. Pharmacologic therapy for OA includes oral, topical, and intra-articular medications. Choice of treatment(s) depends upon individualized assessment, with particular attention to comorbidities, concomitant medications, and especially adverse effects of the treatments. See Principles of Therapeutics for details on the medications used in OA.

Oral and Topical Agents

Oral agents include acetaminophen, NSAIDs, duloxetine, and tramadol. Recent systematic reviews and meta-analyses suggest that acetaminophen provides no benefit for hip or knee OA. NSAIDs are efficacious in OA, but their side-effect profiles make sustained use problematic, especially in the elderly and those with comorbidities. If used, the proper choice of an NSAID, considering drug pharmacokinetics as well as gastrointestinal and cardiovascular effects, may improve tolerance and minimize risk. Duloxetine, a serotonin-norepinephrine reuptake inhibitor with central nervous system activity, has shown efficacy for knee OA pain, implicating the role of central sensitization in OA pain modulation. A 2018 randomized controlled trial demonstrated that opioids were not superior to nonopioid medications for improving pain-related function for chronic back pain or OA-related hip or knee pain; pain intensity was significantly improved in the nonopioid group. Tramadol may be useful in some patients who cannot take other analgesics, but has substantial adverse effects.

Topical NSAIDs are an alternative to oral NSAIDs and may be beneficial for those who should avoid or cannot tolerate oral NSAIDs, including those who are ≥75 years old, have a history of peptic ulcer disease, or have chronic kidney disease. However, topical NSAIDs are associated with more skin reactions and are more expensive than oral NSAIDs. Other topicals such as capsaicin, lidocaine, and methyl salicylate preparations may also be used as adjunctive measures, especially when NSAIDs are either ineffective or not tolerated.

The oral alternative therapies glucosamine and chondroitin sulfate are frequently used by patients; although they appear to be safe, the quality of evidence for their efficacy is poor.

Intra-Articular Injections

Patients with knee or hip OA who have inefficacy, intolerance, or contraindication to oral and topical therapies may benefit from intra-articular glucocorticoid or hyaluronic acid injections. There is no formal evidence for the utility of intra-articular therapy in joints other than the knee and hip.

Intra-articular glucocorticoids are efficacious in knee and hip OA and are supported by multiple treatment guidelines. Long-term harm has not been demonstrated; however, benefit is usually short term and usually wanes within 3 months. Injections can be administered repeatedly but are not usually given more often than every 3 months. A recent 2-year study has called the efficacy and long-term safety of intra-articular glucocorticoid injections into question, with possible negative effects on cartilage thickness, an outcome with unclear clinical meaning.

Patients with inadequate response to intra-articular glucocorticoids may benefit from intra-articular hyaluronic acid injection. The quality of trials assessing intra-articular hyaluronan efficacy is low, and the degree of benefit is unclear. Nonetheless, intra-articular hyaluronans are widely used, especially when other treatments have failed and surgery is not a feasible option. When benefit is seen, it is usually more gradual and more persistent than that of intra-articular glucocorticoids.

Surgical Therapy

Surgery for OA is considered when nonpharmacologic and pharmacologic approaches fail to control pain or functional limitation. Multiple high-quality studies have shown that arthroscopic surgery for knee OA provides no better outcomes than conservative management unless there is joint buckling, instability, or locking or a concomitant and symptomatic mechanical disorder.

In contrast, total joint replacement is a "curative" option for those who have failed conservative therapies, providing pain relief and functional improvement. Overall, long-term outcomes are excellent, although hardware loosening and late infection may occur.

Recent studies suggest that for morbidly obese patients with knee OA, bariatric surgery may result in significant improvement in pain and function even without further OA management.

KEY POINTS

HVC • Nonpharmacologic therapy for osteoarthritis includes education, an exercise regimen, weight loss, proper footwear, and assistive devices as appropriate.

HVC • Recent systematic reviews and meta-analyses suggest that acetaminophen provides no benefit for hip or knee osteoarthritis; NSAIDs and duloxetine are efficacious.

• Pharmacologic therapy for osteoarthritis includes oral, topical, and intra-articular medications; choice of treatment(s) depends upon individualized assessment, with particular attention to comorbidities and concomitant medications.

HVC • Arthroscopic surgery is not indicated in patients with osteoarthritis unless there is joint buckling, instability, or locking, or a concomitant and symptomatic mechanical disorder.

• Total joint replacement provides pain relief and functional improvement in patients with osteoarthritis who have failed conservative therapies.

Fibromyalgia
Epidemiology and Pathophysiology

Fibromyalgia is characterized by widespread pain, fatigue, disturbed sleep, and cognitive dysfunction. It is common (prevalence, 2%-3%), particularly among individuals of lower socioeconomic status and/or educational level. Prevalence increases with age, peaking around the seventh decade. The female-to-male ratio is approximately 3:1.

Early paradigms of fibromyalgia as an inflammatory or psychosomatic condition have yielded to an understanding of fibromyalgia as a disorder of pain processing. It is likely a form of "central sensitization," in which the pain centers of the brain and spinal cord are hyperresponsive. Allodynia (a heightened sensitivity to stimuli that are not normally painful) and hyperalgesia (an increased response to painful stimuli) are common. An additional characteristic feature is "wind-up," or temporal summation. When repeatedly exposed to a mildly uncomfortable stimulus, patients with fibromyalgia experience progressively additive pain, indicating that the stimuli are both persistent and inadequately damped.

The underlying changes seen in the neurologic system are complex. Ascending fibers from the dorsal root ganglia convey inappropriately strong or persistent signals to hypothalamic pain centers. Patients with fibromyalgia have higher cerebrospinal fluid levels of the pain-promoting neurotransmitters substance P and glutamate, along with sensitization of glutamate receptors. Concurrently, descending inhibitory pathways utilizing adrenergic neurotransmitters (serotonin, norepinephrine) are impaired. The resultant circuit of chronic pain is self-sustaining but may be amplified by both psychic distress and peripherally generated tissue pain (such as arthritic joint pain). Genetic influences are a focus of ongoing investigation.

Diagnosis

The characteristic clinical features of fibromyalgia are widespread chronic pain (including hypersensitivity to painful stimuli), fatigue, and sleep disorders (both disrupted and nonrestorative sleep). These are frequently accompanied by impaired cognitive function, mood disorders, and symptoms such as headache, gastrointestinal symptoms, and paresthesia. Although the diagnosis of fibromyalgia traditionally centered on the presence of specific tender points elicited on physical examination, tender point examination is subject to physician expertise (such as appropriate application of force). In addition, male patients report tender point pain less frequently than female patients, leading to possible underdiagnosis. The 2010 American College of Rheumatology Preliminary Diagnostic Criteria forgo physical examination to emphasize a careful characterization of symptoms (**Table 16**). Many physicians rely on these diagnostic criteria but perform tender point assessment as part of the examination.

Treatable alternative diagnoses that may provoke or be mistaken for fibromyalgia include hypothyroidism, hypoadrenalism, and depression.

Management

Optimal management of fibromyalgia requires a holistic approach, including education, exercise, and psychosocial support. Pharmacotherapy is often warranted, although nonpharmacologic measures remain a cornerstone of treatment.

TABLE 16. Comparison of the 1990 ACR Classification Criteria and the 2010 ACR Diagnostic Criteria for Fibromyalgia

1990 ACR Classification Criteria	2010 ACR Preliminary Diagnostic Criteria
Widespread pain by self-report	Widespread pain by the Widespread Pain Index (WPI; 19-point scale) assessing the number of regions in which the patient has pain[a,b]
≥11 tender points on digital palpation or using a dolorimeter	Symptom severity by the Symptom Severity (SS) Scale (12-point scale) assessing 1) fatigue; 2) nonrestorative sleep; 3) cognitive symptoms[a,b]
	Duration of symptoms ≥3 months
	No other disorder explaining the pain

ACR = American College of Rheumatology.

[a]Fibromyalgia is diagnosed in the setting of WPI ≥7 plus SS score ≥5, or WPI ≥3 plus SS score ≥9.

[b]The Widespread Pain Index and the Symptom Severity Scale can be viewed at https://www.rheumatology.org/Portals/0/Files/2010%20Fibromyalgia%20Diagnostic%20Criteria_Excerpt.pdf.

Patients should be educated regarding the disease, with validation that the symptoms are real and that the painful areas are not injured and will not lose function. Aerobic exercise can improve well-being and function as well as reduce pain. Because patients initially experience postexercise pain that may threaten their willingness to continue, exercise must be introduced gradually and supported encouragingly. Strength training may also be helpful. Although the evidence base supporting their use is modest, alternative medicine approaches, including yoga, tai chi, acupuncture, and massage, may also help alleviate symptoms.

Patients with fibromyalgia should be assessed for psychosocial stressors and psychiatric illness, including a history of trauma. If present, referral for psychological care is mandatory, because psychic distress may both promote and result from fibromyalgia. Cognitive behavioral therapy has shown modest benefit in reducing pain, negative mood, and disability.

Choice of pharmacologic therapy is based on symptom profile, patient comorbidities, and medication side effects because few trials directly compare the efficacy of medications. Effective pharmacologic therapies target the underlying pathophysiology and inhibit the ascending pain pathways, enhance the descending inhibitory pathways to the dorsal roots, or inhibit release of the pain-promoting neurotransmitter glutamate.

The antiepileptic agents gabapentin and pregabalin (the latter FDA approved) inhibit $\alpha_2\delta$ calcium channels to inhibit glutamate release. They have been shown to improve quality of life and decrease pain.

Tricyclic antidepressants (TCAs) (such as amitriptyline) raise norepinephrine levels and have documented benefit, although efficacy may wane with time. TCAs induce drowsiness, with potential benefit for disordered sleep. The muscle relaxant cyclobenzaprine, another tricyclic, may be useful in patients with muscle spasms. Selective serotonin reuptake inhibitors have little benefit alone but may complement the activity of TCAs.

Among the more effective fibromyalgia therapies are the dual serotonin-norepinephrine reuptake inhibitors (SNRIs),

including the FDA-approved agents duloxetine and milnacipran. They or a TCA may be particularly appropriate in the patient with concomitant depression.

Tramadol, which has a complex mechanism of action, has shown some benefit and may be considered as a second-line approach. Finally, in some cases, combination pharmacologic therapy may be helpful.

Evidence does not support the benefit of NSAIDs for fibromyalgia, and pure opioids should not be used.

Fibromyalgia is a chronic disease, and the patient and physician should understand that the benefit of treatment will likely be partial and palliative, rather than complete or curative. Nonetheless, proper treatment can help most patients manage and cope with their symptoms as well as maintain function and autonomy.

KEY POINTS

- The characteristic features of fibromyalgia are widespread chronic pain, fatigue, and sleep disorders, which are frequently accompanied by impaired cognitive function, mood disorders, and symptoms such as headache, gastrointestinal symptoms, and paresthesia.

- The diagnosis of fibromyalgia is no longer based upon physician examination findings but a careful characterization of symptoms using a validated scoring tool. **HVC**

- Nonpharmacologic therapy (education, exercise, psychosocial support) remains a cornerstone of treatment for fibromyalgia, although pharmacotherapy is often warranted. **HVC**

Spondyloarthritis
Overview

Spondyloarthritis refers to a group of arthritic disorders that tends to involve the spine and sacroiliac joints and share genetic, pathophysiologic, and clinical features. HLA-B27 is variably expressed but is more frequently present in this group of patients than in the general population. Peripheral arthritis, enthesitis (inflammation of the insertion points of tendons and ligaments onto bone), inflammatory eye disease, psoriatic rashes, and gastrointestinal and genitourinary inflammation may occur in varying degrees.

Pathophysiology

Pathophysiologic processes involved in these disorders include T-cell activation and proliferation; elaboration of cytokines, particularly tumor necrosis factor (TNF)-α and the interleukins (IL)-1 and -23/17; and bony proliferation and destruction. Although the exact trigger for these processes is unknown, genetic and environmental factors are likely to play a role.

Genetic Factors

The most important genetic risk factor for spondyloarthritis is the presence of HLA-B27. The prevalence of HLA-B27 is high among Northern Europeans (about 6%) and low in Africans; accordingly, spondyloarthritis is seen with greater frequency in the former group. However, only 5% to 6% of those carrying HLA-B27 develop spondyloarthritis, and not all patients with spondyloarthritis are positive for HLA-B27. For these reasons, HLA-B27 should not be used as a screening test for these disorders, although its presence in a patient with a high pretest probability can support the diagnosis.

Several theories have been advanced to explain the relationship between HLA-B27 and the spectrum of disease observed. The arthritogenic peptide theory suggests that the presentation of an unknown peptide(s), perhaps of bacterial origin, activates cytotoxic T lymphocytes in the context of HLA-B27. Other theories propose that HLA-B27 molecules on antigen-presenting cells can either directly activate natural killer and T cells even in the absence of antigen or can induce a proinflammatory environment. Similarly, HLA-B27 expression on intestinal epithelium may interact with the gut microbiome to favor inflammation. Finally, tissue-specific chronic inflammation triggered by bacterial or mechanical stress may underlie a more autoinflammatory rather than autoimmune role for HLA-B27.

Other genes that have been identified as risk factors for spondyloarthritis include those associated with the TNF receptor signaling pathway as well as IL-1α and IL-23 receptor polymorphisms.

Environmental Factors

Considerable interest has focused on the role of the microbiome, particularly because gut inflammation is prevalent in many forms of spondyloarthritis. It is hypothesized that microbe-associated intestinal inflammation could cause loss of integrity of the bowel epithelium, permitting macrophage stimulation, increases in IL-23, and Th17 cell activation. However, specific causative pathogen exposure has not been identified except in some cases of reactive arthritis.

KEY POINTS

- Spondyloarthritis refers to a group of arthritic disorders that tends to involve the spine and sacroiliac joints and share genetic, pathophysiologic, and clinical features.

- The most important genetic risk factor for spondyloarthritis is the presence of HLA-B27; however, only 5% to 6% of patients carrying HLA-B27 develop spondyloarthritis, and not all patients with spondyloarthritis are positive for HLA-B27.

Classification

Spondyloarthritis is divided into five categories based on the predominant clinical features, although overlap of clinical features among these categories is common (**Table 17**):

1. Ankylosing spondylitis: Spinal involvement is the defining feature.

2. Psoriatic arthritis: Psoriasis co-occurs with spinal and/or peripheral arthritis.

3. Inflammatory bowel disease–associated arthritis: Clinically apparent intestinal inflammation is present along with spinal and/or peripheral arthritis.

4. Reactive arthritis: Inflammatory synovitis (primarily peripheral) occurs following specific gastrointestinal or genitourinary infections.

5. Undifferentiated spondyloarthritis: Spondylitis occurs in the absence of diagnostic features (including radiographic changes) that would permit diagnosis of one of the other categories of disease.

Clinical features common to all forms of spondyloarthritis are back pain, enthesitis, and dactylitis. Back pain is often the presenting symptom for spondyloarthritis, although spondyloarthritis only accounts for about 5% of chronic low back pain. Unlike most forms of back pain, the pain in spondyloarthritis is inflammatory and typically occurs in patients under the age of 40 years. It is characterized by an insidious onset, duration of more than 3 months, presence at rest and at night (waking the patient), morning stiffness lasting more than 30 minutes, and improvement with exercise. Enthesitis, or inflammation at the site where a ligament or tendon attaches to bone, presents as pain and tenderness in areas such as the Achilles tendon (**Figure 10**). Dactylitis ("sausage digits") is a diffuse fusiform swelling of the fingers or toes, consistent with tendon and ligament involvement beyond the points of insertion (**Figure 11**).

Although the categories listed here are extremely helpful in identifying and diagnosing disease, recently developed classification criteria emphasize the commonalities rather than the differences among the various forms of spondyloarthritis (for example, Assessment of SpondyloArthritis international Society [ASAS] criteria for peripheral and axial disease). Such criteria may permit diagnosis and treatment at an earlier stage

TABLE 17. Clinical Features of Spondyloarthritis

	Ankylosing Spondylitis	Psoriatic Arthritis	IBD-Associated Arthritis	Reactive Arthritis
Musculoskeletal				
Axial involvement	Axial involvement predominates; initially symmetrically involves the SI joints and lower spine, progressing cranially; does not skip regions	May occur at any level; may start in the cervical spine; may skip regions	May be asymptomatic but can follow a course similar to ankylosing spondylitis; SI involvement often asymmetric; axial arthritis does not parallel IBD activity	Less common than in other forms of spondyloarthritis
Peripheral involvement	Enthesitis; may have asymmetric large-joint oligoarthritis, including hips and shoulders; hip involvement can cause significant functional limitation; dactylitis uncommon	Five subtypes (symmetric polyarthritis; asymmetric oligoarthritis; DIP-predominant; spondyloarthritis; arthritis mutilans); also, enthesitis, dactylitis, and tenosynovitis	Acute polyarticular peripheral arthritis: especially knee; early; can parallel IBD activity Chronic polyarticular peripheral arthritis: of PIPs, MCPs, wrists, elbows, shoulders, knees, ankles, and MTPs; does not parallel IBD; dactylitis; enthesitis	Enthesitis and asymmetric large-joint oligoarthritis; usually self-limited; nonerosive; some patients experience recurrent or persistent arthritis; may develop features of other forms of spondyloarthritis
Dermatologic	Skin findings not characteristic, but psoriatic-like lesions may occasionally occur	Psoriasis typically precedes joint involvement; nail pitting; onychodystrophy	Pyoderma gangrenosum; erythema nodosum	Keratoderma blennorrhagicum (psoriasiform rash on soles, toes, palms); circinate balanitis (psoriasiform rash on penis)
Ophthalmologic	Anterior uveitis (unilateral, recurrent)	Conjunctivitis more common than anterior uveitis (can be bilateral, insidious, or chronic)	Anterior uveitis (can be bilateral, insidious, or chronic); conjunctivitis, keratitis, and episcleritis are rare	Conjunctivitis more common than anterior uveitis
Gastrointestinal	Asymptomatic intestinal ulcerations (rare)	—	Crohn disease; ulcerative colitis	Prior GI infection in some patients
Genitourinary	Urethritis (rare)	—	Nephrolithiasis	Prior GU infection in some patients; sterile urethritis; prostatitis; cervicitis; salpingitis
Cardiovascular	Aortic valve disease; aortitis; conduction abnormalities; CAD	Association with traditional CAD risk factors	Thromboembolism	—
Pulmonary	Restrictive lung disease from costovertebral rigidity; apical fibrosis (rare)	—	—	—
Bone quality	Falsely elevated bone mineral density from syndesmophytes; increased risk of spine fracture	Increased risk of fracture (multifactorial)	High risk for vitamin D deficiency, low bone density, and fracture	Localized osteopenia

CAD = coronary artery disease; DIP = distal interphalangeal; GI = gastrointestinal; GU = genitourinary; IBD = inflammatory bowel disease; MCP = metacarpophalangeal; MTP = metatarsophalangeal; PIP = proximal interphalangeal; SI = sacroiliac.

of disease before the unique features of the condition become well defined.

Ankylosing Spondylitis

Ankylosing spondylitis is a chronic inflammatory disease affecting the axial skeleton, entheses, and peripheral joints. In contrast to other forms of spondyloarthritis, sacroiliac joint involvement is considered an essential feature of ankylosing spondylitis. Ankylosing spondylitis has a strong familial predilection and the strongest association with HLA-B27 among the forms of spondyloarthritis, being present in up to 95% of patients. Although a male predominance of 2-3:1 has been

described, women usually have milder and underappreciated disease; prevalence may actually be similar between genders. Disease can begin as early as adolescence, but peak age of diagnosis is between 20 and 30 years.

Symptoms of inflammatory back pain are most frequently the presenting complaint. Spinal involvement begins in the lumbar region and tends to ascend. Buttock pain may indicate sacroiliac joint involvement, which is characteristically bilateral. About one third of patients develop hip joint involvement and about one third develop peripheral arthritis elsewhere, often in the shoulders. Enthesitis most often manifests as Achilles tendinitis. Dactylitis occurs in fewer than 10% of patients.

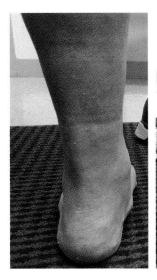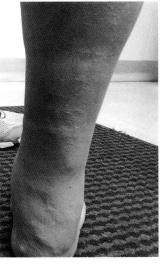

FIGURE 10. Marked thickening of the distal right Achilles tendon and Achilles insertion on the calcaneus as the result of chronic Achilles tendinitis in a patient with psoriatic arthritis (normal contralateral Achilles insertion).

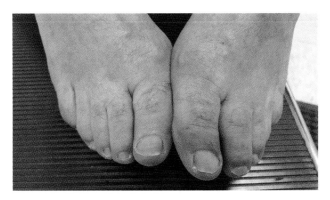

FIGURE 11. Diffuse swelling of the first and second toes of the left foot due to dactylitis in a patient with psoriatic arthritis resulting in a "sausage digit" appearance.

Physical examination, particularly in more advanced disease, can be highly characteristic. With active inflammation, tenderness over the sacroiliac joints is often the first sign of disease. Over time, marked reduction in spinal mobility can occur in all planes, and chest expansion becomes reduced. Flexion deformity at the neck and thoracic hyperkyphosis may lead to a hunched posture. A loss of lumbar lordosis and restricted range of motion in the hips may also be evident.

Extra-articular manifestations of ankylosing spondylitis are not uncommon (see Table 17). Cardiac and pulmonary manifestations, including aortic valve disease, cardiac conduction abnormalities, and restrictive lung disease, are more common in ankylosing spondylitis than other forms of spondyloarthritis. In addition, vertebral compression fractures may occur with little to no trauma as the disease progresses. The cervical spine is the most common site for fractures and can be associated with neurologic complications. ◩

The course of ankylosing spondylitis is variable; progression may occur over many years. Markers of a poorer prognosis include a longer duration of disease, the presence of hip joint involvement, elevation of inflammatory markers, and the presence of radiographic changes in the spine. Mortality is increased in men and correlates with disease activity.

Psoriatic Arthritis

Psoriatic arthritis is an inflammatory joint disease associated with psoriasis. Estimates of the frequency of psoriatic arthritis among patients with psoriasis vary from 7% to 42%. Men and women are equally affected, and the usual age of onset is between 30 to 50 years. Psoriasis precedes or co-occurs with arthritis symptoms in about 90% of patients with psoriatic arthritis; less commonly, the rash may follow the arthritis, with a latency period as long as a decade. Skin involvement may be subtle, involving only areas such as the umbilicus, perineum, or gluteal cleft. There is no correlation between the extent of skin involvement and the severity of joint symptoms. In addition to skin lesions, nail pitting and onychodystrophy are seen; nail involvement is a risk factor for developing joint disease, particularly of the distal interphalangeal joints (**Figure 12**).

Five clinical subtypes of psoriatic arthritis, which may overlap, are recognized as follows: symmetric polyarthritis; asymmetric oligoarthritis; distal interphalangeal–predominant disease; spondyloarthritis; and arthritis mutilans. Arthritis mutilans represents the rare end stage of progressive, destructive arthritis in the small joints of the hands. It results in subluxation, ligamentous laxity, and telescope-like retraction of the fingers. Additional joints usually become involved over time.

Enthesitis, tenosynovitis, and dactylitis often occur. Common locations for enthesitis include the Achilles tendon (see Figure 10), the calcaneal insertion of the plantar fascia, and ligamentous insertions into the pelvic bones. Dactylitis typically involves one or two digits; the feet are more commonly affected than the hands (see Figure 11).

Symptomatic and radiographic spine involvement is unusual at disease onset but increased over long-term follow-up,

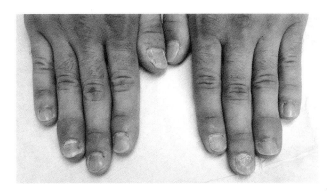

FIGURE 12. Dystrophic nail changes, including onycholysis and pitting, and inflammatory arthritic changes in the distal interphalangeal joints in a patient with psoriasis and psoriatic arthritis.

particularly in the cervical spine. The presence of sacroiliitis is associated with an increased likelihood for HLA-B27 positivity. In contrast to the almost universally bilateral sacroiliitis of ankylosing spondylitis, sacroiliitis is not always present in psoriatic arthritis and is more likely to be unilateral. Extra-articular manifestations are listed in Table 17.

Poor prognostic factors in psoriatic arthritis include the presence of polyarticular or erosive disease at the time of diagnosis. Patients additionally have an increased risk for cardiovascular disease.

Inflammatory Bowel Disease–Associated Arthritis

Inflammatory bowel disease (IBD), including Crohn disease and ulcerative colitis, may be associated with inflammatory arthritis in 6% to 46% of patients. Onset of arthritis may occur at any time in the course of the bowel disease.

IBD-associated arthritis occurs in three patterns:

1. Sacroiliitis/spondylitis: occurs in up to 26% of patients; 50% to 75% are positive for HLA-B27; men are more frequently affected than women; radiographic abnormalities of the sacroiliac joints may be seen in the absence of symptoms.

2. Acute polyarticular peripheral arthritis: self-limited; affects 5% of patients and occurs early in the course of IBD; the presence of arthritis is not as highly associated with HLA-B27 as in axial disease; the knee is most frequently involved; flares of joint symptoms may parallel exacerbations of bowel disease, but 90% resolve within 6 months.

3. Chronic polyarticular peripheral arthritis: affects less than 5% of patients; men and women are equally affected; the presence of arthritis is not as highly associated with HLA-B27 as in axial disease; the metacarpophalangeal joints, knees, ankles, elbows, shoulders, wrists, proximal interphalangeal, and metatarsophalangeal joints may be affected; flares of arthritis may recur repeatedly over years and last for months, but joint symptoms are unrelated to bowel disease activity.

See Table 17 for information on extra-articular manifestations.

Reactive Arthritis

Reactive arthritis is a rare cause of inflammatory arthritis that can occur following specific genitourinary and gastrointestinal infections, including *Chlamydia trachomatis* and *Ureaplasma urealyticum* in the urethra and *Campylobacter, Escherichia coli, Salmonella, Shigella,* and *Yersinia* in the intestine. Reactive arthritis occurs following 2% to 33% of cases of bacterial dysentery, with a higher incidence reported after single source outbreaks. About 90% of *Yersinia*-related cases occur in patients who are HLA-B27 positive, whereas only 30% to 50% of patients with reactive arthritis associated with other infectious agents are HLA-B27 positive.

Symptoms of inflammatory arthritis typically appear 2 to 3 weeks postinfection. Arthritis is asymmetric and may be monoarticular or oligoarticular; joints commonly affected include the knee, ankle, and wrist. Enthesitis is especially common; Achilles tendinitis and plantar fasciitis occur in up to 90% of cases. Dactylitis can also occur. The spine and sacroiliac joints are less commonly involved. In about half of patients, symptoms self-resolve within 6 months; most other cases self-resolve within 1 year, with a small proportion of cases converting to chronic disease. Extra-articular manifestations are described in Table 17. A subset of patients may demonstrate the "complete triad" of conjunctivitis, arthritis, and urethritis.

KEY POINTS

- Ankylosing spondylitis is a chronic inflammatory disease affecting the axial skeleton (including sacroiliac joints), entheses, and peripheral joints; HLA-B27 is present in up to 95% of patients.

- Psoriatic arthritis is an inflammatory joint disease associated with psoriasis, multiple possible joint patterns, enthesitis, tenosynovitis, and dactylitis.

- Inflammatory bowel disease–associated arthritis occurs in three patterns: sacroiliitis/spondylitis, acute polyarticular peripheral arthritis, and chronic polyarticular peripheral arthritis; only the acute polyarticular form is related to flares of bowel disease.

- Reactive arthritis can occur 2 to 3 weeks following specific gastrointestinal and genitourinary infections; an asymmetric monoarticular or oligoarticular arthritis, dactylitis, and enthesitis can occur.

Diagnosis
Laboratory Studies

Spondyloarthritis is considered seronegative because rheumatoid factor and other autoantibodies are typically absent. HLA-B27 is present in many patients, particularly those with ankylosing spondylitis and spinal involvement; however, it cannot independently confirm or exclude a diagnosis. With active disease, evidence of systemic inflammation may be diagnostically helpful, including elevations of erythrocyte sedimentation rate and C-reactive protein as well as normochromic, normocytic anemia. Each of these findings, however, is nonspecific and may be normal even in the presence of active disease. Several other laboratory findings are suggestive of the underlying disorder but are of limited utility diagnostically. Elevated IgA levels have been reported in patients with ankylosing spondylitis and psoriatic arthritis, consistent with increased mucosal immune activity. Serum alkaline phosphatase may be elevated in ankylosing spondylitis. Serum urate levels may be high in psoriatic arthritis, and these patients are at increased risk for co-occurrence of gout. Synovial fluid may show an elevated leukocyte count with a predominance of neutrophils.

In cases of suspected reactive arthritis, stool and urine cultures, genital swabs, nucleic acid amplification testing, and rising serum antibody titers against the suspected causative organism can be helpful in establishing the diagnosis. Pathogens can generally not be cultured from joint fluid in these patients, and antecedent infection is verified in less than half of affected individuals.

Imaging Studies

Radiography of the sacroiliac joints is an essential part of the initial evaluation of patients being assessed for spondyloarthritis but may be normal early in the course of disease. Radiographic evidence of sacroiliitis includes pseudo-widening of the joints, erosions, sclerosis, and ankylosis. In the spine, bony proliferation between vertebral bodies can result in formation of syndesmophytes (bony bridges) that can lead to a "bamboo spine" appearance in 10% to 15% of affected patients with ankylosing spondylitis (**Figure 13**). Other changes in the spine include vertebral squaring, disk calcification, and vertebral and facet joint ankylosis. In psoriatic arthritis, the syndesmophytes are often described as less delicate, more "chunky," patchy, and asymmetric compared with those associated with ankylosing spondylitis.

Plain radiography of peripheral joints may aid in the diagnosis of spondyloarthritis, particularly when erosive and proliferative changes are present concurrently. Bony proliferative changes at entheseal sites may be seen in any spondyloarthritis. Features particularly characteristic of psoriatic arthritis include asymmetric distribution, distal interphalangeal joint involvement, osteolysis leading to pencil-in-cup deformity (**Figure 14**), and proliferative new bone formation along the shaft of metacarpal or metatarsal bones. There are no characteristic findings of reactive arthritis on plain radiographs.

Although plain radiography remains the cornerstone of radiographic diagnosis in spondyloarthritis, MRI is increasingly

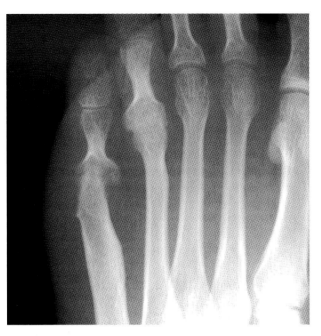

FIGURE 14. Radiograph showing pencil-in-cup deformity of the fifth metatarsal joint and ankylosis of the fourth metatarsal joint in a patient with psoriatic arthritis.

recognized as a useful diagnostic and prognostic modality. MRI is more sensitive for detecting early spine and sacroiliac joint inflammation and may be indicated in the evaluation of suspected spondyloarthritis if plain radiographs are negative. MRI can also detect inflammatory changes even in the absence of bony lesions. For example, the presence of bone marrow edema, although nonspecific, can suggest active inflammation in the sacroiliac joints. MRI can also detect soft-tissue abnormalities (such as bursitis and enthesitis), erosions, sclerosis, and ankylosis.

In older patients, the diagnostic specificity of radiographic evaluation for spondyloarthritis may decline. Other conditions such as osteitis condensans ilii, osteoarthritis, degenerative disk disease, and diffuse idiopathic skeletal hyperostosis (DISH) may cause sclerotic changes of the sacroiliac joints and osteophytes that may be difficult to distinguish from the syndesmophytes of ankylosing spondylitis. In particular, DISH typically causes multilevel bridging osteophytes. In ankylosing spondylitis, however, the bony bridges tend to be thinner and more vertically oriented than those seen in DISH.

KEY POINTS

HVC

- In patients with spondyloarthritis, rheumatoid factor and other autoantibodies are typically absent; HLA-B27 is positive in many patients, but it cannot independently confirm or exclude a diagnosis.

- Markers of systemic inflammation such as erythrocyte sedimentation rate and C-reactive protein may be normal even in the presence of active spondyloarthritis.

(Continued)

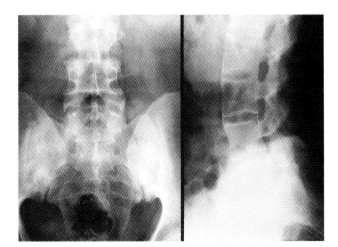

FIGURE 13. Spinal features of ankylosing spondylitis. *Left,* Sacroiliac erosive disease, characterized by areas of joint-space narrowing in some locations, apparent relative widening in others, and secondary bony sclerosis. Although the left sacroiliac joint is more severely involved, both sides are affected. *Right,* Delicate (gracile) syndesmophytes bridging lumbar vertebral bodies, leading to a "bamboo spine" appearance. Note that the syndesmophytes are "flowing" (contiguous without skipping any vertebral joints).

- Radiography of the sacroiliac joints is essential in patients with suspected spondyloarthritis; radiographic evidence of sacroiliitis includes pseudo-widening of the joints, erosions, sclerosis, and ankylosis.

HVC
- MRI is more sensitive for detecting early spine and sacroiliac joint inflammation and may be indicated in the evaluation of suspected spondyloarthritis if plain radiographs are negative.
- Radiographic changes in psoriatic arthritis can include asymmetric distribution, distal interphalangeal joint involvement, osteolysis leading to a pencil-in-cup deformity, and proliferative new bone formation along the shaft of metacarpal or metatarsal bones.

Management

General Considerations

Management goals in spondyloarthritis are to control pain and inflammation, preserve function, and prevent progressive structural damage, including spine and joint ankyloses (fusion). Patient education regarding the course, treatment, and prognosis of disease, as well as the importance of general health, avoiding smoking, and participating in regular exercise are critical components of the overall treatment program.

Ankylosing Spondylitis

NSAIDs are recommended as first-line treatment in ankylosing spondylitis and remain important in management throughout the course of disease. Patients with ankylosing spondylitis are more likely to respond to NSAIDs and to do so more rapidly and completely than patients with chronic low back pain from other causes. Several studies suggest that, in contrast to most forms of arthritis, continuous use of NSAIDs may help slow disease progression in ankylosing spondylitis. Oral glucocorticoids are not recommended, but intra-articular glucocorticoid injections, including in the sacroiliac joints, can help alleviate pain. Nonbiologic disease-modifying antirheumatic drugs (DMARDs) such as methotrexate have no efficacy in axial disease and limited efficacy in peripheral disease.

In patients with persistent symptoms on NSAID therapy, TNF-α inhibitors have efficacy in reducing signs and symptoms of ankylosing spondylitis, with about half of those treated improving by 50%. Whether TNF-α inhibitors can slow radiographic progression in ankylosing spondylitis remains an area of ongoing investigation. These agents are also effective in treating ankylosing spondylitis–associated anterior uveitis.

Physical therapy is the most important nonpharmacologic intervention in ankylosing spondylitis. The goals of therapy include improving pain and stiffness, maintaining range of motion, and reducing disability; transition to an ongoing daily exercise program is optimal.

Total hip arthroplasty can be highly effective in reducing pain and restoring function in the management of progressive hip involvement and may be indicated at an earlier age than in patients with osteoarthritis.

Psoriatic Arthritis

Treatment choices in psoriatic arthritis take into account the extent of both skin and joint involvement. NSAIDs may be effective for mild joint disease. Methotrexate is the most commonly used DMARD for psoriatic arthritis. Although benefit can be demonstrated in control of skin disease and joint pain, methotrexate has not been shown to reduce progression of joint damage. Sulfasalazine and leflunomide can also improve joint symptoms. Apremilast is modestly effective for psoriasis and psoriatic arthritis.

In more severe psoriatic arthritis, TNF-α inhibitors have been shown to have superior efficacy in the management of joint symptoms and to slow the progression of radiographic damage, including joint-space narrowing and erosions.

The biologic agents ustekinumab (anti-IL-12/23 antibody) and secukinumab (anti-IL-17A antibody) have also been approved for treating both psoriasis and psoriatic arthritis, and can improve dactylitis and enthesitis.

Inflammatory Bowel Disease-Associated Arthritis

Various pharmacologic agents may be useful in the treatment of both intestinal and peripheral arthritis related to Crohn disease and ulcerative colitis, including sulfasalazine, azathioprine, 6-mercaptopurine, methotrexate, glucocorticoids, and the TNF-α inhibitors infliximab and adalimumab. NSAIDs can provide symptomatic relief of arthritis symptoms but may occasionally exacerbate IBD.

Reactive Arthritis

Treatment of the antecedent infection is indicated in patients with reactive arthritis who have an identifiable cause. However, most patients present postinfection, and antibiotics are not usually effective in treating the arthritis. Most patients have self-limited disease, and short-term use of daily NSAIDs often improves symptoms until the condition resolves. If relief is incomplete, intra-articular glucocorticoid injections and oral glucocorticoids can be used. If symptoms persist beyond 3 to 6 months, the use of DMARDs such as sulfasalazine, methotrexate, or TNF-α inhibitors may be necessary for symptom control and to prevent joint erosion. Therapy is discontinued 3 to 6 months following disease remission.

- In ankylosing spondylitis, NSAIDs are recommended as first-line treatment and may help slow disease progression; physical therapy is the most important nonpharmacologic intervention. **HVC**

(Continued)

- In more severe psoriatic arthritis, tumor necrosis factor α inhibitors have been shown to have superior efficacy in the management of joint symptoms and to slow the progression of radiographic damage.

- Treatment options for both intestinal and peripheral arthritis related to Crohn disease and ulcerative colitis include sulfasalazine, azathioprine, 6-mercaptopurine, methotrexate, glucocorticoids, infliximab, and adalimumab.

HVC • Antibiotics are not usually effective in treating reactive arthritis, but short-term NSAIDs can be used to improve symptoms in this typically self-limited disease.

Systemic Lupus Erythematosus

Epidemiology and Pathophysiology

Systemic lupus erythematosus (SLE) is a multisystem autoimmune disease characterized by a heterogeneous constellation of organ involvement and the presence of antinuclear antibodies (ANA) and other autoantibodies.

In SLE, a complex and varying interaction of genes, environment, and random events leads to a breakdown of self-tolerance and autoimmunity. Defects in cellular apoptosis result in inadequate clearance of intracellular proteins, especially nuclear antigens, promoting the generation of self-directed T and B cells and the initiation/propagation of autoimmunity. Cytokine generation supports the autoreactivity, with type-1 interferons playing a major role. Autoantibodies may directly induce tissue damage or promote the formation of immune complexes that lead to complement activation and tissue inflammation and damage. Inheritance of SLE risk is polygenic, including major histocompatibility complex.

The risk of SLE developing in genetically predisposed individuals increases at puberty and peaks in the third decade. Approximately 90% of adult patients are women. The disease is more common, and perhaps more severe, in black, Asian, and Hispanic ethnicities.

KEY POINTS

- Systemic lupus erythematosus is a multisystem autoimmune disease characterized by a heterogeneous constellation of organ involvement and the presence of antinuclear antibodies and other autoantibodies.

- Approximately 90% of adult patients with systemic lupus erythematosus are women.

Clinical Manifestations

Mucocutaneous Involvement

Skin disease occurs in up to 90% patients with SLE and is classified as acute, subacute, or chronic.

Acute cutaneous lupus erythematosus (ACLE) presents as an erythematous, macular, patchy eruption, sometimes with desquamation. The facial eruption of ACLE (malar or butterfly rash) is characterized by erythema/edema over the cheeks and bridge of the nose, sparing the nasolabial folds; it occurs in about 50% of patients with SLE (**Figure 15**). Less characteristically, ACLE can also involve the neck, upper chest, and dorsum of the arms and hands; it affects the skin between the fingers but spares the knuckle pads. In some patients, a bullous eruption can occur. ACLE usually responds to therapy and heals without scarring or atrophy.

Subacute cutaneous lupus erythematosus (SCLE) is a photosensitive rash occurring especially on the arms, neck, and face (**Figure 16**). It consists of erythematous annular/polycyclic or patchy papulosquamous lesions, often with a fine scale, that may leave postinflammatory hypo- or hyperpigmentation. SCLE is associated with anti-Ro/SSA autoantibodies (prevalence >75%) and can occur in isolation or as a manifestation of underlying SLE.

Discoid lupus erythematosus (DLE) is the most common chronic cutaneous manifestation of SLE, occurring in 20% of patients (**Figure 17**). DLE presents as hypo- or hyperpigmented patches or plaques, with erythema during active disease, which may be variably atrophic or hyperkeratotic. Unlike ACLE and SCLE, DLE can cause scarring, atrophy, and permanent alopecia. DLE also occurs as an isolated finding in the absence of SLE. Isolated DLE is usually limited to the neck, face, and scalp, whereas discoid lesions in SLE are more diffusely distributed. Patients with isolated DLE tend to be ANA negative and usually do not progress to SLE. It is important to differentiate isolated DLE from DLE as a manifestation of

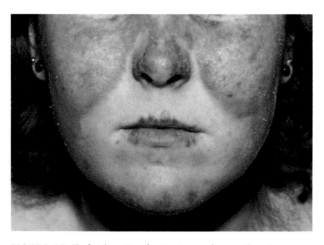

FIGURE 15. The facial eruption of acute cutaneous lupus erythematosus (malar or butterfly rash). This patient has fixed erythematous raised lesions over the malar eminences, the bridge of the nose with sparing of the nasolabial folds, and the chin.

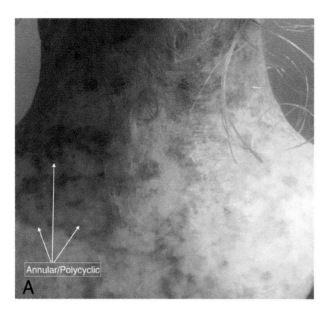
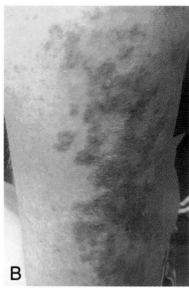

FIGURE 16. Subacute cutaneous lupus erythematosus is characterized by erythematous, macular, or patchy skin lesions that are scaly and can evolve as (*A*) annular/polycyclic lesions or (*B*) papulosquamous plaques.

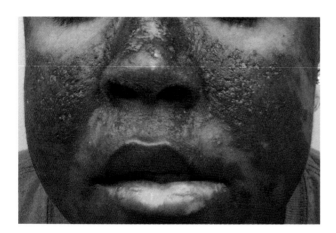

FIGURE 17. Discoid lupus erythematosus. This patient has hyperpigmented, raised patches with keratotic scaling and follicular plugging involving the malar and perioral areas as well as the bridge of the nose. Areas of atrophic scarring are also present.

underlying SLE when making therapeutic and prognostic decisions.

Painless oral or nasopharyngeal ulcerations occur in 5% of patients with SLE, with involvement of hard palate suggestive of the diagnosis. Rarely, DLE can be associated with painful ulcers. Nonscarring alopecia is a common feature of active SLE, with hair regrowth a sign of disease control. Raynaud phenomenon occurs frequently, reflecting arterial vasospasm of digital arteries.

See MKSAP 18 Dermatology for more information.

Musculoskeletal Involvement

Joints are affected in 90% of patients with SLE. The most common involvement is polyarthralgia, with frank arthritis occurring in 40%. Typical distribution is small peripheral joints, but large joints are also affected. In contrast to rheumatoid arthritis, SLE arthritis is nonerosive, but reducible subluxation of the digits, swan neck deformities, and ulnar deviation (Jaccoud arthropathy) can occur.

A serious complication of SLE is osteonecrosis, which most commonly affects the hips but can also involve other large joints, and should be suspected when there is otherwise unexplained pain and/or reduced range of motion. Chronic prednisone doses (>20 mg/d), severe/active SLE, and vasculitis are all associated with increased risk. MRI is the modality of choice for sensitive evaluation of early disease, with plain radiography useful to diagnose and follow later stages. Small lesions can improve and resolve spontaneously, but larger lesions usually lead to bony collapse and structural sequelae.

Myalgia and subjective weakness are common; frank myositis is rare. Assessment is complicated by the potential effect on muscle of antimalarials (rarely) and glucocorticoids (commonly), which must be differentiated from active SLE disease. Fibromyalgia is a common comorbidity (30%); symptoms may be similar to active SLE disease.

Kidney Involvement

Kidney disease occurs frequently among patients with SLE (70%) and was the major cause of SLE mortality prior to the advent of dialysis. Lupus nephritis can present with minimal laboratory abnormalities (non-nephrotic proteinuria, hematuria), frank nephritis (hypertension, lower extremity edema, active urine sediment, and elevated serum creatinine), and/or nephrosis (nephrotic-range proteinuria, dependent edema, and thrombosis). Untreated active disease may progress to kidney failure.

All patients with SLE should be regularly evaluated for kidney disease by assessing serum creatinine and urine for

CONT.

protein and microscopic evaluation. Patients with significant abnormalities, including proteinuria greater than 500 mg/24 h or active urine sediment, should be urgently evaluated for active disease. Anti–double-stranded DNA antibody titers are a marker for risk, and complement consumption is a common phenomenon during active kidney disease.

Kidney biopsy defines both the histological subtype and the activity/chronicity of disease and is usually essential to make therapeutic decisions. Indications for kidney biopsy include an otherwise unexplained rise in serum creatinine, proteinuria greater than 1000 mg/24 h, proteinuria greater than 500 mg/24 h with hematuria, or an active urine sediment.

Patients who have SLE with hypercoagulable states (for example, nephrosis or antiphospholipid syndrome) may be at risk for renal artery or vein thrombosis.

See MKSAP 18 Nephrology for information on the classes and treatment of lupus nephritis.

Neuropsychiatric Involvement

Neuropsychiatric systemic lupus erythematosus (NPSLE) may involve the central and/or peripheral nervous systems and has 19 defined manifestations. NPSLE prevalence is high (75%), with the most common manifestations being headache, mild cognitive dysfunction, and mood disorder. Peripheral neuropathy occurs in 10% to 14% of patients. Severe acute presentations, including seizures and psychosis, happen infrequently (<5%) but require aggressive symptomatic as well as disease-specific treatment.

Patients with suspected serious central NPSLE such as meningitis, stroke, and psychosis should undergo central nervous system imaging (CT, MRI, or PET) and cerebrospinal fluid analysis as appropriate. In some patients with severe disease, measurement of cerebrospinal fluid for NPSLE-associated autoantibodies (antineuronal, anti-*N*-methyl-D-aspartate receptor, antiribosomal P, and others) may be useful. For patients with suspected peripheral neuropathies, electromyography and nerve conduction studies should be performed. Neuropsychologic testing may help distinguish organic versus functional cognitive changes.

Cardiovascular Involvement

Asymptomatic pericarditis is the most frequent cardiac manifestation of SLE (40%). When symptomatic, features include chest pain, exudative effusion, and rarely tamponade or chronic constriction. Patients with SLE have a 2- to 10-fold increased prevalence of coronary artery disease (CAD), the most common cause of death among older patients. High SLE disease activity and prednisone doses greater than 10 mg/d are independent risk factors for future CAD.

Valvular abnormalities occurring in SLE include those associated with antiphospholipid syndrome (nonspecific thickening of the mitral and aortic valve leaflets, vegetations, regurgitation, and stenosis). Libman-Sacks endocarditis (noninfectious verrucous vegetations) preferentially affects the mitral valve and can cause embolic complications. Myocarditis

occurs in 5% to 10% of patients with SLE and usually presents as insidious heart failure but can be acute.

Pulmonary Involvement

Pulmonary involvement is common in SLE, with most patients presenting with pleuritis (45%-60%). Pleural effusions occur in approximately half of these patients and are typically exudative; fluid analysis may reveal a lymphocytic pleocytosis and mildly depressed glucose levels.

Parenchymal lung involvement occurs in less than 10% of patients with SLE. A nonspecific interstitial pneumonia pattern is most common, and evaluation centers on assessing SLE activity and excluding other causes of diffuse parenchymal lung disease. Two rare but potentially life-threatening complications of SLE lung disease are acute lupus pneumonitis (presenting as fever, cough, dyspnea, hypoxemia, pleuritic chest pain, and infiltrates) and diffuse alveolar hemorrhage (presenting with dyspnea, hypoxemia, diffuse alveolar infiltrates, a dropping hematocrit, and a high D_{LCO}). Both carry a high mortality rate (>50%); early recognition, rapid evaluation (CT and/or bronchoscopy with bronchoalveolar lavage or biopsy), and aggressive respiratory support combined with high-dose glucocorticoids and immunosuppression are required. With new pulmonary infiltrates, differentiation between these disorders and infection can be difficult, and antibiotics and immunosuppressive therapy are often administered simultaneously until the diagnosis is clear.

Shrinking lung syndrome is a rare but characteristic syndrome consisting of pleuritic chest pain and dyspnea, with progressive decrease in lung volumes. The cause is uncertain, but pleuropulmonary disease and/or diaphragmatic dysfunction may contribute. Immunosuppression may reverse the process in some patients.

Hematologic Involvement

In patients with SLE, a normocytic, normochromic inflammatory anemia is common; autoimmune hemolytic anemia occurs in approximately 10% and correlates with SLE activity. Lymphopenia/leukopenia is also common but usually mild. Thrombocytopenia occurs in 30% to 50%, and approximately 10% of patients develop severe thrombocytopenia (<50,000/µL [50 × 10⁹/L]) in isolation or in conjunction with hemolytic anemia.

The cytopenias in SLE may be caused by immune and nonimmune destructive mechanisms (including microangiopathy), medications, and kidney and liver disease. Moderate and severe or rapidly progressive cytopenias require prompt evaluation with serologic studies and/or bone marrow biopsy. An exact cause of cytopenias may be difficult to ascertain, and a trial of medication adjustment in concert with evaluation for other causes is often necessary.

Antiphospholipid antibodies/lupus anticoagulant (APLA/LAC) are frequently present in patients with SLE (about 40%) and may be associated with a false-positive rapid plasma reagin test for syphilis. Most patients are asymptomatic.

CONT.

Thrombotic events occur in about 30% and are associated with moderate or high titer of the antibodies; these include venous and arterial thrombosis, miscarriage, stillbirth, livedo reticularis, and cardiac valve thickening/vegetations. The highest risk of thrombosis occurs in the presence of triple positivity for LAC, anti-β_2-glycoprotein I, and anticardiolipin antibodies. Patients with SLE are at increased risk for thrombotic events even in the absence of APLA.

See MKSAP 18 Hematology and Oncology for more information. H

Gastrointestinal Involvement

Gastrointestinal disease is a common (40%) and frequently underrecognized SLE manifestation. Serositis presents as abdominal pain, is usually associated with active disease, and improves with treatment. Mesenteric vasculitis, inflammation of the small and large bowel, pancreatitis, protein-losing enteropathy, and diffuse peritonitis are uncommon but may be severe and associated with cutaneous vasculitis. Patients with APLA can present with mesenteric thrombosis.

Noninfectious hepatitis can occur and is associated with the presence of antiribosomal P antibodies. Patients with SLE who have Raynaud phenomenon and anti-U1-ribonucleoprotein antibodies can develop esophageal disease and reflux.

Medications used to treat SLE (NSAIDs, prednisone, mycophenolate, azathioprine) also frequently affect the gastrointestinal system and may cause esophagitis, gastritis, pancreatitis, and other manifestations.

KEY POINTS

- The facial eruption of acute cutaneous lupus erythematosus (malar or butterfly rash) is characterized by erythema/edema over the cheeks and bridge of the nose, sparing the nasolabial folds.

- Polyarthralgia of the small peripheral joints is the most common joint manifestation in systemic lupus erythematosus; a nonerosive arthritis occurs in 40% of patients.

- All patients with systemic lupus erythematosus should be regularly evaluated for kidney disease by assessing serum creatinine and urine for protein and microscopic evaluation.

- The most common manifestations of neuropsychiatric systemic lupus erythematosus are headache, mild cognitive dysfunction, and mood disorder.

- Patients with systemic lupus erythematosus (SLE) have a 2- to 10-fold increased prevalence of coronary artery disease (CAD); high SLE disease activity and prednisone doses greater than 10 mg/d are independent risk factors for developing CAD.

Association with Malignancy

The greatest malignancy risk among patients with SLE is non-Hodgkin lymphoma, presumably due to chronic B-cell activation and/or medications (azathioprine or cyclophosphamide). Other hematologic malignancies, including Hodgkin lymphoma and leukemia, are also increased. Lung cancer rates are increased slightly compared with the general population, probably related to smoking. Cervical cancer risk is increased, likely due to immunosuppression and increased prevalence of human papillomavirus.

KEY POINT

- The greatest malignancy risk among patients with systemic lupus erythematosus is non-Hodgkin lymphoma.

Diagnosis
General Considerations

The diagnosis of SLE should be considered in any patient with unexplained symptoms affecting multiple organ systems or with any individual manifestation of SLE, especially in young women. At initial presentation, skin and joint manifestations are most common, along with constitutional symptoms (fever, weight loss, or severe fatigue). Patients with subjective complaints of fatigue, myalgia, and/or arthralgia, but lacking objective findings, most likely have an alternative diagnosis and should not be evaluated for SLE.

Classification criteria for SLE were developed by the American College of Rheumatology (ACR) in 1982 and revised in 1997; although intended for accruing homogenous SLE populations for research studies, they can also be used to suggest a clinical diagnosis of SLE (**Table 18**). In 2012, the Systemic Lupus International Collaborating Clinics (SLICC) proposed and validated alternative SLE classification criteria that are similar to the ACR criteria but require the following: 1) fulfillment of at least four criteria, with at least one clinical criterion and one immunologic criterion; or 2) biopsy-proven lupus nephritis as sufficient clinical criterion in the presence of ANA or anti–double-stranded DNA antibodies. When compared with the ACR classification criteria, the SLICC classification criteria are associated with fewer misclassifications and have greater sensitivity but less specificity.

Laboratory Studies

Initial evaluation for SLE includes routine laboratory testing to establish organ-specific involvement, including complete blood count, chemistry panel, and urinalysis with microscopy.

ANA should be obtained to screen for nuclear-directed autoantibodies. The most appropriate methodology for testing ANA is the indirect immunofluorescence assay, which is highly sensitive (95%) for SLE. ANA tests should be interpreted in the context of the probability of disease because ANA may be present in other autoimmune diseases, and low-titer positivity may be seen with aging and even in healthy individuals.

If ANA is positive, SLE-specific autoantibodies (anti–double-stranded DNA, anti-Smith, anti-U1-ribonucleoprotein, anti-Ro/SSA, and anti-La/SSB), as well as tests for other autoimmune diseases under consideration, should be obtained

TABLE 18. American College of Rheumatology Criteria for the Classification of Systemic Lupus Erythematosus

Criteria[a]	Definition
Malar rash	Fixed erythema, flat or raised, over the malar eminences
Discoid rash	Erythematous, circular, raised patches with keratotic scaling and follicular plugging; atrophic scarring may occur
Photosensitivity	Rash after exposure to ultraviolet light
Oral ulcers	Oral and nasopharyngeal ulcers (observed by physician)
Arthritis	Nonerosive arthritis of ≥2 peripheral joints, with tenderness, swelling, or effusion
Serositis	Sterile pleuritis, pericarditis, or peritonitis (documented by electrocardiogram, rub, or evidence of effusion or ascites)
Kidney disorder	Urinalysis: 3+ protein or urine protein >500 mg/24 h; cellular casts
Neurologic disorder	Seizures or psychosis (without other cause)
Hematologic disorder	Hemolytic anemia or leukopenia (<4000/μL [4.0 × 10⁹/L]) or lymphopenia (<1500/μL [1.5 × 10⁹/L]) or thrombocytopenia (<100,000/μL [100 × 10⁹/L]) in the absence of offending drugs
Immunologic disorder	Anti–double-stranded DNA, anti-Smith, and/or antiphospholipid antibodies
ANA	An abnormal titer of ANA by immunofluorescence or an equivalent assay at any point in the absence of drugs known to induce ANA

ANA = antinuclear antibodies.

[a]Any combination of 4 or more of the 11 criteria, well documented at any time during a patient's history, makes it likely that the patient has systemic lupus erythematosus (specificity and sensitivity are 95% and 75%, respectively).

From Hochberg MC. Updating the American College of Rheumatology revised criteria for the classification of systemic lupus erythematosus. Arthritis Rheum. 1997;40(9):1725. [PMID: 9324032] Copyright 1997, American College of Rheumatology. Adapted with permission from John Wiley & Sons, Inc.

to further characterize the disease (**Table 19**). A small percentage of patients with SLE are negative for ANA but positive for anti-Ro/SSA antibodies. A negative ANA plus a negative anti-Ro/SSA essentially rules out SLE.

Disease activity markers (complements C3 and C4) should be assessed initially and regularly thereafter. Complement levels are reduced during SLE activity, reflecting immune complex formation and complement consumption. Anti–double-stranded DNA antibody levels may rise with SLE kidney disease activity. Other SLE autoantibodies, including the ANA test, do not reflect disease activity and need not be repeated. Erythrocyte sedimentation rate (ESR) and C-reactive protein (CRP) are variably associated with disease activity; some patients with SLE do not generate CRP during SLE flares, which may be helpful in distinguishing flares from infection. **H**

Differential Diagnosis

The differential diagnosis of SLE includes multisystem diseases, acute and chronic infections, medication effect, malignancies (particularly hematologic), and neurologic diseases (for example, multiple sclerosis). Multisystem autoimmune diseases (ANCA-associated vasculitis, rheumatoid arthritis, adult-onset Still disease, dermatomyositis, Sjögren syndrome, and mixed connective tissue disease) have overlapping features but may be distinguished through a careful assessment of their unique manifestations.

SLE should also be distinguished from undifferentiated connective tissue disease, which presents with milder symptoms and objective abnormalities that cannot be categorized or diagnosed as a specific connective tissue disease (see Mixed Connective Tissue Disease).

TABLE 19. Common Autoantibodies in Systemic Lupus Erythematosus

Autoantibody	Frequency in SLE	Comments
Antinuclear	>95%	Useful as an initial screening test; assesses multiple antigens simultaneously
Anti-double-stranded DNA	50%-60%	Found in more severe disease, especially kidney disease; antibody levels commonly follow disease activity and are useful to monitor
Anti-Ro/SSA	30%	Associated with photosensitive rashes, discoid lupus erythematosus, and neonatal lupus erythematosus; also common when secondary Sjögren syndrome is present
Anti-U1-ribonucleoprotein	35%	Associated with Raynaud phenomenon and esophageal dysmotility; also seen in MCTD
Anti-Smith	30%	Specific for SLE; often associated with more severe disease
Anti-La/SSB	20%	Common in Sjögren syndrome; less common in SLE and neonatal lupus erythematosus
Antiribosomal P	15%	Associated with CNS lupus and lupus hepatitis

CNS = central nervous system; MCTD = mixed connective tissue disease; SLE = systemic lupus erythematosus.

Certain medications can cause drug-induced lupus erythematosus (DILE), which mimics SLE (**Table 20**). The syndrome is usually mild with symptoms of malaise, fever, arthritis, and rash associated with a transient positive ANA and antihistone antibodies. Symptoms resolve after discontinuing the offending agent. Kidney and central nervous system disease are uncommon. Patients with SLE are at no more risk of DILE than the general population, and there is no contraindication to using medications associated with DILE in patients with SLE.

KEY POINTS

- Patients with systemic lupus erythematosus typically initially present with skin and joint manifestations, along with fever, weight loss, or severe fatigue.

- Initial evaluation for systemic lupus erythematosus includes antinuclear antibody testing as well as routine laboratory testing to establish organ-specific involvement, including complete blood count, chemistry panel, and urinalysis with microscopy.

(Continued)

KEY POINTS *(continued)*

- If antinuclear antibody testing is positive, autoantibodies specific to systemic lupus erythematosus (anti–double-stranded DNA, anti-Smith, anti-U1-ribonucleoprotein, anti-Ro/SSA, and anti-La/SSB) should be obtained to further characterize the disease.

Management

SLE management requires close monitoring of disease activity and frequent adjustment of therapy. Pharmacologic therapy is almost always required and is usually directed toward specific organ involvement (**Table 21**).

Hydroxychloroquine should be initiated in every patient who can tolerate it, because evidence suggests it reduces disease-associated damage, prevents disease flares, and improves kidney and overall survival. Hydroxychloroquine can be used alone for mild disease (especially skin and joints) and in combination with other agents in severe disease. In addition, hydroxychloroquine may reduce the risk of thrombosis, liver

TABLE 20. Medications Commonly Associated with Drug-Induced Lupus Erythematosus

Medication	Antibodies Detected	Comments
Procainamide	ANA (75%); antihistone	20% develop DILE; fever; arthritis; serositis
Hydralazine	ANA (20%); antihistone	5%-8% develop DILE; fever; arthritis; rare vasculitis and kidney disease
Minocycline	ANA; ANCA; anti-dsDNA rare	Arthritis; vasculitis; autoimmune hepatitis
Antithyroid drugs	ANA; ANCA; antihistone	Vasculitic rash; rare pulmonary and kidney disease
Statins	ANA; antihistone; anti-dsDNA	SLE, SCLE, dermatomyositis, and polymyositis all reported
Calcium channel blockers	ANA; anti-Ro/SSA; antihistone rare	SCLE
Thiazide diuretics	ANA; anti-Ro/SSA; antihistone rare	SCLE
ACE inhibitors	ANA; anti-Ro/SSA; antihistone rare	SCLE
TNF-α inhibitors	ANA (23%-57%); chromatin and anti-dsDNA common; antihistone rare	DILE most common with infliximab, uncommon for etanercept; SLE, SCLE, DLE all reported

ANA = antinuclear antibodies; DILE = drug-induced lupus erythematosus; DLE = discoid lupus erythematosus; dsDNA = double-stranded DNA; SCLE = subacute cutaneous lupus erythematosus; SLE = systemic lupus erythematosus; TNF = tumor necrosis factor.

TABLE 21. Medications Commonly Used to Treat Systemic Lupus Erythematosus

Medication	Common Uses in SLE	Important Side Effects
NSAIDs	Arthritis; pain; fever	Hypertension; GI bleeding; AKI
Prednisone	Used for all manifestations in varying doses	Hypertension; glucose intolerance; weight gain; infection; osteonecrosis
Hydroxychloroquine	Used in all patients; especially useful for skin involvement and to prevent disease flares	GI intolerance; rash; blurry vision; retinopathy; vacuolar myopathy
Mycophenolate mofetil	Moderate to severe disease; as effective as cyclophosphamide for remission induction for nephritis	Bone marrow suppression; elevation of liver enzymes; infection
Azathioprine	Moderate to severe disease	Bone marrow suppression; elevation of liver enzymes; hematologic malignancy
Cyclophosphamide	Severe organ or life-threatening disease	Bone marrow suppression; hemorrhagic cystitis; infection; malignancy; infertility
Belimumab	Add-on therapy for moderate to severe disease	Infusion reactions; infections

AKI = acute kidney injury; GI = gastrointestinal; SLE = systemic lupus erythematosus.

disease, and myocardial infarction; improve lipid profiles; and improve outcomes in high-risk pregnancies.

Glucocorticoids are a mainstay of SLE management, particularly in acute disease. The glucocorticoid dose should be determined by the level of disease activity and organ systems threatened. For severe disease activity (including profound cytopenias, class III/IV nephritis, and NPSLE), high-dose glucocorticoids are recommended. For life- or organ-threatening disease (such as rapidly progressive glomerulonephritis or seizures), high-dose intravenous glucocorticoids are given followed by high-dose daily prednisone. After disease stability is achieved, glucocorticoids are tapered to the lowest effective dose, ideally to eventual discontinuation.

Immunosuppressive therapy is usually initiated concurrently with glucocorticoids to achieve and maintain disease control and to allow tapering of glucocorticoids. Intravenous cyclophosphamide is used as induction therapy for severe or refractory disease (for example, severe active nephritis, acute central nervous system lupus, diffuse alveolar hemorrhage, or myocarditis) followed by maintenance therapy with mycophenolate mofetil or azathioprine. Mycophenolate mofetil is currently the preferred oral agent for lupus nephritis and is as effective as cyclophosphamide for induction therapy. The biologic agent belimumab is FDA approved for patients with incomplete response to conventional treatments and has been shown to be useful in skin/joint involvement and moderate/severe disease. ■

NSAIDs can be used as adjunct therapy for arthritis and pleuropericarditis, but are not disease modifying and may adversely affect kidney function and blood pressure.

See Principles of Therapeutics for information on SLE medication toxicities, monitoring parameters, and more. See MKSAP 18 Nephrology for details on the treatment of lupus nephritis.

KEY POINTS

HVC
- Hydroxychloroquine should be initiated in every patient with systemic lupus erythematosus who can tolerate it, because it can reduce disease-associated damage, prevent disease flares, and improve kidney and overall survival.

- Glucocorticoids are a mainstay of systemic lupus erythematosus management, particularly in acute disease; after disease stability is achieved, glucocorticoids are tapered to the lowest effective dose, ideally to eventual discontinuation.

- In systemic lupus erythematosus, immunosuppressive therapy is usually initiated concurrently with glucocorticoids to achieve and maintain disease control and to allow tapering of glucocorticoids.

Pregnancy and Childbirth Issues

SLE is associated with a five- to eightfold increase in miscarriage, stillbirth, premature delivery, and intrauterine growth retardation. Outcomes are worse in patients with active disease, nephritis, or anti–Ro/SSA and/or APLA antibodies. The best time to consider pregnancy is when SLE is quiescent, and conception should be considered only after at least 6 months of adequate disease control.

Proteinuria may increase during pregnancy in patients with SLE, making distinction between SLE and preeclampsia/eclampsia a challenge. Increases in anti–double-stranded DNA antibody levels, decreasing complement levels, or the development of active urine sediment suggests SLE as the cause. In contrast, serum urate levels are increased in preeclampsia but not during SLE flares.

Fetuses of women who have anti–Ro/SSA or anti–La/SSB antibodies are at risk for neonatal lupus erythematosus, which is characterized by rash and congenital heart block (CHB). Although the risk of CHB in the offspring of an anti–Ro/SSA–positive woman is only 2%, it is associated with significant fetal and neonatal morbidity and mortality. After a woman bears a child with neonatal lupus erythematosus, the risk of CHB is substantially increased (20%) in subsequent pregnancies. Hydroxychloroquine may reduce the overall risk.

Management of medications during SLE pregnancy is complicated. Hydroxychloroquine and low-dose glucocorticoids can be started during or continued throughout the pregnancy. Higher-dose glucocorticoids can be used to treat flare-ups or end-organ involvement. The preferred immunosuppressive agent for SLE during pregnancy is azathioprine, which should be used only if absolutely necessary. Belimumab, methotrexate, mycophenolate mofetil, and cyclophosphamide should be avoided. Cyclophosphamide is associated with age- and dose-dependent infertility. See Principles of Therapeutics for information on medications and pregnancy.

KEY POINTS

- Systemic lupus erythematosus is associated with a five- to eightfold increase in miscarriage, stillbirth, premature delivery, and intrauterine growth retardation.

- The best time to consider pregnancy is when systemic lupus erythematosus is quiescent, and conception should be considered only after at least 6 months of adequate disease control.

- Fetuses of women who have anti–Ro/SSA or anti–La/SSB antibodies are at risk for neonatal lupus erythematosus (rash and congenital heart block).

- Hydroxychloroquine and low-dose glucocorticoids can be started during or continued throughout the pregnancy.

Prognosis

The prognosis in SLE has improved significantly, and there is now a 90% 5-year survival rate. Early mortality is usually related to SLE disease and infections, and late mortality related to cardiovascular disease. Factors adversely affecting survival include myocarditis, nephritis, low socioeconomic status, male gender, and age over 50 years at diagnosis. SLE tends to be a chronic waxing and waning disease with only 2% of patients achieving remission at 5 years.

- Factors adversely affecting survival in systemic lupus erythematosus include myocarditis, nephritis, low socioeconomic status, male gender, and age over 50 years at diagnosis.

Sjögren Syndrome

Epidemiology and Pathophysiology

Sjögren syndrome is an autoimmune exocrinopathy affecting salivary and lacrimal glands. It is more prevalent in women and white persons and commonly presents in the fourth and fifth decades. Primary Sjögren syndrome occurs in isolation; secondary Sjögren syndrome occurs in the setting of other rheumatologic diseases, most commonly rheumatoid arthritis and systemic lupus erythematosus. Whereas the prevalence of primary Sjögren syndrome ranges from 0.5 to 5 patients per thousand, secondary Sjögren syndrome is common (10%-30%) among populations with predisposing rheumatologic conditions. Sjögren syndrome etiology remains unclear, although genetic associations include several HLA subtypes.

Clinical Manifestations

The most common presentation of Sjögren syndrome is sicca, consisting of dryness of the eyes (keratoconjunctivitis sicca) and mouth (xerostomia). Patients report gritty eyes or a foreign body sensation. Oral dryness can cause caries and difficulty eating unmoistened food. Symmetric parotid and lacrimal swelling is common, as is skin and vaginal dryness.

Extraglandular manifestations may also occur (**Table 22**). Arthralgia and arthritis are common; the joint distribution and presentation resemble rheumatoid arthritis but without bone erosions (Jaccoud arthropathy). Patients with Sjögren syndrome are at increased risk for non-Hodgkin lymphoma, presumably related to chronic lymphocyte activation.

Diagnosis

A diagnosis of Sjögren syndrome is typically triggered by a complaint of sicca and requires objective confirmation of exocrinopathy along with demonstration of autoimmunity (**Table 23**). Dry eyes can be assessed using the Schirmer test, in which a strip of filter paper is placed under the lower eyelid and wetting is measured; less than 5 mm in 5 minutes indicates dryness. More formally, dryness and corneal damage are ascertained by slit-lamp examination

TABLE 22. Extraglandular Clinical Manifestations of Sjögren Syndrome

Site/Organ	Manifestation/Frequency
General	Fatigue (70%), fever (6%)
Skin	Dry skin (xerosis), cutaneous vasculitis: 10%-16%
Joint	Arthralgia/arthritis: 36%
Lung	Interstitial pneumonitis: 5%-9%
Kidney	Interstitial nephritis, distal (type 1) renal tubular acidosis, glomerulonephritis: 5%-6%
Neurologic	Central nervous system (CNS): demyelinating disease, myelopathy, cranial nerve neuropathy
	Peripheral nervous system: small-fiber neuropathy, mononeuritis multiplex, peripheral neuropathy
	8%-27% for CNS and peripheral
Gastrointestinal	Autoimmune hepatitis, primary biliary cirrhosis: 3%-20%
Hematologic	Lymphoma, cytopenia: 2%
Other	Systemic vasculitis (7%), cryoglobulinemia (4%-12%), Raynaud phenomenon (16%), thyroid disease (10%-15%)

TABLE 23. American College of Rheumatology/European League Against Rheumatism Classification Criteria for Primary Sjögren Syndrome[a]

The presence of a subjective finding of Sjögren syndrome (e.g., sicca complaint) plus any combination of the following resulting in a score of ≥4:

Item	Score
Salivary gland biopsy with ≥1 foci of lymphocytic infiltrate/4 mm^2	3
Anti-Ro/SSA autoantibodies	3
Ocular staining score ≥5 in at least one eye	1
Schirmer test ≤5 mm/5 min in at least one eye	1
Unstimulated whole saliva flow rate ≤0.1 mL/min	1

[a]Exclusion criteria include prior head/neck radiation and history of active hepatitis C virus infection, AIDS, sarcoidosis, amyloidosis, graft-versus-host disease, and IgG4-related disease.

From Shiboski CH, Shiboski SC, Seror R, Criswell LA, Labetoulle M, Lietman TM, et al; International Sjögren's Syndrome Criteria Working Group. 2016 American College of Rheumatology/European League Against Rheumatism Classification Criteria for Primary Sjögren's Syndrome: A Consensus and Data-Driven Methodology Involving Three International Patient Cohorts. Arthritis Rheumatol. 2017 Jan;69(1):35-45. doi: 10.1002/art.39859. [PMID: 27785888]. Copyright 2016, American College of Rheumatology. Adapted with permission from John Wiley & Sons, Inc.

by an ophthalmologist using fluorescein and lissamine green dyes. Dry mouth is assessed by direct examination, with dental caries and a lack of saliva suggesting the diagnosis. Measurement of salivary flow (sialography) is easily done but is less commonly performed. Salivary gland imaging with MRI or ultrasonography may assist in identifying characteristic abnormalities and provide additional support for the diagnosis.

Multiple autoantibodies may be present. Antinuclear antibodies and/or rheumatoid factor are often present at high titers; their coexpression is more suggestive of Sjögren syndrome than if only one is positive. The presence of anti-Ro/SSA autoantibodies is specific in the setting of primary Sjögren syndrome; their presence is less specific for secondary Sjögren syndrome because these antibodies are also common in systemic lupus erythematosus. The presence of anti-La/SSB autoantibodies is also characteristic of Sjögren syndrome, although these are not currently included in formal disease classification criteria. When initial evaluation is uninformative, a lip (minor salivary gland) biopsy should be considered. Characteristic histologic features include aggregate foci (>50 cells/aggregate) of CD4 T cells, B cells, and plasma cells surrounding secretory ducts.

The differential diagnosis of Sjögren syndrome typically relates to the presence of sicca and/or parotid and lacrimal enlargement. Sarcoidosis, IgG4-related disease, granulomatosis with polyangiitis, lymphoma, and viruses such as mumps, hepatitis C, and HIV may be associated with similar findings. Ocular and oral dryness may also occur with aging or in response to drugs such as anticholinergics.

Management

Management of sicca is centered on preservation of moisture and relief of symptoms. Eyes are treated with artificial tears and/or topical cyclosporine. The use of glasses with side panels to prevent surface drying may be helpful, as may be plugging of the lacrimal ducts to promote tear retention. For oral dryness, meticulous dental care is essential. Sugar-free candies can stimulate saliva flow. Artificial saliva may be used, but its effects may be too transient to be useful. Vaginal symptoms may be treated with topical lubricants or estrogen. Pharmacologic therapies include the muscarinic agonists pilocarpine and cevimeline, although these may not be well tolerated and are contraindicated in narrow-angle glaucoma.

Patients with extraglandular involvement are treated with immunosuppression. Evidence-based guidelines are limited, and decisions are often empiric. Options include hydroxychloroquine and methotrexate for arthritis, and cyclophosphamide and rituximab for severe or systemic central nervous system disease. Some of these agents may have benefit for sicca as well.

Prognosis

The prognosis for primary Sjögren syndrome is favorable, with no overall increase in mortality. Management of sicca reduces the risk of corneal damage or loss of teeth. In rare instances, end-organ involvement can be life-threatening. Secondary Sjögren syndrome may be associated with significant morbidity from the primary condition. An increased risk of lymphoma is present in both forms of the syndrome.

Inflammatory Myopathies

Overview

The inflammatory myopathies include polymyositis (PM), dermatomyositis (DM), immune-mediated necrotizing myopathy (IMNM), and inclusion body myositis (IBM). Although the pathogenesis of these disorders is disparate, they all include immune-mediated muscle inflammation and destruction.

Evaluation of the Patient with Muscle Pain or Weakness

The differential diagnosis of muscle disease is broad and includes hereditary, environmental, infectious, and acquired muscle disease (**Table 24**). The inflammatory myopathies commonly present with symmetric proximal muscle weakness without substantial muscle pain or tenderness. Serum creatine kinase is almost universally elevated in the inflammatory myopathies and is a marker of muscle damage. The presence of pain or tenderness, however, should prompt considerations of other causes of myopathy. Muscle pain is more common with overexertion, muscle cramps, and injury. Muscle tenderness should prompt consideration of infectious, thyroid, or drug-induced myopathies. Medications and drugs are common causes of myopathy and should be considered in the differential diagnosis of the inflammatory myopathies (**Table 25**).

Weakness is often caused by conditions other than myopathy. Cardiopulmonary disease, malignancy, depression, and deconditioning frequently lead to generalized weakness. Although uncommon, primary neurologic disorders such as spinal muscle atrophies, amyotrophic lateral sclerosis, and myasthenia gravis may cause weakness. These diseases are distinguished by involvement of muscle groups other than the proximal muscles, nerve involvement on electromyography (EMG), and a normal serum creatine kinase. Finally, the presence of exercise-induced weakness may point to a metabolic etiology rather than an inflammatory myopathy.

TABLE 24. Differential Diagnosis of Myopathy

Myopathy	Common Examples	Comments
Inflammatory myopathies	Dermatomyositis (DM); polymyositis (PM); immune-mediated necrotizing myopathy (IMNM); inclusion body myositis (IBM)	DM and PM: acute-subacute onset, symmetric, proximal; DM: pathognomonic rash; IMNM: acute onset, symmetric, proximal; IBM: insidious onset, proximal and distal
Systemic rheumatologic disease	Systemic lupus erythematosus; systemic sclerosis; mixed connective tissue disease	Prominent extramuscular features typical of underlying disorder
Muscular dystrophies	Duchenne muscular dystrophy; Becker muscular dystrophy	Childhood onset; cardiomyopathy possible
Metabolic myopathies	Glycogen storage diseases; carnitine palmitoyltransferase deficiency	Exercise intolerance
Mitochondrial myopathies	Kearns-Sayre syndrome; Leigh syndrome	Variable age of presentation and features; isolated myopathy or with neurologic, multisystem disease
Endocrine disorders	Hypothyroidism; hyperthyroidism; adrenal insufficiency	Prominent myalgia
Infection induced	Bacterial: pyomyositis; viral: influenza; parasitic: trichinosis	Prominent myalgia; sometimes accompanied by fever

TABLE 25. Drug-Induced Myopathies

Drug	Time Course	Clinical Presentation
Alcohol	Increased with long-term use	Asymptomatic elevations of serum creatine kinase; chronic muscle atrophy; acute, severe rhabdomyolysis with kidney failure
Antimalarials	Can occur after prolonged use	Infrequent elevation of serum creatine kinase (30%); muscle weakness (50%); myopathic electromyogram findings (100%); cardiomyopathy can occur
Cocaine	Can occur after single use	Asymptomatic elevations of serum creatine kinase; acute, severe rhabdomyolysis with kidney failure
Colchicine	Usually months to years; increased risk with coadministration of cytochrome P450 inhibitors	Proximal muscle weakness with elevations of serum creatine kinase; mild sensory symptoms; reduced reflexes
Glucocorticoids	Increased with long-term use	Proximal muscle weakness in the absence of elevations of serum creatine kinase
Statins	Usually weeks to months but can occur at any time; increased risk with preexisting neuromuscular disease, hypothyroidism, kidney failure, and/or coadministration of cytochrome P450 inhibitors; may also trigger immune-mediated necrotizing myopathy	Elevations of serum creatine kinase with myalgia and weakness
Zidovudine	Variable; may be more common after long-term use	Elevations of serum creatine kinase with myalgia and weakness

Epidemiology and Pathophysiology of Inflammatory Myopathies

The annual incidence of inflammatory myopathies is between 2 and 10 cases per million. Two peaks of onset occur, with the first in childhood and the second in middle age. A female adult predominance is approximately 2:1 with the exception of IBM, which preferentially affects men.

Genetic factors contribute to the risk of inflammatory myopathies. The clearest association is with HLA DRB1*0301, but alleles vary in populations throughout the world. Except for IMNM, environmental factors have not been clearly implicated. Immune mechanisms that contribute include the presence of T lymphocytic infiltrates in muscle tissue and the expression of autoantibodies in many patients. T- and B-cell proliferation and activation, as well as increased cytokine and chemokine levels in muscle, also occur.

KEY POINTS

- The inflammatory myopathies commonly present with symmetric proximal muscle weakness without substantial muscle pain or tenderness; serum creatine kinase is almost universally elevated and is a marker of muscle damage.

- Muscle tenderness should prompt consideration of infectious, thyroid, or drug-induced myopathies.

Polymyositis

Clinical Manifestations

Muscle Involvement

The symptoms of PM usually progress slowly over months, although a more rapid onset may occur. Progressive, symmetric, proximal muscle weakness is the classic and dominant feature. Activities such as arising from a chair, stair climbing, and lifting objects above shoulder height are typically affected. Neck flexors are also commonly involved. Muscle pain and tenderness, if present, are mild. Muscle atrophy is a late manifestation. Weakness of respiratory muscles may also occur.

Cardiopulmonary Involvement

Interstitial lung disease, most commonly nonspecific interstitial pneumonitis, occurs in about 10% of patients with PM. It is particularly prominent in the subset of patients with antisynthetase syndrome (also seen in association with dermatomyositis). In addition to interstitial lung disease and myositis, antisynthetase syndrome is characterized by the presence of Raynaud phenomenon, nonerosive arthritis, and mechanic's hands, a dermatologic manifestation characterized by rough, cracked, scaly skin along the lateral aspects of the digits and palms with horizontal lines resembling the weathered hands of a laborer (See MKSAP 18 Dermatology). It can occasionally present as rapidly progressive respiratory failure. Antisynthetase syndrome is associated with autoantibodies against anti–aminoacyl-tRNA synthetases, most commonly anti–Jo-1 antibodies.

Cardiac involvement includes conduction system abnormalities that can result in arrhythmias and sudden death. Pericarditis can occur, and pericardial tamponade has been reported. Patients are also at increased risk for myocardial infarction and heart failure, which represent an important cause of morbidity and mortality in PM.

Gastrointestinal Involvement

The striated muscle of the upper two thirds of the esophagus can be affected by PM, leading to dysphagia, dysmotility, and increased risk of aspiration pneumonia. ▣

Dermatomyositis

Clinical Manifestations

In DM, muscle involvement is clinically similar to PM but is almost universally accompanied by a unique constellation of skin findings.

Cutaneous Involvement

Cutaneous involvement of DM can be virtually pathognomic and serve as an indicator of response to therapy (**Table 26**). Most typical is the Gottron rash (Gottron papules and Gottron sign), erythematous to violaceous areas over the metacarpophalangeal and proximal interphalangeal joints (**Figure 18**). See MKSAP 18 Dermatology for more information.

Muscle Involvement

Similar to PM, the insidious onset of symmetric proximal muscle weakness is most common in DM. Some patients present initially with rash and develop weakness later.

A small percentage of patients may present with skin rash only and never develop muscle involvement (amyopathic DM). At least 6 months without evidence of muscle involvement is necessary before the diagnosis of amyopathic DM can be established.

Cardiopulmonary Involvement

Cardiopulmonary involvement is similar to that seen in PM, but interstitial lung disease is more common in DM (20%-25%). Arrhythmias, complete atrioventricular block, heart failure, myocardial infarction, and pericarditis have been reported. ▣

Gastrointestinal Involvement

Gastrointestinal involvement in DM resembles that in PM.

Immune-Mediated Necrotizing Myopathy

IMNM occurs in a small subset of patients with inflammatory myopathy who demonstrate prominent myonecrosis on biopsy

TABLE 26.	Cutaneous Manifestations of Dermatomyositis	
Cutaneous Sign	**Location**	**Clinical Appearance**
Gottron rash (Gottron papules and Gottron sign)	Metacarpophalangeal and proximal interphalangeal joints; occasionally on distal interphalangeal joints, elbows, knees	Erythematous to violaceous papules; occasional scale; can ulcerate; atrophic scars may occur
Heliotrope rash	Eyelids	Subtle pink to deep purple or brown discoloration; may be associated with edema of eyelids or periorbital edema
V sign	V of neck	Erythematous to violaceous papules to patches
Shawl sign	Base of posterior neck to upper back	Erythematous to violaceous papules to patches
Fixed erythema	Malar area (may cross nasolabial folds); flanks of trunk	Erythematous to violaceous papules to patches
Nail area changes	Periungual area; cuticles	Periungual erythema; capillary dilatation and dropout; cuticular hypertrophy; cuticular infarcts
Mechanic's hands	Lateral aspects of digits and palms	Hyperkeratotic fissuring of the palmar and lateral surfaces of the fingers resembling the hands of a laborer

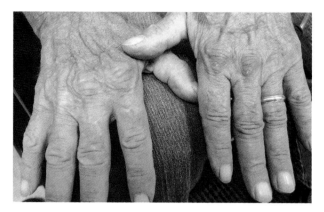

FIGURE 18. Gottron rash. Erythema and mild scaling are seen most prominently over the second and third metacarpophalangeal joints, and more subtle erythema is present over the proximal interphalangeal joints of both hands. The cracked and thickened skin on the lateral surfaces of the second digit bilaterally is consistent with mechanic's hands.

CONT.

without the inflammatory changes typical of the other inflammatory myopathies. An immune-mediated mechanism is suggested by the presence of antibodies to signal recognition particles (SRPs) or 3-hydroxy-3-methylglutaryl-coenzyme A (HMG-CoA) reductase. Although statin exposure may result in antibodies to HMG-CoA reductase and IMNM, most patients with statin-induced myopathies have processes other than IMNM (see Table 25).

Clinical Manifestations

Patients with IMNM experience severe, rapidly progressive weakness, very high serum creatine kinase levels, and few (if any) extramuscular manifestations.

Muscle Involvement

The characteristic symptom of IMNM is severe proximal muscle weakness, making it difficult to distinguish from PM and DM. Rapidity of onset may provide a clue. In patients with statin-triggered IMNM, the weakness may persist or progress even after statins are discontinued.

Other Organ Involvement

Cardiopulmonary involvement in IMNM is rare. Gastrointestinal involvement has not been reported. ⊞

Inclusion Body Myositis

IBM is a uniformly insidious condition and is usually easily distinguishable from PM, DM, and IMNM because of its very slow onset and pattern of muscle involvement.

Clinical Manifestations
Muscle Involvement
Patients typically report a history of preexisting weakness averaging 5 years. Although proximal muscle involvement is present, distal muscle involvement also occurs, distinguishing

it from PM and DM. Muscle distribution is typically symmetric, but asymmetry may occur. On physical examination, muscle weakness and atrophy are often present in the hip flexors, quadriceps, finger flexors, and forearm flexors. Serum creatine kinase levels are elevated but are lower than levels seen in PM and DM.

Gastrointestinal Involvement

Up to half of patients with IBM have cricopharyngeal muscle involvement, leading to dysphagia and increased risk of aspiration.

KEY POINTS

- Polymyositis and dermatomyositis are characterized by progressive, symmetric, proximal muscle weakness, leading to decline in physical function; dermatomyositis is further defined by cutaneous involvement.
- Gottron rash (Gottron papules and Gottron sign) is the characteristic rash of dermatomyositis, and is defined as erythematous to violaceous areas over the metacarpophalangeal and proximal interphalangeal joints.
- Immune-mediated necrotizing myopathy is characterized by severe, rapidly progressive proximal muscle weakness, very high serum creatine kinase levels, and few extramuscular manifestations.
- Inclusion body myositis is a uniformly insidious condition that involves both the proximal and distal muscles; although typically symmetric, muscle distribution may be asymmetric.

Inflammatory Myopathies and Malignancy

There is an association between risk of malignancy and DM (3- to 12-fold that of age-matched populations) as well as, to a lesser extent, PM. IMNM may occasionally be a paraneoplastic syndrome, but IBM is not strongly associated with malignancy. The risk of malignancy is greatest in the 3 years following the diagnosis of DM or PM. Common associated cancers are ovarian, lung, pancreas, stomach, colon, and lymphoma. Age- and sex-appropriate cancer screening is indicated at the time of diagnosis of DM or PM. Many experts advocate CT of the chest, abdomen, and pelvis, particularly in patients with DM.

KEY POINT

- Because of the malignancy risk associated with polymyositis and dermatomyositis, age- and sex-appropriate cancer screening is indicated at the time of diagnosis. **HVC**

Diagnosis
Muscle-Related Enzymes ⊞

Elevations of serum muscle enzymes are particularly useful in differentiating intrinsic muscle disease from neurologic causes

CONT.

of weakness. Elevated serum creatine kinase levels are the most sensitive serum indicator of muscle pathology, and levels parallel the severity of involvement. Aldolase can occasionally be elevated when serum creatine kinase levels are normal. Serum aminotransferases and serum lactate dehydrogenase may also be elevated but are nonspecific. **H**

Autoantibodies

Various autoantibodies are used to help diagnose inflammatory myopathies. Some, such as antinuclear antibodies, lack specificity. Others, often termed *myositis-specific antibodies*, have more diagnostic and prognostic value (**Table 27**).

Imaging Studies

Although not required to diagnose inflammatory myopathies, MRI is potentially useful in identifying areas of muscle inflammation as an appropriate site for muscle biopsy. MRI is also helpful at identifying muscle atrophy; follow-up with MRI may provide a noninvasive technique to assess therapeutic efficacy.

Electromyography

EMG may show findings highly characteristic of active myositis, although no single finding is pathognomonic. The procedure, however, is invasive and uncomfortable. It may also be normal in the presence of active disease due to the patchy distribution of muscle inflammation (that is, sampling error).

Muscle Biopsy

Muscle biopsy is valuable in diagnosing inflammatory myopathies and for excluding metabolic myopathies, mitochondrial disease, and infection. In PM and DM, features include inflammatory cell infiltrates, muscle fiber necrosis, degeneration, and regeneration.

Muscle biopsy findings in IBM include mononuclear cell infiltrates with unique "rimmed" vacuoles without muscle cell necrosis; electron microscopy may show inclusion bodies.

Skin Biopsy

Skin biopsy is useful in diagnosing DM. Light microscopy findings include mild epidermal atrophy, vacuolar changes at the dermal-epidermal junction, perivascular lymphocytic infiltrates, and increased dermal mucin. However, these findings may be similar to those of systemic lupus erythematosus.

Diagnosis of amyopathic DM is made with skin biopsy confirmation of DM in the setting of at least 6 months of normal muscle strength, muscle enzymes, normal EMG, and, if performed, normal muscle biopsy.

KEY POINTS

- Elevated serum creatine kinase levels are the most sensitive serum indicator of muscle pathology, and levels parallel the severity of involvement.

- Antibodies against aminoacyl-tRNA synthetases, particularly anti-Jo-1 (anti-histidyl-tRNA synthetase antibodies), have been associated with antisynthetase syndrome (interstitial lung disease, Raynaud phenomenon, arthritis, and mechanic's hands).

- In patients with inflammatory myopathies, MRI can be helpful to locate a site for muscle biopsy, identify muscle atrophy, and assess therapeutic efficacy.

- Muscle biopsy is valuable in diagnosing inflammatory myopathies and for excluding metabolic myopathies, mitochondrial disease, and infection.

Management

Glucocorticoids are the cornerstone of therapy for the inflammatory myopathies except for IBM. Prolonged exposure to high-dose glucocorticoids, particularly in the elderly, can be associated with the appearance of steroid-induced myopathy that may cause new proximal muscle weakness in a patient who had previously been improving; reduction in dose is appropriate management.

Additional immunosuppressives are often required to control inflammation or to serve as glucocorticoid-sparing agents; methotrexate and azathioprine are most frequently used. DM and PM are most responsive to immunosuppression, although DM is more responsive than PM. For patients with statin-induced IMNM, statin discontinuation is mandatory but not sufficient, and immunosuppressive treatment is required. IBM

TABLE 27. Autoantibodies in Inflammatory Myopathies		
Autoantibody	**Disease Association**	**Clinical Association**
Antinuclear	DM; PM	Seen in up to 80%; nonspecific
Anti-aminoacyl-tRNA synthetase; most commonly anti-Jo-1 (anti-histidyl tRNA synthetase)	DM	Antisynthetase syndrome (ILD, Raynaud phenomenon, nonerosive arthritis, mechanic's hands)
Anti-cytoplasmic 5'-nucleotidase 1A	IBM	Insidious onset
Anti-HMG Co-A reductase	IMNM	Typically but not always in the setting of statin exposure; may also be seen in patients with statin exposure without IMNM
Anti-Mi 2	DM	Seen in up to 30%; associated with acute onset, typical rash
Anti-signal recognition protein	IMNM	Severe, treatment-resistant disease and myofiber necrosis but little to no inflammation on muscle biopsy

DM = dermatomyositis; IBM = inclusion body myositis; ILD = interstitial lung disease; IMNM = immune-mediated necrotizing myopathy; PM = polymyositis.

CONT.

usually does not respond to immunosuppression, and therapeutic trials should be undertaken only in selected patients and discontinued if benefit is not appreciated. Other immunosuppressives, including mycophenolate mofetil and rituximab, have been used in refractory DM, PM, and IMNM. Intravenous immunoglobulin may be a reasonable alternative in DM. **H**

Physical therapy may help maintain muscle function and should be used in all patients.

Prognosis

The prognosis in DM/PM varies from near-complete resolution to severe, treatment-resistant disease with marked functional impairment and early mortality. Prolonged symptoms prior to treatment, greater weakness at presentation, extensive multisystem disease, and the co-occurrence of malignancy confer a poorer prognosis. The degree of serum creatine kinase elevation is not predictive of outcome. Myositis-specific antibodies may have prognostic value. Patients with anti–Jo-1 antibodies have worse outcomes (due to interstitial lung disease), whereas those with anti-Mi-2 antibodies often respond completely, despite a rapidly progressive course of DM.

Patients with IMNM frequently respond well to statin discontinuation (if appropriate) and immunosuppression.

Given the lack of effective treatment, patients with IBM typically demonstrate a slow and gradual loss of function, with progression to wheelchair dependence within 10 to 15 years.

KEY POINTS

- Initial treatment for most inflammatory myopathies consists of glucocorticoids, with additional immunosuppressives (most commonly methotrexate and azathioprine) often required to control inflammation or serve as glucocorticoid-sparing agents.

- Inclusion body myositis often does not respond to immunosuppression, and therapeutic trials should be discontinued if benefit is not appreciated.

- In patients with dermatomyositis or polymyositis, prolonged symptoms prior to treatment, greater weakness at presentation, extensive multisystem disease, and the co-occurrence of malignancy confer a poorer prognosis.

- Patients with inclusion body myositis typically demonstrate a slow and gradual loss of function, with progression to wheelchair dependence within 10 to 15 years.

Systemic Sclerosis

Epidemiology and Pathophysiology

Systemic sclerosis (SSc) is a multiorgan disease characterized by fibrosis and vasculopathy. The skin is the principal target, but internal organs are also affected. SSc is relatively rare, with a prevalence of 275 cases per million, and an annual incidence of 19 cases per million. It is more common among women and black persons.

Vascular injury, vascular and visceral fibrosis, and innate and adaptive immune activation with autoantibody production play an interactive role in SSc. One of the earliest SSc manifestations is Raynaud phenomenon, suggesting that vascular injury precedes the fibrotic reaction. With vascular damage, the endothelial cells release endothelin-1, a potent vasoconstrictor that also induces vascular smooth muscle proliferation and fibroblast activation. Platelet activation occurs concurrently with subsequent release of growth factors that promote further vasoconstriction, fibroblast activation, and collagen production.

B-cell activation results in production of interleukin (IL)-6, which directly stimulates fibroblasts as well as various autoantibodies. The end result is increased collagen production and deposition by activated scleroderma fibroblasts, along with a progressive obliterative vasculopathy.

Classification

Although intended for research studies, the 2013 American College of Rheumatology/European League Against Rheumatism SSc classification criteria can be useful when a patient presents with features suggesting SSc (**Table 28**).

Classically, SSc is divided into three subtypes based on the extent of skin involvement: limited cutaneous systemic sclerosis (LcSSc), diffuse cutaneous systemic sclerosis (DcSSc), and systemic sclerosis sine scleroderma (internal organ involvement only). These subtypes have clinical and prognostic utility because specific long-term complications may be more likely in one subtype than another; however, overlap is common. Importantly, LcSSc is less commonly accompanied by fibrosis of internal organs, but is most commonly associated with pulmonary arterial hypertension and CREST (calcinosis, Raynaud phenomenon, esophageal dysmotility, sclerodactyly, and telangiectasia) syndrome.

Various disorders may present with skin thickening and other manifestations that overlap with the findings of SSc; these conditions should be considered in the differential diagnosis of SSc (**Table 29**). Importantly, these conditions are not typically associated with Raynaud phenomenon, and the absence of Raynaud phenomenon in a patient with skin thickening makes SSc unlikely.

KEY POINTS

- Systemic sclerosis is a multiorgan disease characterized by fibrosis and vasculopathy; the skin is the principle target, with Raynaud phenomenon being one of the earliest manifestations.

- Systemic sclerosis is divided into three subtypes based on the extent of skin involvement: limited cutaneous systemic sclerosis, diffuse cutaneous systemic sclerosis, and systemic sclerosis sine scleroderma.

(Continued)

TABLE 28. American College of Rheumatology/European League Against Rheumatism Classification Criteria for Systemic Sclerosis

Manifestation	Additional Manifestations	Weight/Score[a]
Skin thickening of fingers of both hands extending proximal to the MCPs	—	9
Skin thickening of the fingers (count higher score only)	Puffy fingers	2
	Sclerodactyly of fingers distal to the MCPs but proximal to PIPs	4
Fingertip lesions	Digital tip ulcers	2
	Fingertip pitting scars	3
Telangiectasia	—	2
Abnormal nailfold capillaries	—	2
Pulmonary hypertension and/or interstitial lung disease (maximum score is 2)	Pulmonary hypertension	2
	Interstitial lung disease	2
Raynaud phenomenon	—	3
SSc-related autoantibodies (maximum score is 3)	Anticentromere	3
	Anti-Scl-70 (antitopoisomerase-1)	3
	Anti-RNA polymerase III	3

MCP = metacarpophalangeal; PIP = proximal interphalangeal; SSc = systemic sclerosis.

[a]A score of 9 or more equates to definite systemic sclerosis.

From van den Hoogen F, Khanna D, Fransen J, Johnson SR, Baron M, Tyndall A, et al. 2013 classification criteria for systemic sclerosis: an American College of Rheumatology/European League Against Rheumatism Collaborative Initiative. Ann Rheum Dis 2013;72:1747-55. doi: 10.1136/annrheumdis-2013-204424. [PMID: 24092682] Copyright 2013, American College of Rheumatology. Adapted with permission from BMJ Publishing Group Ltd.

KEY POINTS *(continued)*

- The absence of Raynaud phenomenon in a patient with skin thickening makes systemic sclerosis unlikely.

Clinical Manifestations and Diagnosis

The diagnosis of SSc is dependent on the presence of specific clinical findings and autoantibodies (present in 90%-95% of patients). In patients with clinical features suggestive of SSc, autoantibody testing should be done (**Table 30**).

Cutaneous Involvement

The skin is the most common organ involved in SSc, with the hands being universally affected. In LcSSc, the skin over the fingers/hands, face, and neck is typically affected. In DcSSc, skin involvement is more extensive and additionally includes the arms, trunk, and lower extremities.

The earliest skin manifestations are often diffusely swollen fingers/hands (sclerodactyly). Skin thickening, especially in LcSSc, may be subtle, and the inability to tent the skin over the fingers may be an important clue. With time, the skin becomes thickened, atrophic, and immobile; skin thickening around the joints can lead to contractures (**Figure 19**).

Vascular complications of the skin include digital infarcts, subungual infections, and ischemic skin ulceration. Another feature is poikiloderma, in which areas of hyperpigmentation mixed with hypopigmentation give the skin a salt-and-pepper appearance.

Facial involvement can lead to limitation of the oral aperture and difficulty eating. The face is also typically devoid of wrinkles, causing patients to sometimes look younger than their age.

Calcinosis occurs in approximately 25% of patients with SSc (**Figure 20**). Present in the hands, forearms, elbows, gluteal region, and iliac crest, these deposits can be seen/felt and are easily detected on radiograph.

Musculoskeletal Involvement

Joint involvement occurs in 12% to 65% of patients with SSc; it has a hand/wrist predominance and is one of the few forms of inflammatory arthritis that affects the distal interphalangeal joints. Between 1% and 5% of patients have a rheumatoid arthritis–SSc overlap, with positive anti–cyclic citrullinated antibodies and classic rheumatoid arthritis manifestations along with those of SSc.

Patients with SSc may develop acro-osteolysis, or resorption of the terminal bony tuft of fingers and less commonly the toes, with prevalence as high as 20% to 25% in more severe disease (**Figure 21**).

SSc-associated myositis occurs in 10% to 15% of patients. Myalgia and proximal muscle weakness are common symptoms. Serum creatine kinase and/or serum aldolase levels are

TABLE 29. Common Manifestations/Features of the Scleroderma Spectrum Disorders

Disorder	Manifestation/Feature	Comments
Systemic Sclerosis		
Diffuse cutaneous systemic sclerosis (DcSSc)	Distal and proximal skin thickening (chest, abdomen, arms proximal to wrists); commonly has visceral organ involvement	Skin involvement is extensive and is commonly accompanied by internal organ fibrosis and ILD
Limited cutaneous systemic sclerosis (LcSSc)	Distal (face, neck, hands), but not proximal, skin thickening; typically not accompanied by internal organ fibrosis	More likely to develop PAH and Raynaud phenomenon early in the disease and more likely to display features of the CREST syndrome
Systemic sclerosis sine scleroderma	Fibrosing organ involvement without skin thickening	Difficult to diagnose; prognosis may be similar to LcSSc
Localized Scleroderma		
Morphea	Focal plaques of skin thickening, generally on the trunk	Systemic manifestations or Raynaud phenomenon is extremely rare
Linear scleroderma	Streaks/lines of thickened skin	Same as morphea
Scleroderma-like Conditions[a]		
Eosinophilic fasciitis	Orange peel induration (peau d'orange) of proximal extremities with sparing of hands and face; peripheral eosinophilia; skin retraction over the superficial veins may be more apparent with elevation of an affected limb	Full-thickness skin biopsy demonstrates lymphocytes, plasma cells, and eosinophils infiltrating the deep fascia; glucocorticoids are the mainstay of treatment
Nephrogenic systemic fibrosis	Secondary to gadolinium in patients with kidney disease; brawny, wood-like induration of extremities, sparing the digits	Skeletal muscle fibrosis with contractures and/or cardiac muscle involvement can occur, with cardiomyopathy and increased mortality; changes in use and formulation of gadolinium have reduced incidence
Scleredema	Indurated plaques/patches on back, shoulder girdle, and neck	Typically seen in long-standing diabetes mellitus
Scleromyxedema	Waxy, yellow-red papules over thickened skin of face, upper trunk, neck, and arms; deposition of mucin with large numbers of stellate fibroblasts in the dermis	Associated with paraproteinemia (IgGλ) and may therefore occur in the setting of multiple myeloma or AL amyloidosis; more frequent in men
Chronic graft-versus-host disease	Lichen planus–like skin lesions, or localized or generalized skin thickening	Occurs most commonly after hematopoietic stem cell transplantation; may occasionally be seen after blood transfusion in an immunocompromised host
Drug and toxin exposure	Can produce scleroderma-like tissue changes	Examples: bleomycin, docetaxel, pentazocine, L-tryptophan, organic solvents

CREST = calcinosis cutis, Raynaud phenomenon, esophageal dysmotility, sclerodactyly, and telangiectasia; ILD = interstitial lung disease; PAH = pulmonary arterial hypertension.

[a]Scleroderma-like skin changes may also occur as a manifestation of systemic endocrine, kidney, or infiltrative disorders.

TABLE 30. Autoantibodies and Their Associations in Systemic Sclerosis

Autoantibody	Clinical Associations	Comments
Antinuclear antibodies	DcSSc; LcSSc	Overall prevalence in SSc: 70%; not associated with specific manifestations
Anticentromere (kinetochore proteins)	LcSSc ± PAH	Overall prevalence in SSc up to 30%; highly associated (>90%) with CREST variant of LcSSc
Anti–Scl-70 (DNA topoisomerase-1)	DcSSc; ILD	Overall prevalence in SSc: up to 30%; highly associated with DcSSc
Anti-RNA polymerase III	DcSSc; scleroderma renal crisis	Useful in DcSSc with negative anti–Scl-70
Anti-U3-RNP (fibrillarin)	DcSSc; PAH; myositis	Associated with poor outcome; more common in black men
Anti-PM-Scl	Myositis	Associated with overlap syndrome and polymyositis
Anti-Ku	Myositis	Rare occurrence
Anti-Th/To	LcSSc; PAH	Rare occurrence

CREST= calcinosis, Raynaud phenomenon, esophageal dysmotility, sclerodactyly, and telangiectasia; DcSSc = diffuse cutaneous systemic sclerosis; ILD = interstitial lung disease; LcSSc = limited cutaneous systemic sclerosis; PAH = pulmonary arterial hypertension; RNP = ribonucleoprotein; SSc= systemic sclerosis.

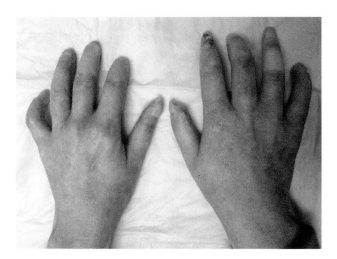

FIGURE 19. A 35-year-old woman with diffuse cutaneous systemic sclerosis. Note shortening of fingers and tight atrophic appearance of the skin. This patient is unable to make a full fist.

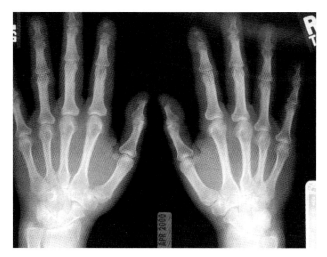

FIGURE 21. A posteroanterior radiograph of the hands in a patient with systemic sclerosis and acro-osteolysis. Note the destruction of the distal phalanges, particularly of the first and second digits, which will eventually result in clinical shortening of the affected digits.

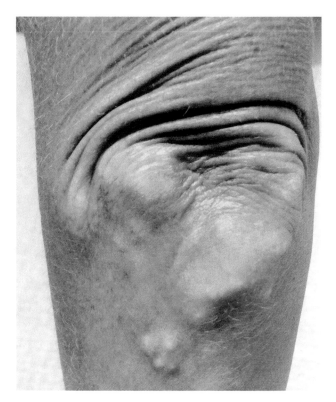

FIGURE 20. Calcinosis seen in CREST (calcinosis cutis, Raynaud phenomenon, esophageal dysmotility, sclerodactyly, and telangiectasia) syndrome in limited cutaneous systemic sclerosis. This patient has deposits of calcium in the subcutaneous tissues around the elbow. Calcinosis often occurs in the hands and forearms but can also affect other locations such as the trunk or lower extremities.

elevated, and electromyogram demonstrates myopathic changes. There is a strong association between SSc-associated myositis and myocardial involvement. The presence of anti-PM-Scl antibodies identifies a group of patients with an overlap between polymyositis and SSc. These patients usually have less skin and gastrointestinal involvement, but have more calcinosis and lung disease.

Tendon rubs can be felt or heard with a stethoscope because fibrosis affects tendons/tendons sheaths, leading to palpable and audible friction.

Vascular Involvement

Raynaud phenomenon occurs in approximately 95% of patients with SSc; it is the most common early manifestation of SSc, typically occurring years before other changes. Initially, Raynaud phenomenon is episodic, but with vascular fibrosis, the blood supply becomes permanently restricted. Approximately 80% of patients with the combination of Raynaud phenomenon, an SSc-associated autoantibody, and nailfold capillary changes in an SSc pattern (**Figure 22**), will develop SSc.

Digital ulcers occur in about 15% of patients with SSc, typically on the extensor surfaces and tips of the fingers and toes but also on the dorsum of hands and feet and even on the lower extremities. Vascular changes in the extremities may be indicative of involvement of the microcirculation of internal organs.

Gastrointestinal Involvement

Symptoms of esophageal dysmotility and reflux are common in all forms of SSc and may offer an early clue to the diagnosis when associated with other symptoms.

Approximately 80% of patients with SSc have involvement of the lower two thirds (smooth muscle portion) of the esophagus. Manifesting primarily as symptoms of dysmotility and/or gastroesophageal reflux disease, esophageal involvement is also associated with an increased risk of Barrett esophagus and adenocarcinoma.

Gastric symptoms also result mainly from dysmotility. Patients describe early satiety and may report nausea and

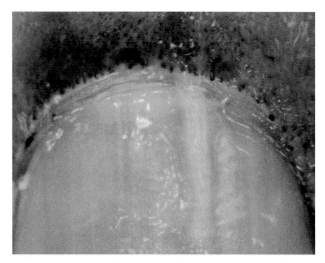

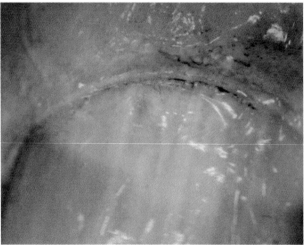

FIGURE 22. Capillary loops in systemic sclerosis. *Top*, Early changes with loss of capillary loop density (or drop out) with marked dilatation of the remaining capillary loops. *Bottom*, Late changes with extensive loss of capillary loops.

Courtesy of Mario Cutolo, MD.

vomiting as a result of delayed gastric emptying. Gastric antral vascular ectasia (GAVE), also known as watermelon stomach, is most common in patients with DcSSc and those with anti-RNA polymerase III antibodies. Bleeding ectasias can occasionally cause significant blood loss.

Small intestine bacterial overgrowth is common and can cause malabsorption and diarrhea. Diagnosis is established by hydrogen breath test, although an empiric trial of antibiotics is often utilized. Small intestine dysmotility can result in pseudo-obstruction. Large intestine dysmotility may lead to constipation, and vascular ectasia can occur in the large intestine (watermelon colon). Some patients may develop fecal incontinence.

Kidney Involvement

One of the most concerning manifestations of SSc is scleroderma renal crisis, which affects 5% of patients and was previously the chief cause of mortality. Risk factors include DcSSc,

use of moderate- to high-dose glucocorticoids, and the presence of anti-RNA polymerase III antibodies. Patients characteristically present with manifestations of hypertensive emergency, including headache, encephalopathy, seizures, and hypertensive retinopathy. Rarely, a normotensive form of scleroderma renal crisis can occur.

Laboratory tests demonstrate microangiopathic hemolytic anemia with schistocytes on peripheral smear, thrombocytopenia, and proteinuria. Serum creatinine is typically elevated and may remain so for some time after controlling blood pressure. Abnormalities in the renin-angiotensin-aldosterone system and endothelin-1 contribute to the pathophysiology.

Lung Involvement

Lung involvement in SSc includes pleuritis and pleural effusions, interstitial lung disease (ILD), pulmonary arterial hypertension (PAH), bronchiolitis, pulmonary veno-occlusive disease, respiratory muscle weakness, and skin involvement of the trunk restricting chest wall movement. Patients are also at increased risk of lung cancer.

Significant ILD occurs in 50% of patients with DcSSc (85% of patients with anti-Scl-70 antibodies) and 35% of patients with LcSSc, and is the main cause of disease-associated mortality. The most common pathology pattern is nonspecific interstitial pneumonitis followed by usual interstitial pneumonitis. In patients with SSc, men are more likely than women to develop ILD, and black persons tend to have more severe disease. An abnormal FVC early in the disease course (first 5 years) is highly predictive of developing more severe disease, as is fibrosis of more than 20% of lung volume on baseline high-resolution CT scan. There is a strong association between ILD and GERD, but whether GERD contributes to ILD (through aspiration) is uncertain. ILD is common enough that all patients should undergo pulmonary function tests (PFTs) and high-resolution CT at the time of initial SSc diagnosis, and PFTs with DLCO should be repeated every 6 to 12 months for 5 years. A decline in the FVC of 10% or the DLCO of 15% within 12 months should raise concern for progression.

PAH has a prevalence of 10% in SSc. Patients present with exertional dyspnea, and with more advanced disease may have chest pain and edema as the right ventricle begins to fail. Patients with SSc should undergo echocardiography annually and more frequently for new or concerning symptoms. PFTs can provide a clue to underlying PAH; an FVC/DLCO ratio of ≥1.6 suggests the diagnosis. Right heart catheterization is required for accurate diagnosis.

Cardiac Involvement

Cardiac involvement with SSc is more common in men. Clinically significant pericarditis occurs in 10% of patients. Myocardial fibrosis is a more significant process caused by vascular vasospasm leading to myocardial ischemia and fibrosis. The result may be heart failure and arrhythmias. Mortality in those with myocardial fibrosis is quite high.

- The earliest skin manifestations of systemic sclerosis are often diffusely swollen fingers/hands (sclerodactyly); with time, the skin becomes thickened, atrophic, and immobile.
- Raynaud phenomenon is the most common early manifestation of systemic sclerosis.
- Symptoms of esophageal dysmotility and reflux are common in all forms of systemic sclerosis and may offer an early clue to the diagnosis when associated with other symptoms.

(Continued)

- Patients with scleroderma renal crisis characteristically present with manifestations of hypertensive emergency; risk factors include diffuse cutaneous systemic sclerosis, use of moderate- to high-dose glucocorticoids, and the presence of anti-RNA polymerase III antibodies.
- Lung involvement in systemic sclerosis includes pulmonary arterial hypertension and interstitial lung disease (ILD); ILD is currently the main cause of disease-associated mortality.

Management

Table 31 outlines treatment options for manifestations of SSc.

TABLE 31. Treatment Options for Common Manifestations of Systemic Sclerosis

Manifestations	Treatment
Cutaneous manifestations	Methotrexate, mycophenolate, cyclophosphamide, and rituximab have been shown to improve skin scores; for pruritus, antihistamines can be tried; low-dose prednisone can also help; laser therapy can be used for telangiectasias.
Musculoskeletal manifestations	NSAIDs, intra-articular or low-dose prednisone, hydroxychloroquine, or methotrexate can be used for arthralgia/arthritis; methotrexate, azathioprine, or mycophenolate can be used for significant myositis.
Raynaud phenomenon	Cold avoidance; gloves; central warmth
	Calcium channel blockers
	Sildenafil; losartan; prazosin
	Topical nitrates; low-dose aspirin
	Digital sympathectomy
Gastroesophageal reflux disease	Avoid eating close to bed time; head of bed elevation
	H$_2$ blockers; proton pump inhibitors
	Surgical fundoplication
Gastrointestinal dysmotility	Metoclopramide (avoid long-term use); domperidone (limited access program)
	Erythromycin; cisapride (limited access program)
Gastric antral vascular ectasia	Ablation laser therapy
Small intestine bacterial overgrowth	Rotating antibiotics
	If fat malabsorption, cholestyramine
Pseudo-obstruction	A promotility agent such as domperidone can be tried
	If resistant, octreotide may be useful
Constipation	Fiber; stool softeners
	Polyethylene glycol
Scleroderma renal crisis	ACE inhibitors (typically captopril)
	Dialysis
Interstitial lung disease	Mycophenolate mofetil
	Cyclophosphamide
	Lung transplantation
Pulmonary arterial hypertension	Supplemental oxygen; treat right-sided heart failure
	Prostanoids; endothelin receptor antagonists; phosphodiesterase-5 inhibitors; soluble guanylate cyclase inhibitors
	Combination therapy
	Lung transplantation

CONT.

ACE inhibitors (typically captopril) can be lifesaving in patients with scleroderma renal crisis and should be titrated to control blood pressure. Dialysis may be needed temporarily. ACE inhibitor therapy should be continued in scleroderma renal crisis even in the presence of a rising serum creatinine and the need for dialysis, as late improvement may occur. In patients at high risk for developing scleroderma renal crisis, the prophylactic use of calcium channel blockers seems to offer some protection. However, prophylactic use of an ACE inhibitor has not been shown to offer protection and may increase mortality.

Cyclophosphamide can be used for stabilizing ILD, but the impact is modest and may not persist beyond 1 year. Recent evidence suggests that mycophenolate mofetil is as useful for stabilizing ILD as cyclophosphamide in SSc but with less toxicity. Mycophenolate mofetil can also be used for long-term therapy, making it the preferred agent for most patients with SSc-associated ILD.

Rituximab is a promising agent in SSc; in case series and one controlled trial, it has stabilized or slightly improved lung function and skin ulcers. Nintedanib (a tyrosine kinase inhibitor) and pirfenidone (a synthetic molecule) were recently approved by the FDA for treatment of idiopathic pulmonary fibrosis; results from clinical trials in SSc are pending. Autologous hematopoietic stem cell transplantation has been studied for several years in patients with severe SSc; one third to one half of patients had significant improvement in skin thickening and antibody status. However, cost and potential toxicity limit the utility of stem cell transplantation at present.

KEY POINTS

- Treatment options for systemic sclerosis are mainly symptomatic and organ system specific.

- ACE inhibitors can be lifesaving in patients with scleroderma renal crisis and should be titrated to control blood pressure even in the presence of rising serum creatinine.

Pregnancy

Pregnant patients with SSc may experience hypertensive disease, preeclampsia, preterm delivery, and low birth weights. In general, pregnancy does not make SSc worse, and some features (for example, digital ulcers) may actually improve. Contraindications to pregnancy in patients with SSc include PAH and severe restrictive lung disease (FVC of <1 L); in the setting of PAH, the hemodynamic changes of pregnancy can put the mother at considerable risk. See Principles of Therapeutics for details on medications and pregnancy.

KEY POINT

- Pregnant patients with systemic sclerosis (SSc) may experience hypertensive disease, preeclampsia, preterm delivery, and low birth weights; contraindications to pregnancy in patients with SSc include pulmonary arterial hypertension and severe restrictive lung disease.

Mixed Connective Tissue Disease
Overview

Despite long-standing attempts to define rheumatologic diseases according to precise classification, some patients express only nonspecific, nondiagnostic signs and symptoms (undifferentiated connective tissue disease [UCTD]), whereas others experience features of more than one disease simultaneously (overlap syndromes). Mixed connective tissue disease (MCTD) is a specific overlap syndrome that includes clinical manifestations of at least two of the following: systemic lupus erythematosus (SLE), polymyositis, and systemic sclerosis. Positive anti-U1-ribonucleoprotein (RNP) antibodies are the primary laboratory feature.

See **Table 32** for a comparison of MCTD, UCTD, and overlap syndromes.

TABLE 32. Comparison of Mixed Connective Tissue Disease, Undifferentiated Connective Tissue Disease, and Overlap Syndrome			
Condition	**Typical Clinical Features**	**Diagnosis**	**Treatment**
Mixed connective tissue disease	Raynaud phenomenon; arthritis; puffy fingers; sclerodactyly; serositis; esophageal dysmotility; myositis; interstitial lung disease; PAH	Positive anti-U1-RNP antibodies Fulfills criteria for at least two of the following: SSc, PM, and SLE	Disease/organ involvement specific Anti-inflammatories for symptoms; DMARDs and/or immunosuppressives for arthritis or other major organ disease Vasodilators for PAH and Raynaud phenomenon PPI for esophageal disease
Undifferentiated connective tissue disease	Variable; most common include Raynaud phenomenon, arthralgia, skin rash, cytopenia, and serositis	Insufficient criteria for any specific connective tissue disease	Same as mixed connective tissue disease
Overlap syndrome	Variable; will have features satisfying two distinct autoimmune diseases (such as SLE, RA, PM, and SSc)	Fulfills criteria for two distinct autoimmune diseases	Same as mixed connective tissue disease

DMARD = disease-modifying antirheumatic drug; PAH = pulmonary arterial hypertension; PM = polymyositis; PPI = proton pump inhibitor; RA = rheumatoid arthritis; RNP = ribonucleoprotein; SLE = systemic lupus erythematosus; SSc = systemic sclerosis.

Epidemiology and Pathophysiology

MCTD is rare, and 80% of patients are women. B-cell abnormalities and an association between anti-U1-RNP antibody titer and disease activity have been described.

Clinical Manifestations and Diagnosis

See Table 32 for details on the clinical manifestations and diagnosis of MCTD. Raynaud phenomenon is a particularly common feature. Pulmonary arterial hypertension is the major cause of death, but severe kidney disease is uncommon. Although antinuclear antibodies, rheumatoid factor, and anti-cyclic citrullinated peptide antibodies are often present, the presence of anti–double-stranded DNA or anti-Smith antibodies make SLE a more likely diagnosis.

Management

Treatment for MCTD is directed at the specific diseases and organ system involvement manifesting in the individual patient (see Table 32).

Prognosis

Prognosis of MCTD varies depending on the spectrum and severity of organ involvement. Patients with initially mild disease may develop new and more severe manifestations over decades, importantly including interstitial lung disease and pulmonary arterial hypertension. As with many other systemic inflammatory disorders, patients are at increased risk of atherosclerotic cardiovascular disease.

UCTD usually remains mild and stable but over time may evolve into a more specific autoimmune disorder, most commonly SLE.

KEY POINTS

- Mixed connective tissue disease includes clinical manifestations of at least two of the following diseases: systemic lupus erythematosus, polymyositis, and systemic sclerosis; anti-U1-ribonucleoprotein antibodies are typically present.
- Treatment for mixed connective tissue disease is directed at the specific diseases and organ systems involved.

Crystal Arthropathies

Gout

Epidemiology

Gout is characterized by intermittent painful inflammatory joint attacks, in response to crystals formed as a consequence of excessive levels of uric acid (hyperuricemia). Gout is increasingly common, with a U.S. prevalence of approximately 4%. Factors contributing to this increase include dietary changes, increasing obesity, and an aging population (the elderly account for the sharpest rise in gout over the past few decades). Nearly all patients with gout have comorbidities, including hypertension, coronary artery disease, hyperlipidemia, diabetes mellitus, and chronic kidney disease (CKD). Comorbidities frequently complicate treatment by posing relative contraindications for appropriate therapeutics (for example, CKD for NSAIDs or colchicine).

Men reach a steady-state serum urate level after puberty, whereas premenopausal women are generally protected from hyperuricemia by estrogenic effects. It is rare for premenopausal women to develop gout, whereas men usually have their first gout attack in the third to fifth decade.

Pathophysiology

Uric acid is the end product of purine metabolism, and about two thirds of urate production derives from cellular turnover of nucleic acids (purine bases); the remainder is derived from dietary purine intake. A small proportion of patients overproduce urate on an inherited metabolic basis. Unlike most mammals, humans do not express uricase, an enzyme that converts urate into highly soluble allantoin. Urate therefore accumulates and can precipitate as crystals in joints and other tissues if serum concentrations exceed the saturation point. At normal body temperature, the saturation point of urate is 6.8 mg/dL (0.40 mmol/L). At lower temperatures (for example, in the extremities), the saturation point is lower.

Nearly all urate is filtered at the glomerulus, but approximately 90% is reabsorbed in the proximal tubule; in most patients with gout, hereditary underexcretion of uric acid contributes to hyperuricemia (**Table 33**). Not all patients with hyperuricemia develop gout; about 20% of the U.S. population is hyperuricemic compared with the 4% prevalence of gout. The factors that lead to the development of gout in hyperuricemia are unclear, but degree of elevation in urate level is predictive. A serum urate level greater than 10 mg/dL (0.59 mmol/L) is associated with a 30% likelihood of an initial attack of gout within 5 years.

Acute gouty arthritis is triggered when tissue macrophages ingest uric acid crystals, leading to the generation of interleukin (IL)-1β. IL-1β is an inflammatory cytokine that causes local vasodilation, triggers production of other inflammatory cytokines (tumor necrosis factor α and IL-6), and both recruits and activates neutrophils. Complement activation on the surface of uric acid crystals also promotes neutrophil recruitment. Neutrophils are primarily responsible for the symptoms and signs of an acute gout attack.

Clinical Manifestations

Three requirements generally must be fulfilled for the onset of clinically apparent gout: 1) hyperuricemia, usually

TABLE 33. Causes of Hyperuricemia
Primary renal uric acid underexcretion (hereditary, renal tubular basis)
Chronic kidney disease of any cause (secondary uric acid underexcretion)
Uric acid overproduction due to primary defect in purine metabolism: PRPP synthetase overactivity; HPRT deficiency
Conditions of increased cell turnover leading to purine/urate generation: leukemia/lymphoma; psoriasis; hemolytic anemia; polycythemia vera
Drug-induced hyperuricemia (agents reducing renal glomerular filtration and/or tubular urate excretion): thiazide and loop diuretics; cyclosporine; low-dose salicylates; ethambutol; pyrazinamide; lead ingestion/toxicity
Diet-induced hyperuricemia (agents high in purines or inducing purine/urate biosynthesis): alcohol; shellfish; red meat; high-fructose corn syrup–sweetened beverages and foods; impact on serum urate generally is limited in the absence of other causes

HPRT = hypoxanthine-guanine phosphoribosyltransferase; PRPP = phosphoribosylpyrophosphate.

long-standing, 2) uric acid deposition in the joints and/or soft tissues, and 3) a reaction to phagocytosed crystals that leads to an acute inflammatory event.

Acute Gouty Arthritis
Initial acute gouty attacks are typically monoarticular, and ≥50% of first attacks in men involve the first metatarsophalangeal (MTP) joint of the great toe (podagra). Inflammatory states such as infection, surgery, and myocardial infarction can provoke gouty attacks, possibly through volume and pH changes. The hallmarks of an attack are pain, tenderness, swelling, redness, and warmth of the affected area. Attacks typically begin at night, and peak within 12 to 24 hours. The pain is often so exquisite that even the touch of a sheet on an affected toe is unbearable. Untreated, most gout attacks self-resolve within days to a few weeks, although with long-standing disease, attacks can persist for months. In men with established disease, attacks eventually affect joints other than the first MTPs, including the proximal feet, ankles, and knees, and later virtually any joint, including the spine. Postmenopausal women may present differently, with initial attacks often involving finger joints already affected by osteoarthritis. For those with more severe or long-standing disease, polyarticular attacks may occur. Soft tissues can also be involved, manifesting as acute bursitis, periarthritis, and gouty panniculitis and cellulitis, the last of which can be misdiagnosed as a refractory bacterial soft-tissue infection.

Intercritical Gout
Intercritical gout is the period between gout attacks. Early in the disease course, the intercritical period can be years, although most patients will have a second gout attack within 2 years. As the disease progresses, the intercritical period can progressively shorten. Even in the absence of acute arthritis, uric acid crystals still reside within joints and soft tissues, and low-grade inflammation persists in the absence of clinically apparent systemic disease.

Chronic Recurrent and Tophaceous Gout
Chronic recurrent gout and tophaceous gout result from a failure to recognize or adequately treat gout at an earlier stage.

In chronic recurrent gout, patients experience increasingly frequent and severe, and often polyarticular, arthritic attacks. These attacks may eventually evolve into a persistent chronic arthritis.

Other patients with long-standing disease develop tophaceous gout. Tophi are solid chalky white masses of uric acid, surrounded by inflammatory cells and a rind of fibrous tissue. They are located around joints and in soft tissues, with a predilection for the extensor surfaces of the elbows, the distal Achilles tendon, the fingers (usually from the proximal interphalangeal joints distally) (**Figure 23**), and the cartilaginous portions of the ears. The size ranges from millimeters to several centimeters in diameter. Tophi are deforming, can interfere with function, and directly erode bone. Ulceration of overlying skin can occur, and accompanying infection can be difficult to treat because tophi are avascular.

Diagnosis
A diagnosis of acute gout should be entertained in any patient with an acute monoarticular or oligoarticular arthritis. The differential diagnosis is listed in **Table 34**. Although designed primarily for research, gout classification criteria are available

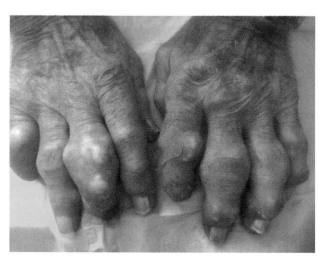

FIGURE 23. Fingers of a patient with numerous bulky tophaceous deposits of monosodium uric acid crystals, a consequence of years of gout with uncontrolled hyperuricemia.

TABLE 34.	Differential Diagnosis of Acute Gouty Arthritis
Condition	**Comments**
Infectious arthritis	Presentation may be identical to gout. Infectious arthritis is usually monoarticular but can be polyarticular. Onset may be less acute than gout. Gout and infectious arthritis can coexist.
Acute calcium pyrophosphate crystal arthritis (pseudogout)	Pseudogout is less likely to present in the great toe, but acute presentations may otherwise be identical to gout. Synovial fluid analysis can distinguish these entities. Gout and pseudogout can coexist.
Basic calcium phosphate deposition	Basic calcium phosphate deposition in articular cartilage and periarticular tissues. Because of their small size, basic calcium phosphate crystals are unlikely to be seen in synovial fluid on light microscopy except as aggregates stained with alizarin red.
Trauma	Trauma can lead to local pain and swelling, with or without a fracture, and can also trigger a gout attack.
Other forms of inflammatory arthritis (e.g., reactive arthritis, rheumatoid arthritis, psoriatic arthritis, acute rheumatic fever)	Clinical context, affected joints, and pattern of arthritis are all helpful in distinguishing these entities. Synovial fluid analysis is particularly important when there is diagnostic uncertainty.

CONT.

for guidance, including as an online calculator (http://goutclassificationcalculator.auckland.ac.nz).

The gold standard for the diagnosis of acute gout is the identification of negatively birefringent, needle-like uric acid crystals within neutrophils in fluid obtained by arthrocentesis. Negatively birefringent means that under polarized light, the crystals appear yellow when parallel and blue when perpendicular to the polarizing axis. Arthrocentesis is not always completed when gout is suspected, but when infection is a concern, joint aspiration for Gram stain and culture is mandatory.

Findings that support an acute gout diagnosis include onset of symptoms over several hours, first MTP joint or midfoot/ankle involvement, and severe pain. The involved joint(s) are warm, red, swollen, and very tender. Low-grade fever may be present. Measuring serum urate at the time of attack is often done but may not be helpful, because levels may drop precipitously during periods of acute systemic inflammation (owing to the uricosuric effects of circulating cytokines). Nonetheless, an elevated serum urate level increases the likelihood of gout. Checking the serum urate 2 weeks after acute gout resolution gives a more accurate measure of baseline level. C-reactive protein and erythrocyte sedimentation rate are elevated but are nonspecific. Joint fluid will have an inflammatory leukocyte count (above 2000/μL [2.0×10^9/L] and occasionally >100,000/μL [100×10^9/L], with neutrophil predominance). Importantly, the diagnosis of acute gout, even when confirmed by the presence of intracellular crystals in synovial fluid, does not definitively rule out a concomitant infection.

Radiographs are not helpful in diagnosing acute gouty arthritis, but the characteristic radiographic changes of established disease (punched-out lesions with overhanging edges of cortical bone) may help confirm a history of previously unrecognized gout (**Figure 24**). Newer imaging modalities (ultrasonography and dual-energy CT) can demonstrate uric acid deposition in joints and are being studied for their possible role in acute diagnosis.

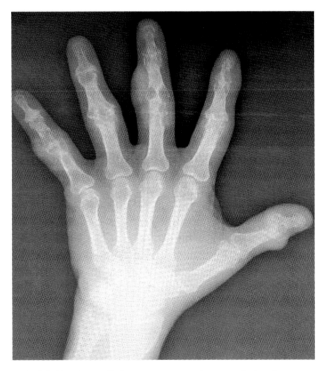

FIGURE 24. Periarticular bony erosions, appearing as punched-out bone lesions with disruption of bone cortex (overhanging edges), represent areas of tophaceous monosodium uric acid deposition and accompanying inflammation in a patient with severe, long-standing, inadequately treated gout.

Courtesy of Elaine Karis, MD.

Management

There are three components to treating gout: 1) treating acute attacks, 2) prophylaxis to prevent future attacks, and 3) urate-lowering therapy. See Principle of Therapeutics for details on the medications described in this section.

Treatment of Acute Gouty Arthritis

Treatment of acute gout focuses on anti-inflammatory therapy; colchicine, NSAIDs, and glucocorticoids are all reasonable options. Treatment choice should be determined by potential drug interactions and patient comorbidities. The simplest is colchicine, 1.2 mg at the first symptoms of a gout attack, followed 1 hour later by a 0.6-mg dose. Colchicine is most effective when used early in attacks (<24 hours after onset) and is less useful when the attack is well established. High-dose NSAID therapy for 5 to 7 days is effective, as are glucocorticoids in any form—intra-articular injection, intramuscular depot injection (for example, depo-methylprednisolone, 40-80 mg), or an oral "burst" of prednisone (for example, 0.5 mg/kg/d, for 5 days).

Most gout attacks respond to a week or less of therapy, although more severe attacks may require a longer course of treatment. For patients with severe and refractory attacks, or with contraindications to other treatments, off-label use of IL-1 inhibitors (anakinra or canakinumab) can be considered. Gouty cellulitis, if present, should be treated as any other acute gout attack.

Urate-Lowering Therapy

Guidelines conflict as to whether patients with gout should receive dietary counseling to reduce serum urate levels. If recommended, patients may limit intake of shellfish, oily fish, red meat, high-fructose foods, and alcohol. Overly strict diets that are unlikely to be complied with are not helpful, however. Weight loss (when appropriate) and increasing dairy intake may also lower serum urate levels. In patients with hypertension, agents other than diuretics should be used; losartan, for example, has mild uricosuric effects.

It is important to note that two recently published guidelines differ regarding the role of pharmacologic urate-lowering therapy in patients with gout. The 2016 American College of Physicians guideline (http://annals.org/aim/article/2578528/management-acute-recurrent-gout-clinical-practice-guide line-from-american-college) notes a lack of evidence supporting a specific target level for urate lowering; this guideline stresses discussing the risks and benefits of urate-lowering therapy with patients and suggests a "treat to avoid symptoms" approach without specifically considering the serum urate levels. The 2016 European League Against Rheumatism (EULAR) recommendations support a "treat-to-target" approach (consistent with the 2012 ACR gout guidelines), reducing the serum urate level to less than 6.0 mg/dL (0.35 mmol/L) in patients without tophi and less than 5.0 mg/dL (0.30 mmol/L) in patients with tophi. Both the ACR and EULAR recommend urate-lowering therapy for patients with gout plus any of the following: (1) ≥ stage 2 CKD; (2) ≥2 acute attacks per year; (3) one or more tophi; or (4) uric acid nephrolithiasis.

 Contrary to prior practice, urate-lowering therapy can be initiated during an acute attack if adequate anti-inflammatory therapy is concurrently started; doing so may improve compliance in some patients.

Three classes of urate-lowering therapy are available: xanthine oxidase inhibitors (reduce urate production), uricosuric agents (decrease renal urate resorption), and pegloticase (a uricase). A xanthine oxidase inhibitor, either allopurinol or febuxostat, is the recommended first-line therapy. Allopurinol is FDA approved for doses up to 800 mg/d. According to the ACR, allopurinol should be initiated at 100 mg/d and titrated in 100-mg increments as needed, and for those with stage 4 or 5 CKD, allopurinol should be initiated at 50 mg/d and titrated in 50-mg increments as needed. An uncommon but serious complication of allopurinol is a hypersensitive rash that may progress to DRESS (drug reaction with eosinophilia and systemic symptoms) syndrome; the drug should therefore be discontinued in most (if not all) patients who develop a rash. Febuxostat is equally or more efficacious than allopurinol. It is less likely to cause hypersensitivity reactions than allopurinol and does not require dose adjustment in mild to moderate CKD, but is expensive. There appears to be an increased risk of heart-related death with febuxostat compared to allopurinol; FDA-mandated safety studies are ongoing.

The uricosuric agent probenecid is infrequently used because it is less effective than xanthine oxidase inhibitors and should be avoided in patients with CKD or nephrolithiasis. Combination therapy with a xanthine oxidase inhibitor and probenecid (or the incidentally uricosuric agents losartan and fenofibrate) may be more effective than a xanthine oxidase inhibitor alone. A more effective uricosuric agent, lesinurad, was recently FDA approved as add-on therapy to allopurinol or febuxostat; reversible kidney insufficiency may develop in some patients.

For patients with severe recurrent and/or tophaceous gout intolerant or resistant to standard therapies, pegloticase is an option. Infused every 2 weeks, pegloticase lowers serum urate to nearly zero, but 30% to 50% of patients develop antibodies to the drug within a month, rendering it ineffective and increasing the likelihood of infusion reactions. Pegloticase should be discontinued in any patient for whom it ceases to work.

Prophylaxis

When initiating urate-lowering therapy, mobilization of uric acid crystals from the joints and soft tissues can provoke acute attacks. Accordingly, patients starting urate-lowering therapy should be placed on anti-inflammatory prophylaxis to prevent flares. For patients without tophi, the ACR recommends continuing prophylaxis for at least 6 months and 3 months after achieving the target serum urate level. In patients with tophi, prophylaxis should be continued for 6 months following achievement of the target serum urate level and resolution of tophi. Most patients tolerate colchicine, 0.6 mg (once or twice daily); for those who do not, low-dose NSAIDs or glucocorticoids are appropriate substitutes.

KEY POINTS

- The gold standard for the diagnosis of acute gout is the identification of negatively birefringent, needle-like uric acid crystals within neutrophils in fluid obtained by arthrocentesis.

- Colchicine, NSAIDs, and glucocorticoids are all reasonable options for treatment of acute gout; choice should be determined by potential drug interactions and patient comorbidities.

(Continued)

HVC
- The 2016 American College of Physicians guideline notes a lack of evidence supporting a specific target level for urate lowering; the guideline stresses discussing the risks and benefits of urate-lowering therapy with patients and suggests a "treat to avoid symptoms" approach without specifically considering the serum urate levels.
- The American College of Rheumatology and the European League Against Rheumatism both recommend a "treat-to-target" approach, reducing the serum urate level to less than 6.0 mg/dL (0.35 mmol/L) in patients without tophi and less than 5.0 mg/dL (0.30 mmol/L) in patients with tophi.
- Patients starting urate-lowering therapy should be placed on anti-inflammatory prophylaxis to prevent flares.

Calcium Pyrophosphate Deposition

Deposition of calcium pyrophosphate (CPP) crystals in and on cartilaginous surfaces can provoke acute inflammatory arthritis that is clinically similar to acute gout. Calcium pyrophosphate deposition (CPPD) is less well characterized than gout, but four subgroups are described: asymptomatic CPPD; acute CPP crystal arthritis; chronic CPP crystal inflammatory arthritis; and osteoarthritis with CPPD.

Epidemiology and Pathophysiology

CPPD primarily affects the elderly, and prior joint damage is a significant risk factor. The risk for cartilage calcification (chondrocalcinosis) doubles for every decade past 60 years, and nearly half of patients in their late 80s have CPPD. For younger patients with CPPD, consideration of contributory metabolic disease (hyperparathyroidism, hemochromatosis, hypophosphatasia, hypomagnesemia) is warranted.

The pathophysiology of CPPD is incompletely understood. Pyrophosphate produced by chondrocytes likely precipitates with calcium to form CPP crystals, which then activate inflammatory pathways resulting in an acute arthritic attack. CPPD may also drive osteoarthritis by inducing proinflammatory activity in chondrocytes and synovial fibroblasts, resulting in cartilage damage. Epidemiologic evidence suggests that cartilage calcification might play a role in osteoarthritis of the knees and wrists, but not at the hip.

Clinical Manifestations and Diagnosis
Asymptomatic Calcium Pyrophosphate Deposition

Asymptomatic CPPD occurs with radiographic changes in the absence of clinical symptoms. Cartilage calcification appears as a linear opacity below the surface of articular cartilage (**Figure 25**). It most commonly occurs in the knees, wrists (triangular fibrocartilage), pelvis (pubis symphysis), and metacar-

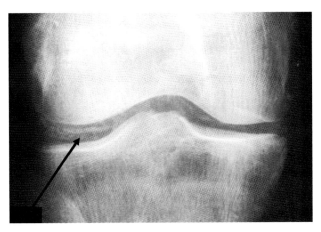
FIGURE 25. Cartilage calcification (chondrocalcinosis) of the knee. This radiograph shows linearly arranged calcific deposits in the articular cartilage (*arrow*).

pophalangeal (MCP) joints, in descending order. Asymptomatic CPPD is common in the elderly and in osteoarthritic joints, and it may be a precursor of osteoarthritis with CPPD.

Acute Calcium Pyrophosphate Crystal Arthritis

Acute CPP crystal arthritis (pseudogout) typically presents as a monoarticular inflammatory arthritis, characterized by sudden onset of swelling, pain, loss of function, tenderness, and warmth of the affected joint, usually a knee or wrist. Similar to acute gout, attacks may be provoked by systemic insults such as major surgery or acute illness. Attacks are usually milder than those of gout, but if untreated can persist for months. Definitive diagnosis requires identification of CPP crystals (along with leukocytes) in synovial fluid; in contrast to uric acid crystals, the CPP crystals are rhomboid shaped and positively birefringent under polarized light. Radiographic evidence of cartilage calcification in elderly patients with acute monoarticular arthritis is suggestive but not diagnostic of acute CPP crystal arthritis.

Chronic Calcium Pyrophosphate Arthropathy

Chronic calcium pyrophosphate arthropathy may be present as two patterns: (1) chronic calcium pyrophosphate (CPP) crystal inflammatory arthritis and (2) osteoarthritis with calcium pyrophosphate deposition (CPPD). Chronic CPP crystal inflammatory arthritis is a polyarthritis involving the wrists and MCP joints ("pseudo–rheumatoid arthritis"); it is rare and difficult to treat. Osteoarthritis with CPPD manifests as typical osteoarthritic findings involving joints not commonly associated with osteoarthritis (such as shoulders or MCP joints); radiographic CPPD often precedes the onset of osteoarthritis, suggesting a causal role for the CPP.

Management

Because there is no known mechanism for dissolving or preventing the formation of articular CPP crystals, treatment aims at abrogating the inflammatory manifestations of the disease (**Table 35**).

TABLE 35. Management of Calcium Pyrophosphate Deposition

Clinical Presentation	Treatment/Comments
Cartilage calcification (chondrocalcinosis)	No specific treatment
Acute calcium pyrophosphate crystal arthritis (pseudogout)	Local treatment: joint aspiration, followed by intra-articular glucocorticoid injection; intramuscular glucocorticoid injection; joint immobilization; ice packs
	Systemic treatment: NSAIDs; colchicine; glucocorticoids (oral or parenteral)
	Prophylaxis if recurrent attacks (three or more annual attacks): low-dose colchicine or daily NSAIDs (with gastrointestinal protection)
Chronic calcium pyrophosphate crystal inflammatory arthritis	Low-dose colchicine or daily low-dose NSAIDs (with gastrointestinal protection); low-dose glucocorticoids
Osteoarthritis with calcium pyrophosphate deposition (CPPD)	Same treatment as osteoarthritis without CPPD (e.g., physical therapy; pain control; local glucocorticoids)

- Asymptomatic calcium pyrophosphate deposition is characterized by radiographic changes, including cartilage calcification (chondrocalcinosis), in the absence of clinical symptoms.

- The presentation of acute calcium pyrophosphate crystal arthritis (pseudogout) resembles gout; however, attacks are usually milder, and crystals are rhomboid shaped and positively birefringent under polarized light.

- Chronic calcium pyrophosphate crystal inflammatory arthritis often involves the wrists and metacarpophalangeal joints ("pseudo–rheumatoid arthritis").

- Osteoarthritis with calcium pyrophosphate deposition causes typical osteoarthritic findings involving joints not commonly associated with osteoarthritis (shoulders, metacarpophalangeal joints).

Basic Calcium Phosphate Deposition

Basic calcium phosphate (BCP) deposition occurs in the elderly and forms in the articular cartilage; in contrast to CPPD, BCP crystals also often deposit periarticularly. BCP is thought to rarely cause inflammatory arthritis and periarthritis, most classically manifesting in elderly women as "Milwaukee shoulder," an inflammatory periarthritis and arthritis of the shoulder, leading to progressive destruction of the rotator cuff and glenohumeral joint. Diagnosis is usually clinical; imaging of BCP crystals requires special stains and/or electron microscopy and is rarely performed.

- Basic calcium phosphate deposition can rarely cause Milwaukee shoulder, an inflammatory arthritis and periarthritis of the shoulder occurring in elderly women that leads to progressive destruction of the rotator cuff and glenohumeral joint; diagnosis is usually clinical.

Infectious Arthritis

Diagnosis

Clinical Manifestations

Infectious arthritis typically presents with pain, swelling, warmth, and erythema of the affected joint, accompanied by fever and constitutional symptoms. Knee infection is common, but any joint may be affected. Previously damaged joints are at increased risk for involvement. Monoarthritis or new inflammation of a single joint in a patient with well-controlled inflammatory arthritis should prompt evaluation for infection.

Physical examination commonly shows functional loss of both active and passive range of motion in addition to signs of inflammation. Skin examination can reveal signs suggesting gonococcal infection (pustular skin lesions) or portals of entry (scratches, bites, or thorns).

Laboratory and Imaging Studies

In patients with suspected infectious arthritis, the most important diagnostic procedure is expeditious arthrocentesis. The synovial fluid should be sent for Gram stain, culture (bacterial and, when indicated, mycobacterial and/or fungal), leukocyte count, and crystal analysis. Synovial fluid levels of glucose, lactate dehydrogenase, and total protein do not aid in diagnosis and should not be obtained. Depending upon the clinical picture, the fluid may be sent for polymerase chain reaction to detect *Mycobacteria* or *Borrelia burgdorferi* DNA.

Bacterially infected synovial fluid is cloudy and less viscous than that seen in noninflammatory arthritis. Elevated synovial fluid leukocyte counts are typically greater than 50,000/µL (50 × 10⁹/L) and often exceed 100,000/µL (100 × 10⁹/L), with a polymorphonuclear cell predominance. Such high leukocyte counts may occur in other conditions (for example, crystal arthropathies) but should be presumed infectious until proven otherwise. Notably, the presence of crystals does not exclude the possibility of co-infection. Patients with gonococcal, mycobacterial, or fungal infections, injection drug users, or those who are immunocompromised may have lower synovial fluid leukocyte counts.

CONT.

A positive Gram stain for bacteria should be considered definitive, but the sensitivity of the test is inadequate for a negative result to rule out infection when suspicion is high. Synovial fluid cultures are usually positive in bacterial infections unless antibiotics were administered prior to arthrocentesis. The peripheral blood leukocyte count, erythrocyte sedimentation rate, and C-reactive protein are often elevated; however, normal levels do not exclude the diagnosis, and elevated levels may occur in inflammatory arthritis and other conditions.

Blood cultures should always be drawn before antibiotic administration. When gonococcal arthritis is suspected, urogenital, rectal, and pharyngeal specimens should also be obtained for nucleic acid amplification testing.

Plain radiographs are usually normal early in the course of the infection, but baseline films are helpful to identify other diseases or contiguous osteomyelitis. Later radiographs (weeks to months) often show nonspecific changes. In advanced infection, periosteal reaction, marginal or central erosions, and subchondral bone destruction may be seen. Bony ankylosis is a late sequel. In joints that are difficult to evaluate clinically or have complex anatomic structures, ultrasonography, CT, and MRI can delineate the extent of the effusion and identify early bony changes. **H**

KEY POINTS

- Infectious arthritis typically presents with pain, swelling, warmth, and erythema of the affected joint, accompanied by fever and constitutional symptoms; monoarthritis or new inflammation of a single joint in a patient with well-controlled inflammatory arthritis should prompt evaluation for infection.

- Diagnosis of infectious arthritis is confirmed by arthrocentesis and evaluation of the synovial fluid for Gram stain, culture, leukocyte count, and crystal analysis.

Causes

See MKSAP 18 Infectious Disease for details on the specific infections and diseases discussed in this section.

Infection with Gram-Positive Organisms

Bacterial arthritis is a medical emergency requiring immediate diagnosis and treatment. Risk factors include an immunocompromised state (including diabetes mellitus), injection drug use, joint surgery, and having a prosthetic joint. A recent "dirty" skin break may be a contributing factor. Infections occur very rarely after invasive procedures such as arthrocentesis or joint injection (**Table 36**). Most joint infections are monoarticular and derive from hematogenous seeding of synovium. Polyarticular infectious arthritis may occur in injection drug users, those with systemic inflammatory disorders such as rheumatoid arthritis, and in patients with overwhelming sepsis.

TABLE 36. Risk Factors for Infectious Arthritis in Adults

General Risk Factors
Age >80 years
Alcoholism
Cutaneous ulcers or skin infections
Diabetes mellitus
End-stage kidney disease
History of intra-articular glucocorticoid injection
Injection drug use
Low socioeconomic status
Malignancy
Patients receiving immunosuppressive agents
Preexisting arthritis or joint damage (e.g., rheumatoid arthritis or osteoarthritis)
Prosthetic joint or recent joint surgery
Sickle cell disease
Risk Factors for Gonococcal Arthritis
Younger, sexually active patients
Risk Factors for Lyme Arthritis
Travel or residence in an endemic area
Documented tick bite or erythema chronicum migrans
Risk Factors for Mycobacterial or Fungal Arthritis
Patients with HIV infection or other immunosuppression
Patients receiving tumor necrosis factor α inhibitors
Travel or residence in an endemic area
Risk Factors for Viral Arthritis
Chronic viral infection (HIV, hepatitis B, hepatitis C)
Exposure to infectious agent or vaccine (e.g., rubella)
Travel or residence in an endemic area
Exposure to affected children (parvovirus, rubella)

Approximately 75% of adult nongonococcal infectious arthritis is caused by gram-positive cocci, with *Staphylococcus aureus* being the most frequent microorganism in both native and prosthetic joints. *Staphylococcus epidermidis* infections occur more commonly in prosthetic than in native joints.

Infection with Gram-Negative Organisms
Disseminated Gonococcal Infection

Neisseria gonorrhoeae most typically occurs in younger, sexually active individuals. Disseminated infection occurs in 1% to 3% of patients infected with *N. gonorrhoeae*, with arthritis a common feature.

Disseminated gonococcal infection may present in one of two ways, although there may be overlap. The first is the arthritis-dermatitis syndrome, a triad of tenosynovitis, dermatitis (usually painless pustular or vesiculopustular lesions)

(Figure 26), and polyarthralgia without frank arthritis. Fever, chills, and malaise are common. Inflammation of multiple tendons of the wrists, fingers, ankles, and toes distinguishes this syndrome from other forms of infectious arthritis. The second presentation is a purulent arthritis, usually without associated skin lesions or fever. Patients present with acute onset of mono- or oligoarthritis; the knees, wrists, and ankles are most commonly involved.

Patients with the arthritis-dermatitis syndrome are more likely to have positive blood cultures, whereas those with purulent arthritis are more likely to have positive synovial fluid cultures. Nucleic acid amplification testing should also be obtained on samples from genital, rectal, and pharyngeal sites.

Nongonococcal Gram-Negative Organisms

Aerobic gram-negative bacilli are the predominant cause of nongonococcal gram-negative joint infections. Predisposing factors include injection drug use, advanced age, and an immunocompromised state. *Pseudomonas aeruginosa* can be seen in infection related to injection drug use. Patients with sickle cell anemia may become infected with *Salmonella*. Gram-negative anaerobes account for only 5% to 7% of bacterial arthritis cases, most commonly in prosthetic joint infections and/or immunocompromised hosts.

Lyme Arthritis

Although arthralgia and myalgia often occur at the earlier stages of Lyme disease, Lyme arthritis is a late-stage manifestation. It is typically monoarticular or oligoarticular, most commonly in the knee. It should be suspected in patients who may have had untreated or incompletely treated Lyme disease, although not all patients will have a history compatible with prior Lyme disease. All patients with Lyme arthritis, however, should have positive enzyme-linked immunosorbent assay (ELISA) and Western blot serologies; this is the major means of establishing the diagnosis of Lyme arthritis. Additionally,

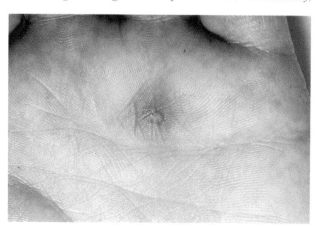

FIGURE 26. Disseminated gonococcal infection can present as a febrile arthritis-dermatitis syndrome with migratory polyarthralgia that may evolve to septic arthritis, tenosynovitis, and painless skin rash that may involve the palms and soles. Skin lesions can vary from maculopapular to pustular, often with a hemorrhagic component.

B. burgdorferi DNA can be detected by polymerase chain reaction in synovial fluid.

Mycobacterium tuberculosis

The most common musculoskeletal manifestation of tuberculosis is vertebral osteomyelitis (Pott's disease), usually resulting from the hematogenous spread of *Mycobacterium tuberculosis* into the cancellous bone tissue of the vertebral bodies. Patients usually have a primary pulmonary focus or extrapulmonary foci such as the lymph nodes. Predisposing factors for skeletal tuberculosis include previous tuberculosis infection, malnutrition, alcoholism, diabetes mellitus, and HIV infection. The onset of symptoms is commonly insidious, and disease progression is slow, sometimes resulting in delayed diagnosis.

Peripheral arthritis may also occur and typically presents with chronic pain in a single weight-bearing joint such as the knee, with only limited swelling. Concurrent pulmonary tuberculosis is present in a minority of these patients. Musculoskeletal tuberculosis infections are chronic and indolent; laboratory indicators of inflammation may be normal. Synovial fluid shows only nonspecific inflammation, and radiographic abnormalities may be delayed. Synovial biopsy is usually necessary for diagnosis because the yield of synovial fluid smear and culture is less than 50%.

Fungal Infections

Fungi are uncommon but important causes of bone and joint infections. Risk factors include immunosuppression and exposure to the fungi in endemic areas. Travel and immigration have broadened the risk of some fungal infections to non-endemic areas. Fungal joint infection may be indolent and more difficult to diagnose than other bone and joint infections. Fungal causes of osteomyelitis and arthritis include coccidioidomycosis, blastomycosis, cryptococcosis, candidiasis, and sporotrichosis. Fungal arthritis is usually a result of hematogenous dissemination but can occur after direct inoculation of the joint. Diagnosis of some fungal infections (for example, blastomycosis and sporotrichosis) can be made by synovial fluid examination and culture, whereas serologic testing and synovial biopsy may be needed for other organisms (such as *Coccidioides*). Synovial fluid leukocyte counts vary. ▣

Viral Infections
HIV

HIV infection is associated with several musculoskeletal disorders, including painful articular syndrome, HIV-associated arthritis, reactive arthritis, infectious arthritis, and diffuse infiltrative lymphocytosis syndrome (DILS). Painful articular syndrome consists of bone and joint pain, especially in the lower extremities in an asymmetric pattern, lasting less than 24 hours. HIV-associated arthritis is a nondestructive arthritis that involves joints of the lower extremity in an oligoarticular pattern and usually lasts less than 6 weeks. Reactive arthritis is the primary form of spondyloarthritis seen in patients with HIV infection and is likely due to a response to other sexually transmitted or enteric infections, rather than the HIV itself. Reactive arthritis in HIV may take a chronic relapsing course and may be accompanied by enthesopathy and mucocutaneous manifestations. Psoriatic arthritis is not more common but is often more severe in patients with HIV infection, with disabling enthesitis and joint erosion as well as axial involvement including sacroiliitis. DILS is a rare condition that resembles Sjögren syndrome but with CD8 rather than CD4 cell infiltration.

Hepatitis

Hepatitis B virus infection causes a self-limited arthritis in up to 25% of infected patients during a prodromal stage prior to the onset of jaundice. Joint involvement can be sudden and severe, with a pattern that is usually symmetric, but can be migratory or additive. Hand and knee joints are most often affected; wrists, ankles, elbows, shoulders, and other large joints may be involved as well. Morning stiffness is common. Fusiform swelling of the small joints of the hand may be found on physical examination. Patients with chronic hepatitis B virus infection may have recurrent but self-limited polyarthralgia or polyarthritis; it is not known to progress or cause joint damage. Both hepatitis B and C virus infection may be accompanied by the presence of rheumatoid factor, which can cause diagnostic confusion.

Acute hepatitis C virus infection can cause acute-onset polyarthritis, including the small hand joints, wrists, shoulders, knees, and hips. One third of patients have an oligoarthritis. Chronic hepatitis C virus infection is often associated with circulating immune complexes, which may produce the clinical syndrome of mixed essential cryoglobulinemia (arthritis, glomerulonephritis, and vasculitis).

Parvovirus B19

Up to 60% of adults with parvovirus B19 experience arthritis. It often presents acutely, is symmetric and polyarticular, and typically involves the proximal small joints of the hands. Parvovirus B19 arthritis should be suspected when appropriate clinical features are present in someone who has exposure to children, such as teachers and caregivers. Acute parvovirus infection is diagnosed by detecting anti-parvovirus IgM antibodies in the serum. Anti-parvovirus IgG antibodies are highly prevalent in the general population and indicate prior infection. Joint symptoms may persist for weeks to months.

Rubella

Arthritis is uncommon in childhood rubella infection, but up to 60% of adults with rubella develop joint symptoms, mainly arthralgia. Joint involvement is usually symmetric and migratory, with resolution of most symptoms within 2 weeks. The small joints of the hands, wrists, elbows, ankles, and knees are most commonly affected. Tenosynovitis and carpal tunnel syndrome also occur. The pathogenesis of rubella arthritis is thought to be due to immune complexes and/or persistence of the virus in synovial cells or joint macrophages. Diagnosis is usually made by detection of IgM antirubella antibodies; the virus may also be cultured from the nasopharynx or joint tissues. Joint fluid findings are inflammatory.

Mosquito-Borne Viruses

Zika, dengue, and chikungunya viruses are transmitted by *Aedes* mosquitos in tropical areas. Zika also can be vertically and sexually transmitted, and localized transmission in the southern United States is now reported. All of these viruses can cause musculoskeletal symptoms in addition to fever, rash, and headache. In chikungunya, arthritis is a predominant feature; patients may experience synovial thickening and tenosynovitis, often involving the fingers and wrists. Zika may also manifest with a symmetric polyarthritis, whereas dengue tends to produce more arthralgia. The musculoskeletal symptoms of Zika and dengue tend to subside within a couple of weeks, whereas those of chikungunya usually continue longer, resembling rheumatoid arthritis (without rheumatoid factor or anti-cyclic citrullinated peptide antibodies) in some cases. Diagnosis of these mosquito-borne diseases is based on clinical features and serologic testing. Polymerase chain reaction testing on blood samples is also available.

Prosthetic Joint Infections

Bacterial infection complicates 1% to 3% of total knee and hip replacements; higher rates are seen in immunocompromised patients and those with rheumatoid arthritis. Infection with gram-positive organisms such as *S. aureus* is most common. Prosthetic joint infections are divided into early onset (<3 months after placement), delayed (3 to 24 months postsurgery), and late onset (>24 months after placement). Early and delayed infections are usually related to surgical contamination at the time of the implantation, whereas late infections result from hematogenous seeding of the joint. Early and late prosthetic joint infections typically present with pain, warmth, effusion, and fever. Peripheral leukocyte count and inflammatory markers are usually elevated. Delayed infections, however, may be more difficult to recognize because symptoms are less severe, and they are often caused by less virulent microorganisms such as coagulase-negative staphylococci and other skin organisms. **H**

> ### KEY POINTS
>
> - Approximately 75% of adult nongonococcal infectious arthritis is caused by gram-positive cocci, with *Staphylococcus aureus* being the most frequent microorganism in both native and prosthetic joints.
>
> - Disseminated gonococcal infection may present as the arthritis-dermatitis syndrome (tenosynovitis, dermatitis, and polyarthralgia) or as a purulent arthritis with pain and swelling but usually without skin lesions or fever.
>
> - Lyme arthritis is a late-stage manifestation of the disease and is typically monoarticular or oligoarticular, most commonly in the knee, and inflammatory; diagnosis should be suspected in patients who may have had untreated or incompletely treated Lyme disease.
>
> *(Continued)*

- *Mycobacterium tuberculosis* arthritis typically presents as chronic pain in a single weight-bearing joint such as the knee, with only limited swelling; concurrent pulmonary tuberculosis is present in a minority of patients.

- Early and late prosthetic joint infections usually present with pain of the joint, warmth, effusion, and fever; delayed infections may be more difficult to recognize because they are often caused by less virulent microorganisms, and symptoms may be less severe.

Management

In patients with suspected infectious arthritis, blood and synovial cultures must be obtained before treatment, but empiric antibiotic therapy should be started while awaiting culture results (**Table 37**). In suspected bacterial arthritis, the initial antimicrobial coverage should be broad and account for host factors such as immunosuppression as well as likely causative microorganisms and regional antibiotic sensitivity data. Antibiotics should initially be given parenterally. Given the high prevalence of methicillin-resistant

TABLE 37. Infectious Arthritis Treatment Based on the Suspected Pathogen			
Likely or Identified Pathogen	**First-Line Therapy**	**Second-Line Therapy**	**Comments**
Gram-Positive Cocci			
If MRSA is a concern (risk factors or known MRSA carrier)	Vancomycin	Clindamycin; daptomycin; linezolid	—
MSSA	Nafcillin or cefazolin	—	Narrow treatment to MSSA coverage based on sensitivity data.
Gram-Negative Bacilli			
Enteric gram-negative bacilli	Third generation cephalosporin (e.g., ceftriaxone or cefotaxime)	Fluoroquinolones	—
Pseudomonas aeruginosa	Ceftazidime; cefepime; piperacillin-tazobactam	Carbapenems; aztreonam; fluoroquinolones	—
Gram-Negative Cocci			
Neisseria gonorrhoeae	IV ceftriaxone for at least 7 days plus 1 gram of oral azithromycin x one dose	Fluoroquinolones (only if culture sensitivities confirm susceptibility)	In the absence of specific culture sensitivity data, "stepping down" to oral therapy of any type is no longer recommended due to increasing resistance of *N. gonorrhoeae* to commonly used oral agents.
Gram Stain Unavailable or Inconclusive			
Likely pathogen depends on patient risk factors: consider MRSA, and gram-negative organism if immunocompromised, at risk for gonococcal infection, or with joint trauma; also consider community patterns of infection.	Vancomycin, or vancomycin + third generation cephalosporin, or antipseudomonal antibiotic if pseudomonas suspected	—	Appropriate to start with broad antibiotic coverage and narrow coverage if culture data become available.
Borrelia burgdorferi (Lyme arthritis)	Oral doxycycline or amoxicillin × 28 days	—	If inadequate response or concurrent neurologic findings, IV ceftriaxone × 28 days.
Mycobacterium tuberculosis	3- to 4-drug treatment (e.g., isoniazid, pyrazinamide, rifampin, ethambutol, streptomycin)	—	Duration may vary from 6 months or longer depending on drug regimen (shorter treatment if rifampin is used).
Fungal infections	Amphotericin B, echinocandin, or azoles (fluconazole, itraconazole, voriconazole, posaconazole), depending on suspected organism or culture data	—	Prolonged treatment courses of several months may be needed; maintenance therapy may be required in high-risk patients.

IV = intravenous; MRSA = methicillin-resistant *Staphylococcus aureus*; MSSA = methicillin-sensitive *Staphylococcus aureus*.

CONT.

S. aureus, vancomycin is often initially used to cover gram-positive cocci. The duration of treatment depends on the causative organism and patient response, but usually lasts 2 to 4 weeks.

An infected joint must also be adequately drained. Needle aspiration is an acceptable approach and should be performed regularly (usually daily) as long as there is an effusion. Ultrasound guidance may improve the ability to fully drain the joint. Surgical drainage is an equally good alternative and is more immediately definitive. Additionally, surgical drainage is required for joints that are not easily accessible for needle aspiration (for example, sternoclavicular, sternomanubrial, shoulder, and hip joints), if there is evidence of soft-tissue extension of infection, or if the clinical response to antimicrobial therapy is inadequate. The goal of surgery is to remove all purulent material and nonviable tissue and, in some cases, to perform synovial biopsy or synovectomy.

Antibiotic treatment is recommended for all patients with Lyme arthritis. Approximately 90% of patients will respond to a 28-day course of oral doxycycline, amoxicillin, or cefuroxime axetil. Patients with incomplete responses may need treatment with a second course or a more aggressive drug regimen, usually intravenous ceftriaxone. Treatment beyond 1 month of ceftriaxone offers no benefit and should not be employed. Antibiotic-refractory Lyme arthritis occurs in ≤10% of patients, probably represents a progression to sterile autoimmune arthritis, and responds to synovectomy or treatment with disease-modifying antirheumatic drugs such as hydroxychloroquine or methotrexate.

Mycobacterial joint infections require at least 6 to 9 months of therapy. Treatment of arthritis associated with viral infections is largely supportive, although specific viral therapy is appropriate for HIV and hepatitis C infection; immunosuppressive therapy with glucocorticoids and rituximab may be needed in refractory hepatitis C–related disease or severe mixed cryoglobulinemia.

Treatment of prosthetic joint infections is challenging and requires early surgical consultation. Orthopedic implants serve as a nidus for microorganisms, and the avascularity of the infected hardware limits antibiotic penetrance. Many patients require removal of the orthopedic device as part of a two-stage procedure, with reimplantation of a new device after an appropriate course of intravenous antibiotics.

KEY POINTS

- In patients with suspected infectious arthritis, blood and synovial cultures must be obtained before treatment, but empiric antibiotic therapy should be started while awaiting culture results.

- In addition to antibiotic therapy, an infected joint must also be adequately drained by needle aspiration or surgical drainage.

- Many patients with prosthetic joint infections require removal of the orthopedic device as part of a two-stage procedure, with reimplantation of a new device after an appropriate course of intravenous antibiotics.

Systemic Vasculitis

Overview

Vasculitis is inflammation of blood vessels, including the capillaries, arteries, and veins. Clinical manifestations result from tissue ischemia associated with the involved vessels. Vasculitis may be primary, secondary to an autoimmune disease, or triggered by other causes (**Table 38**). Mimics of vasculitis must also be considered in the differential diagnosis (**Table 39**). Primary autoimmune vasculitis disorders are discussed in this section.

TABLE 38. Causes of Secondary Vasculitis
Medications
Common causes: antimicrobial agents (e.g., minocycline, sulfadiazine); antithyroid agents (mostly propylthiouracil [80%-90%], methimazole, carbimazole, and benzylthiouracil [10%-20%]); other cardiovascular drugs (hydralazine); tumor necrosis factor α inhibitors
Rare causes: vaccines; antiepileptic agents; antiarrhythmic agents; diuretics; anticoagulants; antineoplastic agents; hematopoietic growth factors; NSAIDs; psychotropic drugs; sympathomimetic agents; allopurinol; interferon alfa; levamisole (associated with cocaine)
Infections
Hepatitis A, B, and C viruses; HIV; bacterial endocarditis; parvovirus B19
Neoplasms
Hairy cell leukemia (associated with polyarteritis nodosa); other hematologic and solid malignancies
Autoimmune Diseases
Systemic lupus erythematosus; rheumatoid arthritis; Sjögren syndrome; inflammatory myopathies; systemic sclerosis; relapsing polychondritis; inflammatory bowel disease; primary biliary cirrhosis

TABLE 39. Differential Diagnosis (Mimics) of Vasculitis

Disease	Comments
Infection (sepsis; endocarditis; hepatitis)	Rash and/or musculoskeletal symptoms can occur.
Drug toxicity/poisoning	Cocaine, amphetamines, ephedra alkaloids, and phenylpropanolamine may produce vasospasm, resulting in ischemia.
Coagulopathy	Thrombotic diseases (disseminated intravascular coagulation; antiphospholipid syndrome; thrombotic thrombocytopenic purpura) can produce ischemic symptoms.
Malignancy	Paraneoplastic vasculitis is rare. Any organ system may be affected, but the skin and nervous system are the most common. Vasculitic symptoms may precede, occur simultaneously with, or follow diagnosis of cancer. Lymphoma occasionally may involve the blood vessels and mimic vasculitis. Consider malignancy in patients with incomplete or no response to therapy for idiopathic vasculitis.
Atrial myxoma	Classic triad of symptoms is embolism, intracardiac obstruction leading to pulmonary congestion or heart failure, and constitutional symptoms (fatigue; weight loss; fever). Skin lesions can be identical to those seen in leukocytoclastic vasculitis. Atrial myxomas are rare but are the most common primary intracardiac tumors. Myxomas can also occur in other cardiac chambers.
Cholesterol emboli	Typically seen in patients with severe atherosclerosis. Embolization may occur after abdominal trauma, aortic surgery, or angiography. May also occur after heparin, warfarin, or thrombolytic therapy. Patients may have livedo reticularis, petechiae and purpuric lesions, and localized skin necrosis.

Large-Vessel Vasculitis

Giant Cell Arteritis

Epidemiology and Pathophysiology

Giant cell arteritis (GCA; temporal arteritis) affects patients over 50 years of age (peak incidence between 70 and 80 years). Most patients are women. GCA is more common in white persons; incidence ranges from 10 to 20/100,000 in Europe. An association with HLA-DRB*04 has been identified.

GCA is characterized by granulomatous inflammation of affected vessels with infiltration of lymphocytes, macrophages, and multinucleated giant cells. Involved vessels include the aorta, its major branches off the arch, and secondary branch vessels, including the external carotid, subclavian, axillary, temporal, ophthalmic, ciliary, occipital, and vertebral arteries. The level of vessel involved dictates the clinical symptoms.

Clinical Manifestations and Diagnosis

Common GCA symptoms include headache, scalp pain, and temporal artery tenderness. Symptoms are frequently unilateral but can be bilateral. Aching and fatigue with chewing (jaw claudication) indicates ischemia of the muscles of mastication. Fever, fatigue, and weight loss may be present. The most feared complication is ischemic optic neuropathy, which can cause amaurosis fugax and blindness. Because blindness is usually permanent, early recognition and treatment of any visual change are critical. Subcranial disease involving great vessels in the chest occurs in 25% of cases, resulting in upper extremity claudication. Severe but uncommon complications include aortic aneurysm and dissection. Dilation of the aortic root may cause aortic valve regurgitation and heart failure. Up to 50% of patients with GCA have polymyalgia rheumatica

(PMR) that may occur before, concurrent with, or following diagnosis of GCA.

Physical examination may reveal scalp or temporal artery tenderness and induration, reduced pulses and bruits, or aortic regurgitation and heart failure. Laboratory findings may include elevated erythrocyte sedimentation rate (ESR) and/or C-reactive protein (CRP), but some have normal values. Nonspecific evidence of inflammation may include anemia and thrombocytosis.

GCA is suspected on the basis of the clinical presentation and is confirmed by temporal artery biopsy and/or imaging of great vessels. New or atypical headache, jaw claudication, or visual changes in a patient over the age of 50 years, especially with concurrent PMR, should raise suspicion. Temporal artery biopsy is diagnostic, but false-negative results are common; bilateral temporal artery biopsy can increase the yield. Importantly, temporal artery biopsy will remain abnormal for up to 2 weeks after initiation of glucocorticoids. Angiography is used to document and follow subcranial disease.

Management

Suspected GCA must be treated immediately to prevent visual loss. Prednisone, 1 mg/kg/d, is recommended. Intravenous pulse methylprednisolone for 3 days is used for acute visual loss, but established blindness is usually irreversible. Symptoms and inflammatory markers usually respond rapidly to glucocorticoids; lack of response should prompt reconsideration of the diagnosis. High-dose prednisone is maintained for 2 to 4 weeks; after symptoms resolve and inflammatory markers normalize, prednisone is tapered by 10% to 20% every 2 weeks. Once a dose of 10 mg/d is reached, the taper is slowed to 1 mg per month. Patients should be carefully monitored for

CONT.

symptom recurrence. ESR and/or CRP should be monitored monthly but should not be the sole indication for adjusting the glucocorticoid dose. Mild flares can be managed with increases of prednisone by 10% to 20% and a slower tapering schedule.

Based on limited data, daily low-dose aspirin may help to reduce the risk of blindness and is recommended for those without contraindication. Glucocorticoid-sparing immunosuppressives such as methotrexate are sometimes used, although little data support their efficacy. The IL-6 inhibitor tocilizumab was recently approved by the FDA for treatment of GCA.

The prognosis for properly treated GCA is good unless aortitis is present. GCA may recur.

Polymyalgia Rheumatica
Epidemiology and Pathophysiology
Although not a vasculitis, polymyalgia rheumatica (PMR) is an inflammatory disorder that frequently accompanies GCA. PMR and GCA likely reflect the clinical spectrum of a single disease process, although PMR occurs 3 to 10 times more frequently. Up to 50% of patients presenting with GCA have PMR, and 20% of patients presenting with PMR have GCA symptoms on questioning.

Clinical Manifestations and Diagnosis
PMR is associated with pain and stiffness of the neck, shoulder, and hip girdle. Pain and stiffness are worse after immobility; 1 hour or more of morning stiffness is common. Inflammation is periarticular (bursitis and tenosynovitis). Synovitis in the hands and feet occasionally occurs. Constitutional symptoms and laboratory findings resemble GCA, but temporal artery biopsy should be performed only if GCA is suspected. Diagnosis of PMR is made clinically. Differential diagnosis includes myopathies, metabolic syndromes (thyroid and parathyroid), and musculoskeletal syndromes (capsulitis, cervical spondylosis, or calcium pyrophosphate deposition).

Management
PMR responds dramatically to low-dose prednisone (12.5-20 mg/d); lack of a rapid response should prompt consideration of alternate diagnoses. Prednisone taper is initiated 1 to 2 months after symptom resolution and requires months to years. Monitoring of recurrence is managed similarly to GCA. For relapses, recent guidelines for the management of PMR (developed by a collaborative effort of the American College of Rheumatology and the European League Against Rheumatism) recommend increasing the prednisone to the last pre-relapse dose at which the patient was doing well, followed by a gradual reduction within 4 to 8 weeks back to the relapse dose. Glucocorticoid-sparing therapies are the same as for GCA. Prognosis is good, although periodic recurrences are common.

Takayasu Arteritis
Epidemiology and Pathophysiology
Takayasu arteritis (TA) causes inflammation of the large vessels, most commonly the aorta, followed by the subclavian, common carotid, and renal arteries; the pulmonary arteries may also be involved. TA is rare (40/million in Japan and 4.7 to 8/million elsewhere). In contrast to GCA, TA predominantly affects younger women. Arterial lesions are often stenotic ("pulseless disease"), and one third contain aneurysms. Histopathology is similar to GCA.

Clinical Manifestations and Diagnosis

TA manifestations include carotodynia, limb claudication, reduced pulses, bruits, and blood pressure discrepancies between the arms. Heart failure related to aortic insufficiency or coronary artery disease may occur. Neurologic manifestations include transient ischemic attack, stroke, and mesenteric ischemia. As with GCA, laboratory studies are nonspecific and reveal anemia as well as elevated ESR and CRP. Angiogram may demonstrate arterial stenosis or aneurysm (**Figure 27**).

Management
Primary treatment of TA is high-dose glucocorticoids (1 mg/kg/d) with a slow taper. Glucocorticoid-sparing medications such as disease-modifying antirheumatic drugs are used but without clear evidence for efficacy. Angioplasty, graft placement, and bypass may be necessary but should be avoided during active inflammation. The leading cause of death is heart failure; stroke and cardiovascular disease also contribute to morbidity. The 10-year survival rate is 90%.

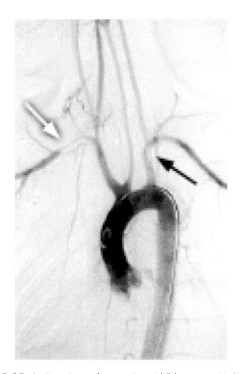

FIGURE 27. Aortic angiogram from a patient with Takayasu arteritis. Note the high-grade stenosis of the proximal right subclavian artery (*white arrow*) as well as the left subclavian artery just below the origin of the left vertebral artery (*black arrow*). Incidentally noted is an anatomic variation with a common origin of the right brachiocephalic artery and the left common carotid artery.

- Giant cell arteritis should be suspected in a patient over the age of 50 years with new or atypical headache, jaw claudication, or visual changes.

HVC
- Suspected giant cell arteritis should be treated immediately with prednisone because of the risk for visual loss; diagnosis is confirmed with temporal artery biopsy, as pathologic findings will persist for up to 2 weeks after initiation of prednisone.

HVC
- Polymyalgia rheumatica is associated with pain and profound stiffness of the neck, shoulder, and hip girdle; it responds dramatically to low-dose prednisone.

- Takayasu arteritis occurs in younger women and causes inflammation of the aorta and other major noncranial vessels; manifestations include carotodynia, limb claudication, reduced pulses, bruits, and blood pressure discrepancies between the arms.

Medium-Vessel Vasculitis

Polyarteritis Nodosa

Epidemiology and Pathophysiology

Polyarteritis nodosa (PAN) is a rare systemic necrotizing vasculitis that affects medium and occasionally small arteries. Prevalence is 31/million but declining. PAN is more common in men than women. Average age of onset is 50 years.

Hepatitis B virus (HBV) infection has been strongly associated with PAN. However, the proportion of patients with HBV-associated PAN has declined from 36% to less than 5% since the advent of the HBV vaccine; thus, most contemporary cases are presumed autoimmune. Activated endothelial cells as well as increased interleukins, T cells, and macrophages have been identified as potential contributors to vessel damage.

Clinical Manifestations and Diagnosis

PAN most commonly affects the skin, neurologic, and musculoskeletal systems. It does not involve the lungs and rarely the heart. Kidney involvement is renovascular rather than glomerular. Cutaneous PAN is a variant confined to the skin. See **Table 40** for the clinical and laboratory findings of PAN.

The gold standard for diagnosis is focal segmental panmural necrotizing inflammation of a medium-sized vessel shown on biopsy. The biopsy is usually performed on an involved, easily accessible area, such as skin or a peripheral nerve/muscle. PAN may also be diagnosed on angiogram; mesenteric or renal arteries show characteristic aneurysms and stenosis, especially at branch points.

Management

Glucocorticoids and cyclophosphamide are indicated for severe organ-threatening disease; glucocorticoids and disease-modifying antirheumatic drugs are used for milder disease. HBV-associated PAN is treated with short-term glucocorticoids, antiviral medication, and plasmapheresis if necessary. The 5-year survival rate for treated PAN is 80%, and the relapse rate is 10% to 20%.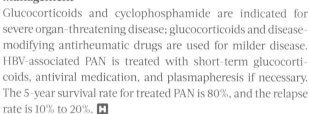

Primary Angiitis of the Central Nervous System

Epidemiology and Pathophysiology

Primary angiitis of the central nervous system (PACNS) is a rare medium-vessel vasculitis of unknown cause that is confined to the central nervous system. Incidence is 2.4/100,000. Median age at onset is 50 years. There are three histologic

Organ System	Symptoms	Frequency	Comments
Constitutional	Fever; malaise; weight loss	65%	—
Musculoskeletal	Arthralgia; myalgia	55%	—
Skin	Purpura; nodules; necrotic ulcers	50%-60%	—
Neurologic	Mononeuritis multiplex; peripheral neuropathy	79%	Wrist drop; foot drop
Kidney	Hypertension; hematuria; proteinuria	40%	Renal artery microaneurysms with tissue infarct/hematoma; no glomerulonephritis
Gastrointestinal	Mesenteric ischemia; intestinal perforation; pancreatitis; cholecystitis; appendicitis; gastrointestinal bleeding	38%	One third of gastrointestinal cases manifest as acute abdomen
Testicular	Orchitis	17%	Usually unilateral, due to testicular artery involvement
Other	Sensorineural hearing loss	Case reports	Bilateral; symmetric; sudden onset; rapidly progressive
Laboratory	Elevated erythrocyte sedimentation rate in 82%; elevated C-reactive protein; leukocytosis; anemia; thrombocytosis; increased liver chemistry tests in 33%	—	—

TABLE 40. Clinical Features of Polyarteritis Nodosa

presentations, all with patchy distribution: granulomatous (58%), lymphocytic (28%), and necrotizing (14%).

Clinical Manifestations and Diagnosis

Patients with PACNS usually present with gradual and progressive symptoms of headache, cognitive impairment, neurologic deficits, transient ischemic attacks, and strokes. Laboratory studies are normal. Cerebrospinal fluid (CSF) is abnormal in 90%, with elevated protein, lymphocytic pleocytosis, and occasional oligoclonal bands. MRI shows nonspecific white and gray matter changes and infarcts. MR angiography and CT angiography have limited usefulness due to poor resolution. Cerebral angiogram may demonstrate vessel "beading" (alternating dilations and stenoses) but has limited sensitivity and specificity. Brain biopsy is the best test for diagnosis, but the patchy distribution of findings results in a 50% false-negative rate.

Evaluation centers on ruling out other conditions, including infection, malignancy, and reversible cerebral vasoconstriction syndrome.

Management

PACNS is treated with high-dose glucocorticoids and cyclophosphamide. Patients often have permanent disability from neurologic damage, and the recurrence rate is 27%.

Kawasaki Disease

Kawasaki disease (KD) is a medium-vessel vasculitis that affects children and is very rare in adults. KD presents as fever, rash, cervical lymphadenopathy, conjunctival congestion, and mucositis. Coronary vessel vasculitis, aneurysm formation, and other cardiac complications (heart failure, pericarditis, arrhythmias) may develop. Treatment is with intravenous immunoglobulin and aspirin.

Many patients recover fully. However, coronary aneurysms may develop, and adults who had KD in childhood may suffer long-term cardiac sequelae. Chronic low-dose aspirin is indicated for coronary artery abnormalities. Clopidogrel may be added for cases with multiple aneurisms; warfarin prophylaxis is recommended for giant aneurysms.

> **KEY POINTS**
>
> - Polyarteritis nodosa most commonly affects the skin, neurologic, and musculoskeletal systems; the gold standard for diagnosis is focal segmental panmural necrotizing inflammation of a medium-sized vessel on biopsy.
> - Patients with primary angiitis of the central nervous system usually present with gradual and progressive symptoms of headache, cognitive impairment, neurologic deficits, transient ischemic attacks, and strokes; treatment consists of high-dose glucocorticoids and cyclophosphamide.
>
> *(Continued)*

> **KEY POINTS** *(continued)*
>
> - Kawasaki disease (KD) affects children; many patients recover fully, but coronary aneurysms may develop, and adults who had KD in childhood may suffer long-term cardiac sequelae.

Small-Vessel Vasculitis

ANCA-Associated Vasculitis

ANCA-associated vasculitis includes three diseases characterized by the presence of ANCA: granulomatosis with polyangiitis, microscopic polyangiitis, and eosinophilic granulomatosis with polyangiitis, along with ANCA-associated glomerulonephritis.

There are two types of vasculitis-associated ANCA: p-ANCA (perinuclear, directed against the neutrophil enzyme myeloperoxidase) and c-ANCA (cytoplasmic, directed against the neutrophil proteinase 3). Perinuclear and cytoplasmic refer to patterns of immunofluorescent staining; enzyme-linked immunosorbent assays are used to confirm antibody positivity.

ANCA may play a direct role in vessel damage by hyperactivating already primed neutrophils, leading to vessel endothelial inflammation and damage. The presence of granulomatous inflammation in some forms of ANCA-associated vasculitis suggests a role for cell-mediated immunity.

See **Table 41** for a comparison of the features of the three forms of ANCA-associated vasculitis.

See MKSAP 18 Nephrology for details on kidney involvement in ANCA-associated vasculitis.

Granulomatosis with Polyangiitis

Epidemiology and Pathophysiology

Granulomatosis with polyangiitis (GPA) is the most common ANCA-associated vasculitis, with an incidence of 7 to 12/million/year. It is more prevalent in Nordic countries and white persons. Typical age of onset is between 45 and 60 years.

Clinical Manifestations and Diagnosis

GPA affects the upper and lower airways, kidneys, eyes, and ears. At least 50% of patients have constitutional symptoms. More than 95% of patients are ANCA positive, overwhelmingly (>90%) directed against proteinase 3 (anti-PR3 antibodies; c-ANCA).

GPA has two forms: systemic and localized. Systemic is more common, involves major organs, and is anti-PR3 positive. Localized has more granulomatous inflammation, has less vasculitis, and is less likely to be anti-PR3 positive. Patients in the localized group are more likely to be younger and female; have mainly ear, nose, and throat involvement; and be more prone to relapse. See Table 41 for GPA clinical features.

In the setting of a classic clinical presentation and positive c-ANCA/anti-PR3, diagnosis of GPA is straightforward. However, because of significant risks of treatment, biopsy of

TABLE 41. Clinical Features of ANCA-Associated Vasculitis Diseases			
	Granulomatosis with Polyangiitis	**Microscopic Polyangiitis**	**Eosinophilic Granulomatosis with Polyangiitis**
ANCA	c-ANCA (antiproteinase-3 antibodies) (>95%)	p-ANCA (antimyeloperoxidase antibodies) (50%-75%)	p-ANCA (antimyeloperoxidase antibodies) (~50%)
Vascular Histology	Pauci-immune necrotizing granulomatous vasculitis	Pauci-immune nongranulomatous necrotizing vasculitis	Pauci-immune necrotizing granulomatous vasculitis with eosinophilic infiltration of vessel walls and tissues; extravascular granulomas
Cardiac	Pericarditis; myocarditis; conduction disorder (<10%)	—	Pericarditis; endomyocarditis; conduction disorder; heart failure (27%-47%)
Ears/Nose/Throat	Crusting; rhinorrhea; sinusitis; otitis media; chondritis of ears and nose with saddle nose deformity; septal perforation (70%-100%)	Sinusitis; sensorineural hearing loss (9%-30%)	Nasal polyps; rhinitis; sinusitis (prodromal)
Gastrointestinal	Ulceration; perforation (5%-11%)	Abdominal pain; bleeding (30%-58%)	Abdominal pain; bleeding
Kidney	Pauci-immune necrotizing glomerulonephritis (40%-100%)	Pauci-immune necrotizing glomerulonephritis (80%-100%)	Pauci-immune necrotizing glomerulonephritis (25%)
Lung	Alveolar hemorrhage; nodules; tracheal/subglottic stenosis (50%-90%)	Alveolar hemorrhage; pulmonary infiltrates; pulmonary fibrosis (25%-55%)	Asthma (prodromal, >90%); nodular opacities; infiltrates (25%-86%)
Ocular	Scleritis; episcleritis; retinal vasculitis; retro-orbital pseudotumor; dacryoadenitis (14%-60%)	—	—
Skin	Palpable purpura; nodules; pyoderma gangrenosum; mucosal ulcerations (10%-50%)	Palpable purpura; livedo reticularis; nodules; necrotic skin ulcers (30%-60%)	Palpable purpura; nodules (60%)
Neurologic	Mononeuritis multiplex, sensorimotor peripheral neuropathy (33%)	Distal symmetric polyneuropathy; mononeuritis multiplex (37%-72%)	Sensorimotor peripheral neuropathy, mononeuritis multiplex (70%)
	Central nervous system involvement (pachymeningitis) (<5%)	Central nervous system pachymeningitis; cerebral hemorrhage; infarcts (<20%)	

CONT.

involved tissue is usually recommended. Histopathology of most tissues demonstrates pauci-immune necrotizing granulomatous vasculitis; pauci-immune necrotizing glomerulonephritis without granulomas is seen on kidney biopsy.

Management

For induction of remission in severe organ-threatening or life-threatening disease, treatment of GPA consists of high-dose glucocorticoids plus cyclophosphamide or rituximab, followed by maintenance therapy with azathioprine, mycophenolate mofetil, or rituximab for at least 12 to 24 months after stable remission has been achieved. Glucocorticoids alone are insufficient to control GPA. Patients with nonsevere forms of GPA (such as arthropathy or upper airway disease) without organ-threatening disease can be treated with glucocorticoids plus either methotrexate or mycophenolate mofetil; such patients should be carefully monitored for treatment failure or the development of renal or other organ-threatening disease, necessitating the more aggressive regimen. Using these approaches, GPA mortality has declined from 90% to around 10%.

Relapses are common (>50% 5 years after initial remission) and may respond better to rituximab than to cyclophosphamide.

Kidney failure and infection are the main causes of mortality.

Microscopic Polyangiitis
Epidemiology and Pathophysiology

The incidence of microscopic polyangiitis (MPA) is estimated at 2.7 to 94/million/year in Europe and lower elsewhere. Average age at onset is between 50 to 60 years with a predilection of men over women (1.8:1). In contrast to GPA, ANCA are less prevalent (50%-75%) and tends to be directed against myeloperoxidase (MPO) rather than PR3.

Clinical Manifestations and Diagnosis

Like GPA, MPA characteristically affects the lungs and kidneys, along with other organ systems. See Table 41 for the clinical features of MPA. Diagnosis is suspected based upon typical clinical findings and positive ANCA, although negative ANCA

CONT.

does not rule out the diagnosis. The diagnostic gold standard is a biopsy demonstrating nongranulomatous necrotizing pauci-immune vasculitis of small vessels or pauci-immune necrotizing crescentic glomerulonephritis in the kidney. Absence of granulomas distinguishes MPA from GPA.

Management

Like GPA, MPA treatment requires high-dose glucocorticoids plus either cyclophosphamide or rituximab, followed by maintenance therapy with azathioprine, mycophenolate mofetil, or rituximab.

Prognosis is worse in the setting of pulmonary hemorrhage or rapidly progressive glomerulonephritis. Survival with treatment is 82% at 1 year and 76% at 5 years.

Eosinophilic Granulomatosis with Polyangiitis

Epidemiology and Pathophysiology

Eosinophilic granulomatosis with polyangiitis (EGPA) is the rarest ANCA-associated vasculitis, with an incidence of 0.11 to 2.66/million/year and a prevalence of 10 to 14/million (France). EGPA has no predisposition for gender or ethnicity. In addition to neutrophil activation, eosinophil infiltration, activation, and degranulation participate in the pathogenesis.

Clinical Manifestations and Diagnosis

The typical patient with EGPA has a history of asthma (96%-100%), nasal polyps, rhinitis, sinusitis, and/or atopy. A prodromal phase (months to years) consisting of arthralgia, myalgia, malaise, fever, and weight loss may occur. An eosinophilic phase with increased peripheral and tissue eosinophilia follows, with migratory pulmonary infiltrates and, less commonly, endomyocardial infiltration and gastrointestinal disease. The subsequent acute vasculitic phase includes mononeuritis multiplex or peripheral sensorimotor neuropathy (70%), kidney (25%), and skin involvement (60%). Paradoxically, the vasculitis phase is often associated with improvement of asthma. See Table 41 for the clinical features of EGPA.

Laboratory findings show peripheral eosinophilia of more than 10%, or more than 1500/μL (1.5×10^9/L). Only 50% of patients have a positive ANCA, mostly directed against MPO.

Diagnosis is based upon typical clinical findings, eosinophilia, and biopsy demonstrating fibrinoid necrosis and eosinophilic infiltration of vessel walls, as well as extravascular granuloma formation.

Management

In EGPA, glucocorticoids alone may be sufficient for mild disease without major organ involvement. With kidney, gastrointestinal, cardiac, or neurologic involvement, cyclophosphamide is indicated.

Mortality for EGPA is the lowest of all the forms of ANCA-associated vasculitis. The 5-year survival is 97%, and the relapse rate is 28%.

- Granulomatosis with polyangiitis typically affects the upper and lower airways, kidneys, eyes, and ears; induction of remission in severe organ-threatening or life-threatening disease consists of high-dose glucocorticoids plus cyclophosphamide or rituximab, followed by maintenance therapy with azathioprine, mycophenolate mofetil, or rituximab.

- Microscopic polyangiitis commonly affects the lungs and kidneys; treatment requires high-dose glucocorticoids plus either cyclophosphamide or rituximab, followed by maintenance therapy with azathioprine, mycophenolate mofetil, or rituximab.

- Eosinophilic granulomatosis with polyangiitis is associated with asthma, nasal polyps, rhinitis, sinusitis, atopy, peripheral and tissue eosinophilia, migratory pulmonary infiltrates, and mononeuritis multiplex; treatment consists of glucocorticoids for mild disease, with cyclophosphamide added for more severe disease.

Immune Complex-Mediated Vasculitis

Immune complexes form from cross-linking of multiple antigens and antibodies. If not cleared, immune complexes deposit in tissue, leading to complement and neutrophil activation with inflammation and tissue damage. Although any tissue or organ may be affected, the classic finding is invariably in the skin. Inflammation and erythrocyte extravasation from involved vessels result in nonblanching palpable purpura, usually in dependent areas (**Figure 28**). Leukocytoclastic vasculitis refers to disintegration of nuclei (nuclear dust) of dead neutrophils along with fibrinoid necrosis of the vessel wall.

Cryoglobulinemic Vasculitis

Cryoglobulins can cause immune complex–mediated small-vessel vasculitis. There are three types of cryoglobulins;

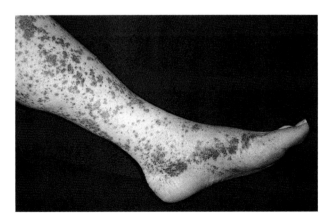

FIGURE 28. Palpable purpura is the classic rash of any small-vessel, immune complex–mediated vasculitis. The lesions are nonblanching and represent extravasations of blood from damaged vessels. Purpuric lesions are typically more prominent on the lower extremities, a consequence of the superimposed effect of gravity on hydrostatic pressure.

discussion here is limited to types II and III ("mixed" types). Both are polyclonal, but type II cryoglobulins include a monoclonal IgM rheumatoid factor, whereas type III cryoglobulins include a polyclonal IgM rheumatoid factor. The ability of rheumatoid factor to directly bind other antibodies facilitates the formation of immune complexes even in the absence of persistent antigen. See MKSAP 18 Hematology and Oncology for details on cryoglobulins and the differentiation from cold agglutinin disease.

Epidemiology and Pathophysiology

Mixed cryoglobulinemia accounts for 85% to 90% of all cases; 90% of mixed cases are related to hepatitis C virus (HCV) infection, which can cause both type II and type III cryoglobulinemia. Autoimmune diseases such as systemic lupus erythematosus and Sjögren syndrome cause type III cryoglobulinemia. Onset is usually in the fifth decade, and women slightly outnumber men.

Clinical Manifestations and Diagnosis

Cutaneous symptoms (palpable purpura, Raynaud phenomenon, ulcers, necrosis, and livedo reticularis) predominate in 70% to 90% of patients with mixed cryoglobulinemia, but any organ may be involved. Peripheral neuropathy (60%), arthritis (40%), and glomerulonephritis (40%) are common. In addition to cryoglobulins, a low C4 complement and positive rheumatoid factor are present. A false-negative cryoglobulin result may occur if the serum sample is not maintained at 37.0 °C (98.6 °F) due to ex vivo cryoprecipitation at room temperature.

HCV infection associated with mixed cryoglobulinemia may go unrecognized for many years before the development of vasculitis. It is therefore important to test for HCV infection in patients with cryoglobulinemia.

Management

When possible, treatment of the underlying cause of cryoglobulinemia is the first priority. For HCV-related disease, antiviral medication is the primary therapy. For severe or refractory disease, the vasculitis must be independently addressed. Glucocorticoids and cyclophosphamide have been used in the past; plasmapheresis and rituximab (provided there is no hepatitis B virus infection) have demonstrated efficacy and may carry less toxicity.

IgA Vasculitis

See MKSAP 18 Nephrology for information on IgA nephropathy and on kidney involvement in IgA vasculitis.

Epidemiology and Pathophysiology

IgA vasculitis (Henoch-Schönlein purpura) is a common vasculitis of childhood that occurs rarely in adults. Estimated incidence in adults is 14/million/year. Onset is often preceded by a viral or streptococcal upper respiratory infection.

Clinical Manifestations and Diagnosis

Patients with IgA vasculitis typically present with a palpable purpura in dependent areas. Gastrointestinal symptoms such

as abdominal pain or bleeding (65%), arthritis and arthralgia (63%), and glomerulonephritis (40%) may be present. Although rare, life-threatening pulmonary hemorrhage may occur.

There are no specific laboratory tests for diagnosis; serum IgA may be elevated but is not sensitive or specific. Diagnosis is confirmed with biopsy. Skin biopsy demonstrates leukocytoclastic vasculitis with heavy deposits of IgA and complement on immunofluorescent staining. Renal histology is identical to IgA nephropathy.

Management

Although IgA vasculitis in children tends to be self-limited, adults are more likely to develop severe persistent disease, especially nephropathy, and may require glucocorticoids and cyclophosphamide.

Hypersensitivity Vasculitis

Epidemiology and Pathophysiology

Hypersensitivity vasculitis is a small-vessel vasculitis mediated by immune complex deposition confined to the skin. It may be triggered by an antigen such as a drug or infection; in 50% of cases, the antigen is unknown.

Clinical Manifestations and Diagnosis

The most common presentation of hypersensitivity vasculitis is palpable purpura in dependent regions, developing 7 to 10 days after exposure to a triggering antigen; lesions appear in "crops" and resolve over a few weeks after the antigen is removed. Internal organs are unaffected. Skin biopsy with immunofluorescence demonstrates leukocytoclastic vasculitis without heavy IgA deposits. Evaluation should be guided by clinical signs and symptoms, and may only require a complete blood count, basic chemistries, and urinalysis.

Management

Removal of the antigen (if identified) and supportive care are usually sufficient. Resolution within a month is the rule. If symptoms persist or recur, anti-inflammatories, topical or low-dose systemic glucocorticoids, colchicine, or dapsone may be helpful.

KEY POINTS

- Mixed cryoglobulinemia is associated with cutaneous symptoms, peripheral neuropathy, arthritis, and glomerulonephritis, with 90% of cases related to hepatitis C virus infection; treatment of the underlying disorder causing cryoglobulinemia is required.

- IgA vasculitis (Henoch-Schönlein purpura) is characterized by palpable purpura and abdominal pain/bleeding and occurs mainly in children; adult disease is rare but more likely to be severe and/or persistent and to require glucocorticoids and cyclophosphamide.

(Continued)

- The most common presentation of hypersensitivity vasculitis is palpable purpura, developing 7 to 10 days after exposure to a triggering antigen; removal of the antigen and supportive care are usually sufficient management.

Other Rheumatologic Diseases

Behçet Syndrome

Behçet syndrome is a systemic disease associated with inflammatory infiltration of multiple organs, as well as small-vessel vasculitis and large-vessel vasculopathy. The characteristic clinical features are recurrent painful oral and genital mucosal ulcerations (**Figure 29**) and inflammatory eye disease (panuveitis, retinal vasculitis). A characteristic clinical finding is pathergy, an inflamed papular or pustular response to local skin injury that is clinically defined by similar lesions appearing 48 hours after skin prick with a sterile needle (**Figure 30**).

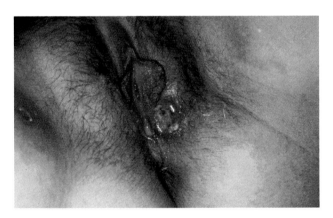

FIGURE 29. Recurrent, painful genital mucosal ulcerations are a characteristic clinical feature of Behçet syndrome. In women, they typically appear on the vulva, as shown, and may heal with disfiguring scaring.

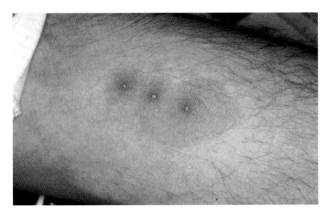

FIGURE 30. Pathergy associated with Behçet syndrome, characterized by pustular-appearing skin lesions occurring 48 hours after skin pricking with a sterile needle.

Other clinical manifestations include venous thrombosis that may affect the large veins, including the vena cava and the dural venous sinuses. Central nervous system (CNS) manifestations include brainstem lesions and aseptic meningitis; the most common CNS symptoms are headache and diplopia. Inflammatory arthritis (usually in the knees), skin lesions, and gastrointestinal inflammation/ulceration indistinguishable from inflammatory bowel disease also occur. Diagnostic criteria are listed in **Table 42**.

Behçet syndrome is most common in Asia, with the highest reported prevalence in Turkey; it is much less common in North America. It is slightly more prevalent in men than women, and men usually have more severe disease. HLA-B51 is strongly associated with the disease and is seen in patients with varied ethnicity.

Treatment for mild disease includes colchicine and low-dose glucocorticoids. The phosphodiesterase-4 inhibitor apremilast appears to be beneficial for oral ulcers. High-dose glucocorticoids and immunosuppressives such as cyclosporine and azathioprine are used for more severe disease. Interferon alfa and tumor necrosis factor (TNF)-α inhibitors may be used for refractory disease. Interleukin (IL)-1 and IL-6 inhibitors have been reported to be beneficial.

- Behçet syndrome is characterized by recurrent painful oral and genital mucosal ulcerations, inflammatory eye disease, and pathergy.

Relapsing Polychondritis

Relapsing polychondritis (RP) is a rare autoimmune disease characterized by inflammation and damage of cartilaginous tissues. Anti-type II collagen antibodies have been identified, but a role in pathogenesis has not been established. RP can be primary or associated with other autoimmune diseases, particularly ANCA-associated vasculitis, Behçet syndrome, and antiphospholipid syndrome. Onset usually occurs between the ages of 40 and 50 years.

TABLE 42.	International Criteria for Behçet Disease
Manifestations	**Points[a]**
Oral ulcers	2
Genital ulcers	2
Pathergy	1
Skin lesions (pseudofolliculitis; skin ulcers; erythema nodosum)	1
Eye lesions (anterior uveitis; posterior uveitis; retinal vasculitis)	2
Central nervous system lesions	1
Vascular lesions (arterial thrombosis; large vein thrombosis; phlebitis)	1

[a]Four or more points are needed for the diagnosis of Behçet syndrome.

Tissues affected include the cartilaginous portions of the external and middle ear (90%), nose (60%), tracheobronchial tree (50%), and joints (65%). Inflammation of noncartilaginous connective tissue also occurs, particularly uveitis and keratitis (65%). Cochlear and/or vestibular dysfunction may rarely occur (10%). Elevated inflammatory markers, anemia, antinuclear antibodies, and other autoantibodies are often observed but are nonspecific. Cartilage biopsy, which is necessary only with atypical presentations in which there is substantial diagnostic uncertainty, typically demonstrates inflammatory cell infiltration of the perichondrium. CT can demonstrate bronchial thickening, strictures, malacia, and air trapping.

Therapy is guided by organ involvement and disease severity. Mild disease may respond to NSAIDs, colchicine, or dapsone. Glucocorticoids and disease-modifying antirheumatic drugs (DMARDs) such as cyclosporine, azathioprine, or methotrexate are used for more severe disease. Biologic drugs such as TNF-α inhibitors have been reported as effective but not on a consistent basis. Surgery (stenting, dilation, extirpation, reconstruction) for airway lesions may be necessary.

KEY POINT

- Relapsing polychondritis is characterized by inflammation and damage of cartilaginous tissues; tissues most commonly affected include the cartilaginous portions of the external and middle ear, nose, tracheobronchial tree, and joints.

Adult-Onset Still Disease

Adult-onset Still disease (AOSD) is a rare disorder that affects multiple organ systems. Symptoms and signs include daily high spiking fever, evanescent salmon-colored rash on the trunk and extremities, arthritis, lymphadenopathy, and leukocytosis. It is most commonly diagnosed in young adults (median age, 36 years) but has been described in older age groups. Some reports indicate a predilection for women. The cause is unknown, but AOSD appears to be a disease of autoinflammation rather than autoimmunity.

See **Table 43** for diagnostic criteria. Diagnosis is clinical, and other infectious, neoplastic, and rheumatologic diseases must be excluded. Rare complications include hemophagocytic lymphohistiocytosis, myocarditis, shock, multiple organ failure, disseminated intravascular coagulation, thrombotic microangiopathy, and fulminant hepatitis. ▣

Treatment includes NSAIDs, glucocorticoids, DMARDs such as methotrexate, and IL-1 inhibitors. TNF-α and IL-6 inhibitors may be beneficial, but more studies are needed to establish their efficacy. Most patients respond to therapy, and prognosis of AOSD with treatment is good.

KEY POINT

- Adult-onset Still disease is characterized by daily high spiking fever, evanescent salmon-colored rash, arthritis, lymphadenopathy, and leukocytosis.

TABLE 43. Yamaguchi Criteria for the Diagnosis of Adult-Onset Still Disease

Major Criteria[a]	Approximate Frequency
Daily spiking fever to 39.0 °C (102.2 °F)	99%
Arthralgia/arthritis >2 weeks	85%
Nonpruritic salmon-colored macular/maculopapular rash on trunk or extremities	85%
Leukocyte count >10,000/μL (10 × 10⁹/L), >80% neutrophils	90%

Minor Criteria	Approximate Frequency
Sore throat	66%
Lymphadenopathy and/or splenomegaly	65%/50%
Elevated AST, ALT, or LDH	70%
Negative ANA and RF	—

ALT = alanine aminotransferase; ANA = antinuclear antibodies; AST = aspartate aminotransferase; LDH = lactate dehydrogenase; RF = rheumatoid factor.

[a]Diagnosis requires five criteria with at least two major criteria included.

Adapted with permission from Yamaguchi M, Ohta A, Tsunematsu T, Kasukawa R, Mizushima Y, Kashiwagi H, et al. Preliminary criteria for classification of adult Still's disease. J Rheumatol. 1992 Mar;19(3):424-30. [PMID: 1578458] Copyright 1992, the Journal of Rheumatology.

Autoinflammatory Diseases

Autoinflammatory diseases (periodic fever syndromes) are a category of rare monogenic conditions characterized by episodic and/or persistent inflammation in the absence of antigenically driven autoimmunity. Pathogenesis involves dysregulation of the innate immune system. The innate immune system represents a process separate and distinct from the antigen-based immune response modulated by lymphocytes. Rather than adaptively responding to antigens, the innate immune system responds to stimuli that it "innately knows" to mandate a response. Examples of such stimuli are "pathogen-associated molecular patterns" such as bacterial cell wall proteins and "damage-associated molecular patterns" or markers of cellular damage such as released uric acid. This process is largely regulated by "inflammasomes," large protein structures that recognize these stimuli. Autoinflammatory diseases involve inherited or spontaneous mutation of genes that encode for inflammasomes, including components of the IL-1β–activating inflammasome and the TNF-α receptor pathway.

See **Table 44** for the features and treatment of select autoinflammatory diseases.

KEY POINT

- Autoinflammatory diseases are characterized by episodic and/or persistent inflammation and involve inherited or spontaneous mutation of genes that encode for inflammasomes.

TABLE 44. Features and Treatment of Select Autoinflammatory Diseases

	FMFª	TRAPS	FCASᵇ	MWSᵇ	NOMID/ CINCAᵇ	Schnitzler Syndrome
Inheritance	AR	AD	AD	AD	AD	Acquired
Gene	MEFV	TNFRSF1A	NLRP3	NLRP3	NLRP3	Unknown
Protein	Pyrin	TNF receptor type 1	Cryopyrin	Cryopyrin	Cryopyrin	MGUS (hallmark but not proven causal)
Age at Onset	65% <10 years of age; 90% <20 years of age	50% <10 years of age; up to fifth decade	<1 year of age	Childhood	Neonatal period	Adult (51 ± 10 years)
Ethnicity	Mediterranean	All	European	European	All	Caucasian/European
Clinical Manifestations						
Attack Duration	12-72 h	Days to weeks	12-24 h	1-2 days	Continuous	Daily
Abdominal	Pain; serositis	Pain; serositis	Nausea	Pain	—	—
Pleuritis	Common	Common	—	Rare	Rare	—
Musculoskeletal	Monoarthritis of lower extremities	Large joints	Arthralgia	Arthralgia; oligoarthritis	Epiphyseal overgrowth; contractures	Arthralgia; arthritis; bone pain
Rash	Erysipeloid on lower legs	Migratory with underlying myalgia	Cold-induced; urticaria-like	Urticaria-like	Urticaria-like	Urticarial rash; neutrophilic
Other	High risk for amyloidosis	Conjunctivitis; periorbital edema	Conjunctivitis; headache; amyloidosis; sensorineural deafness	Sensorineural deafness; conjunctivitis; amyloidosis	Sensorineural deafness; aseptic meningitis; mental retardation; amyloidosis	Leukocytosis; lymphadenopathy; hepatospleno-megaly; MGUS (usually IgM kappa); may later develop Waldenstrom macroglobulinemia
Treatment	Colchicine	Glucocorticoids; TNF-α inhibitors	IL-1β inhibition	IL-1β inhibition	IL-1β inhibition	IL-1Ra or IL-1β inhibition

AD = autosomal dominant; AR = autosomal recessive; CINCA = chronic infantile neurologic, cutaneous, articular syndrome; FCAS = familial cold autoinflammatory syndrome; FMF = familial Mediterranean fever; IL = interleukin; IL-1Ra = interleukin-1 receptor antagonist; MGUS = monoclonal gammopathy of uncertain significance; MWS = Muckle-Wells syndrome; NOMID = neonatal-onset multisystem inflammatory disease; TNF = tumor necrosis factor; TRAPS = tumor necrosis factor receptor-associated periodic syndrome.

ªFMF is the most common autoinflammatory disease.

ᵇThe cryopyrin-associated periodic syndromes (CAPS) include familial cold autoinflammatory syndrome, Muckle-Wells syndrome, and neonatal-onset multisystem inflammatory disease (chronic infantile neurologic, cutaneous, articular syndrome).

Sarcoidosis

Sarcoidosis is an inflammatory disease of unknown cause characterized by formation of noncaseating granulomas in multiple organs and tissues. Sarcoidosis most commonly affects the lungs, which is discussed in MKSAP 18 Pulmonary and Critical Care Medicine. Rheumatologic manifestations are discussed in this section.

In patients with sarcoidosis, a periarthritis involving multiple joints may occur, typically affecting the ankles but also potentially the knees, wrists, and small joints of the hands and feet. Erosive damage, deformity, and dactylitis may develop. Bone involvement has been reported in 1% to 15% of patients; it most commonly accompanies multiorgan disease and is associated with a chronic disease course and poorer prognosis.

Typical radiographic findings include cystic or sclerotic lesions and a lacy pattern of multiple lesions (**Figure 31**). Sarcoid myopathy is histologically present in 25% to 75% of patients but is symptomatic in only 0.5% to 5%. The most common clinical presentation is chronic proximal weakness with development of atrophy or contractures. Biopsy may show inflammatory muscle disease or destruction of muscle by granuloma formation. Glucocorticoids, DMARDs, and TNF-α inhibitors may be used to treat arthritis, bone disease, and myopathy.

Rarely, sarcoidosis can cause Heerfordt syndrome (uveoparotid fever), a combination of fever, uveitis, and parotitis with or without cranial nerve VII palsy. This can lead to sicca symptoms and can mimic Sjögren syndrome.

Löfgren syndrome is a sarcoidosis triad of bilateral hilar lymphadenopathy, erythema nodosum, and migratory

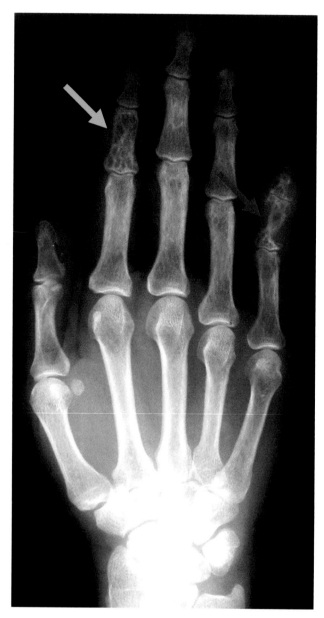

FIGURE 31. Hand radiograph showing the typical cystic lesions (*red arrow*) and a lacy pattern (*green arrow*) characteristic of sarcoidosis.

polyarthralgia. Fever is frequently present. When all three parts of the triad are present, there is a 95% diagnostic specificity for sarcoidosis, obviating the need for biopsy. Löfgren syndrome has a good prognosis and usually remits in 2 to 16 weeks. The goal of treatment is symptom reduction; NSAIDs are usually adequate, but low-dose glucocorticoids, colchicine, and hydroxychloroquine can all be helpful. **H**

KEY POINTS

- Rheumatologic manifestations of sarcoidosis include arthritis involving multiple joints that may develop erosive damage, deformity, and dactylitis; bone disease; and myopathy.

(Continued)

KEY POINTS *(continued)*

- Löfgren syndrome is a sarcoidosis triad of bilateral hilar lymphadenopathy, erythema nodosum, and migratory polyarthralgia; the presence of all three findings has a 95% diagnostic specificity for sarcoidosis. **HVC**

Genetic Diseases of Connective Tissue

Mutations in genes encoding for collagen, fibrillin, and other components of connective tissue can lead to poorly functional skin and integument. Common clinical findings include skin and joint laxity, skeletal fractures, and cardiovascular complications related to involvement of the aorta and cardiac valves. The three most common syndromes are Ehlers-Danlos syndrome (EDS), Marfan syndrome (MFS), and osteogenesis imperfecta (OI). See **Table 45** for a summary of clinical findings and management of these syndromes.

Vascular monitoring is necessary in MFS and several types of EDS. Patients with MFS should undergo echocardiography to assess the aortic root and ascending aorta at the time of diagnosis and at 6 months to ensure stability. Follow-up studies should be completed at least annually; MRI and/or CT are often used to further delineate risk. The best means of vascular surveillance in vascular EDS is unclear, and all patients should undergo expert consultation. See MKSAP 18 Cardiovascular Medicine for more information.

KEY POINTS

- Common clinical findings of genetic diseases of connective tissue include skin and joint laxity, skeletal fractures, and cardiovascular complications related to involvement of the aorta and cardiac valves.

- Regular vascular monitoring is required for patients with Marfan syndrome and several types of Ehlers-Danlos syndrome.

IgG4-Related Disease

Several previously ill-defined illnesses have been brought under the banner of IgG4-related disease (IgG4-RD) (**Table 46**). Most of these conditions are characterized by infiltration and tumefaction of the affected tissue with resultant organ enlargement, fibrosis, and dysfunction. Patients commonly present with a sentinel organ enlargement, but careful evaluation often reveals more extensive disease.

Currently, IgG4 is hypothesized not to be pathologic, but instead to act as a blocking antibody in patients with atopic disease, preventing allergens from interacting with IgE on mast cell surfaces. Consistent with this model, IgG4 elevations accompany loss of clinical responses to allergens in atopic individuals.

TABLE 45. Findings and Management of Genetic Diseases of Connective Tissue

	Ehlers-Danlos Syndrome				Marfan Syndrome	Osteogenesis Imperfecta
	Hypermobility	**Classic**	**Kyphoscoliotic**	**Vascular**		
Genetic Testing Available	Gene is unknown	*COL5A1; COL5A2*	*PLOD1*	*COL3A1*	*FBN1*	*COL*
Inheritance	AD	AD	AR	AD	AD	AD or AR
Clinical Findings						
Musculoskeletal	Joint laxity; joint instability; musculoskeletal pain; early osteoarthritis	Hypermobility; joint dislocations; pes planus	Hypermobility; progressive scoliosis; marfanoid habitus	Hypermobility; joint dislocations	Hypermobility; tall stature; dolichosteno-melia[a]; arachnodactyly; pectus excavatum/carinatum; scoliosis	Bone fractures; short stature
Skin	Easy bruising; mild laxity	Smooth, velvety; easy bruising; hyperextensible; striae atrophicae (widened stretch marks)	Easy bruising; hyperextensible	Thin; translucent; easy bruising	Hyperextensible	—
Cardiovascular	No risk of organ rupture or dissection	Mitral/tricuspid valve prolapse; aortic root dilation (rare); arterial rupture (rare)	Medium-size arterial rupture; mitral/tricuspid valve prolapse	Arterial rupture; aneurysm; dissection	Aortic aneurysm/dissection; mitral valve prolapse	—
Other	—	Muscular hypotonia; delayed motor development	Muscular hypotonia; scleral fragility with risk of globe rupture; restrictive lung disease; recurrent pneumonia; heart failure	Organ rupture (uterus, bowel, rarely spleen, liver); pneumothorax; gingival recession	Myopia (most common feature [60%]); ectopia lentis; high arched palate; pneumothorax; blue sclerae	Dentinogenesis imperfecta[b]; hearing loss; blue sclerae
Management[c]	Joint protection; supportive care	Joint protection; echo/vascular monitoring; preconception counseling	Joint protection; echo/vascular monitoring; preconception counseling; physical therapy; bracing	Joint protection; echo/vascular monitoring; preconception counseling	Annual ophthalmic examination; periodic aortic arch imaging; β-blockers[d]; joint protection; pregnancy counseling/monitoring	Bisphospho-nates; audiology assessments; joint and bone protection; dental evaluations

AD = autosomal dominant; AR = autosomal recessive.

[a]Dolichostenomelia describes when the extremities are disproportionately long for the size of the trunk.

[b]Dentinogenesis imperfecta is defined as discolored (blue/gray or yellow/brown), translucent, weak teeth prone to breakage.

[c]Genetic consultation is appropriate for all listed conditions.

[d]Slow rate of aortopathy.

Most patients with IgG4-RD are men over the age of 50 years; history of atopic disease is common. Clinical signs include painless enlargement of lymph nodes or the thyroid, parotid, or submandibular glands; proptosis with orbital pseudo-tumor; back or chest pain from aortic involvement; and abdominal pain from pancreatic or biliary tree disease. Systemic symptoms such as fever or weight loss are uncommon.

IgG4-RD can affect vascular structures directly, including the carotid, pulmonary, coronary, and iliac arteries as well as the aorta, in particular the thoracic aorta. The affected vessels can develop aneurysms, dissection, and stenosis. A periarteritis

TABLE 46. Select Conditions Associated with IgG4-Related Disease

Condition	Organ Involved
Hypertrophic pachymeningitis	Dura mater
Lymphocytic hypophysitis	Pituitary gland
Idiopathic orbital inflammatory disease	Periorbital often with involvement of the ocular adnexal tissues
Mikulicz disease	Parotid glands
Dacryoadenitis	Lacrimal glands
Küttner tumor	Submandibular glands
Riedel thyroiditis	Thyroid
Inflammatory aortitis/vasculitis	Aorta/arteries
Autoimmune pancreatitis	Pancreas
Ormond disease (retroperitoneal fibrosis)	Periaortic mass
Tubulointerstitial nephropathy	Kidneys
Sclerosing cholangitis	Biliary tract

primarily affecting the infrarenal aorta in conjunction with retroperitoneal fibrosis may also develop.

Diagnosis is by tissue biopsy, which demonstrates a dense lymphoplasmacytic infiltrate, CD4-positive T cells and plasma cells in germinal centers, IgG4-staining plasma cells, storiform fibrosis, obliterative phlebitis or arteritis, and tissue eosinophilia.

IgG4 levels are elevated in the serum in 70% to 80% of patients; therefore, a normal serum level does not rule out the disease. A ratio of the IgG4 level to total IgG of more than 8% is suggestive of the diagnosis. PET scan can identify involvement that is not clinically apparent and can be used to document response.

Initial treatment is prednisone, 0.5-0.6 mg/kg/d, for 2 to 4 weeks with a slow taper over 3 to 6 months; some experts advocate subsequent low-dose (5 mg/d) therapy for several years. Rituximab has shown significant benefit and appears to affect IgG4 production more than other IgG subtypes. Methotrexate may be a useful agent to maintain remission in patients treated with prednisone or rituximab. Azathioprine and mycophenolate mofetil have also been used as glucocorticoid-sparing agents. Treatment response may be influenced by the amount of fibrosis present prior to therapy initiation.

See MKSAP 18 Gastroenterology and Hepatology for information on IgG4-related pancreatitis.

KEY POINT

- The conditions comprising IgG4-related disease are characterized by infiltration and tumefaction of the affected tissue with resultant organ enlargement, fibrosis, and dysfunction; diagnosis is by tissue biopsy.

Bibliography

Approach to the Patient with Rheumatologic Disease

Brown AK. How to interpret plain radiographs in clinical practice. Best Pract Res Clin Rheumatol. 2013;27:249-69. [PMID: 23731934] doi:10.1016/j.berh.2013.03.004

Castro C, Gourley M. Diagnostic testing and interpretation of tests for autoimmunity. J Allergy Clin Immunol. 2010;125:S238-47. [PMID: 20061009] doi:10.1016/j.jaci.2009.09.041

Colglazier CL, Sutej PG. Laboratory testing in the rheumatic diseases: a practical review. South Med J. 2005;98:185-91. [PMID: 15759949]

Courtney P, Doherty M. Joint aspiration and injection and synovial fluid analysis. Best Pract Res Clin Rheumatol. 2013 Apr;27(2):137-69. [PMID: 23731929]

Iagnocco A, Ceccarelli F, Perricone C, Gattamelata A, Finucci A, Ricci E, et al. The use of musculoskeletal ultrasound in a rheumatology outpatient clinic. Med Ultrason. 2014;16:332-5. [PMID: 25463887]

Man A, Shojania K, Phoon C, Pal J, de Badyn MH, Pi D, et al. An evaluation of autoimmune antibody testing patterns in a Canadian health region and an evaluation of a laboratory algorithm aimed at reducing unnecessary testing. Clin Rheumatol. 2013;32:601-8. [PMID: 23292519] doi:10.1007/s10067-012-2141-y

Qaseem A, Alguire P, Dallas P, Feinberg LE, Fitzgerald FT, Horwitch C, et al. Appropriate use of screening and diagnostic tests to foster high-value, cost-conscious care. Ann Intern Med. 2012;156:147-9. [PMID: 22250146] doi:10.7326/0003-4819-156-2-201201170-00011

Yazdany J, Schmajuk G, Robbins M, Daikh D, Beall A, Yelin E, et al; American College of Rheumatology Core Membership Group. Choosing wisely: the American College of Rheumatology's top 5 list of things physicians and patients should question. Arthritis Care Res (Hoboken). 2013;65:329-39. [PMID: 23436818] doi:10.1002/acr.21930

Principles of Therapeutics

Cheng L, Xiong Y, Qin CZ, Zhang W, Chen XP, Li J, et al. HLA-B*58:01 is strongly associated with allopurinol-induced severe cutaneous adverse reactions in Han Chinese patients: a multicentre retrospective case-control clinical study [Letter]. Br J Dermatol. 2015;173:555-8. [PMID: 26104483] doi:10.1111/bjd.13688

da Costa BR, Reichenbach S, Keller N, Nartey L, Wandel S, Jüni P, et al. Effectiveness of non-steroidal anti-inflammatory drugs for the treatment of pain in knee and hip osteoarthritis: a network meta-analysis. Lancet. 2017;390:e21-e33. [PMID: 28699595] doi:10.1016/S0140-6736(17)31744-0

Hochberg MC, Altman RD, April KT, Benkhalti M, Guyatt G, McGowan J, et al; American College of Rheumatology. American College of Rheumatology 2012 recommendations for the use of nonpharmacologic and pharmacologic therapies in osteoarthritis of the hand, hip, and knee. Arthritis Care Res (Hoboken). 2012;64:465-74. [PMID: 22563589]

Hwang YG, Saag K. The safety of low-dose glucocorticoids in rheumatic diseases: results from observational studies. Neuroimmunomodulation. 2015;22:72-82. [PMID: 25228230] doi:10.1159/000362727

Kavanaugh A, Mease PJ, Gomez-Reino JJ, Adebajo AO, Wollenhaupt J, Gladman DD, et al. Treatment of psoriatic arthritis in a phase 3 randomised, placebo-controlled trial with apremilast, an oral phosphodiesterase 4 inhibitor. Ann Rheum Dis. 2014;73:1020-6. [PMID: 24595547] doi:10.1136/annrheumdis-2013-205056

Kroon FP, van der Burg LR, Ramiro S, Landewé RB, Buchbinder R, Falzon L, et al. Non-steroidal anti-inflammatory drugs (NSAIDs) for axial spondyloarthritis (ankylosing spondylitis and non-radiographic axial spondyloarthritis). Cochrane Database Syst Rev. 2015:CD010952. [PMID: 26186173] doi:10.1002/14651858.CD010952.pub2

McGrory BJ, Weber KL, Jevsevar DS, Sevarino K. Surgical management of osteoarthritis of the knee: evidence-based guideline. J Am Acad Orthop Surg. 2016;24:e87-93. [PMID: 27355286] doi:10.5435/JAAOS-D-16-00159

McInnes IB, Mease PJ, Kirkham B, Kavanaugh A, Ritchlin CT, Rahman P, et al; FUTURE 2 Study Group. Secukinumab, a human anti-interleukin-17A monoclonal antibody, in patients with psoriatic arthritis (FUTURE 2): a randomised, double-blind, placebo-controlled, phase 3 trial. Lancet. 2015;386:1137-46. [PMID: 26135703] doi:10.1016/S0140-6736(15)61134-5

Mielenz TJ, Xiao C, Callahan LF. Self-management of arthritis symptoms by complementary and alternative medicine movement therapies. J Altern Complement Med. 2016;22:404-7. [PMID: 27058260] doi:10.1089/acm.2015.0222

Mok CC, Ying KY, Yim CW, Siu YP, Tong KH, To CH, et al. Tacrolimus versus mycophenolate mofetil for induction therapy of lupus nephritis: a randomised controlled trial and long-term follow-up. Ann Rheum Dis. 2016;75:30-6. [PMID: 25550339] doi:10.1136/annrheumdis-2014-206456

Omair MA, Alahmadi A, Johnson SR. Safety and effectiveness of mycophenolate in systemic sclerosis. A systematic review. PLoS One. 2015;10:e0124205. [PMID: 25933090] doi:10.1371/journal.pone.0124205

Singh JA, Saag KG, Bridges SL Jr, Akl EA, Bannuru RR, Sullivan MC, et al. 2015 American College of Rheumatology guideline for the treatment of rheumatoid arthritis. Arthritis Rheumatol. 2016;68:1-26. [PMID: 26545940] doi:10.1002/art.39480

van der Goes MC, Jacobs JW, Bijlsma JW. The value of glucocorticoid co-therapy in different rheumatic diseases-positive and adverse effects. Arthritis Res Ther. 2014;16 Suppl 2:S2. [PMID: 25608693] doi:10.1186/ar4686

Wang C, Schmid CH, Iversen MD, Harvey WF, Fielding RA, Driban JB, et al. Comparative effectiveness of tai chi versus physical therapy for knee osteoarthritis: a randomized trial. Ann Intern Med. 2016;165:77-86. [PMID: 27183035] doi:10.7326/M15-2143

Rheumatoid Arthritis

Aletaha D, Neogi T, Silman AJ, Funovits J, Felson DT, Bingham CO 3rd, et al. 2010 Rheumatoid arthritis classification criteria: an American College of Rheumatology/European League Against Rheumatism collaborative initiative. Arthritis Rheum. 2010;62:2569-81. [PMID: 20872595] doi:10.1002/art.27584

Bakker MF, Jacobs JW, Welsing PM, Verstappen SM, Tekstra J, Ton E, et al; Utrecht Rheumatoid Arthritis Cohort Study Group. Low-dose prednisone inclusion in a methotrexate-based, tight control strategy for early rheumatoid arthritis: a randomized trial. Ann Intern Med. 2012;156:329-39. [PMID: 22393128] doi:10.7326/0003-4819-156-5-201203060-00004

Moreland LW, O'Dell JR, Paulus HE, Curtis JR, Bathon JM, St Clair EW, et al; TEAR Investigators. A randomized comparative effectiveness study of oral triple therapy versus etanercept plus methotrexate in early aggressive rheumatoid arthritis: the treatment of Early Aggressive Rheumatoid Arthritis Trial. Arthritis Rheum. 2012;64:2824-35. [PMID: 22508468] doi:10.1002/art.34498

Scher JU, Littman DR, Abramson SB. Microbiome in Inflammatory Arthritis and Human Rheumatic Diseases. Arthritis Rheumatol. 2016;68:35-45. [PMID: 26331579] doi:10.1002/art.39259

Schiff MH, Jaffe JS, Freundlich B. Head-to-head, randomised, crossover study of oral versus subcutaneous methotrexate in patients with rheumatoid arthritis: drug-exposure limitations of oral methotrexate at doses ≥15 mg may be overcome with subcutaneous administration. Ann Rheum Dis. 2014;73:1549-51. [PMID: 24728329] doi:10.1136/annrheumdis-2014-205228

Singh JA, Saag KG, Bridges SL Jr, Akl EA, Bannuru RR, Sullivan MC, et al. 2015 American College of Rheumatology guideline for the treatment of rheumatoid arthritis. Arthritis Rheumatol. 2016;68:1-26. [PMID: 26545940] doi:10.1002/art.39480

Smolen JS, Aletaha D, McInnes IB. Rheumatoid arthritis. Lancet. 2016;388:2023-2038. [PMID: 27156434] doi:10.1016/S0140-6736(16)30173-8

Soubrier M, Barber Chamoux N, Tatar Z, Couderc M, Dubost JJ, Mathieu S. Cardiovascular risk in rheumatoid arthritis. Joint Bone Spine. 2014;81:298-302. [PMID: 24880190] doi:10.1016/j.jbspin.2014.01.009

Stoffer MA, Schoels MM, Smolen JS, Aletaha D, Breedveld FC, Burmester G, et al. Evidence for treating rheumatoid arthritis to target: results of a systematic literature search update. Ann Rheum Dis. 2016;75:16-22. [PMID: 25990290] doi:10.1136/annrheumdis-2015-207526

Osteoarthritis

Bannuru RR, Schmid CH, Kent DM, Vaysbrot EE, Wong JB, McAlindon TE. Comparative effectiveness of pharmacologic interventions for knee osteoarthritis: a systematic review and network meta-analysis. Ann Intern Med. 2015;162:46-54. [PMID: 25560713] doi:10.7326/M14-1231

da Costa BR, Reichenbach S, Keller N, Nartey L, Wandel S, Jüni P, et al. Effectiveness of non-steroidal anti-inflammatory drugs for the treatment of pain in knee and hip osteoarthritis: a network meta-analysis. Lancet. 2017;390:e21-e33. [PMID: 28699595] doi:10.1016/S0140-6736(17)31744-0

Derry S, Moore RA, Rabbie R. Topical NSAIDs for chronic musculoskeletal pain in adults. Cochrane Database Syst Rev. 2012:CD007400. [PMID: 22972108] doi:10.1002/14651858.CD007400.pub2

Fernandes L, Hagen KB, Bijlsma JW, Andreassen O, Christensen P, Conaghan PG, et al; European League Against Rheumatism (EULAR). EULAR recommendations for the non-pharmacological core management of hip and knee osteoarthritis. Ann Rheum Dis. 2013;72:1125-35. [PMID: 23595142] doi:10.1136/annrheumdis-2012-202745

Fransen M, McConnell S, Harmer AR, Van der Esch M, Simic M, Bennell KL. Exercise for osteoarthritis of the knee. Cochrane Database Syst Rev. 2015;1:CD004376. [PMID: 25569281] doi:10.1002/14651858.CD004376.pub3

Hochberg MC, Altman RD, April KT, Benkhalti M, Guyatt G, McGowan J, et al; American College of Rheumatology. American College of Rheumatology 2012 recommendations for the use of nonpharmacologic and pharmacologic therapies in osteoarthritis of the hand, hip, and knee. Arthritis Care Res (Hoboken). 2012;64:465-74. [PMID: 22563589]

McAlindon TE, Bannuru RR, Sullivan MC, Arden NK, Berenbaum F, Bierma-Zeinstra SM, et al. OARSI guidelines for the non-surgical management of knee osteoarthritis. Osteoarthritis Cartilage. 2014;22:363-88. [PMID: 24462672] doi:10.1016/j.joca.2014.01.003

McAlindon TE, LaValley MP, Harvey WF, Price LL, Driban JB, Zhang M, et al. Effect of intra-articular triamcinolone vs saline on knee cartilage volume and pain in patients with knee osteoarthritis: a randomized clinical trial. JAMA. 2017;317:1967-1975. [PMID: 28510679] doi:10.1001/jama.2017.5283

Machado GC, Maher CG, Ferreira PH, Pinheiro MB, Lin CW, Day RO, et al. Efficacy and safety of paracetamol for spinal pain and osteoarthritis: systematic review and meta-analysis of randomised placebo controlled trials. BMJ. 2015;350:h1225. [PMID: 25828856] doi:10.1136/bmj.h1225

Messier SP, Mihalko SL, Legault C, Miller GD, Nicklas BJ, DeVita P, et al. Effects of intensive diet and exercise on knee joint loads, inflammation, and clinical outcomes among overweight and obese adults with knee osteoarthritis: the IDEA randomized clinical trial. JAMA. 2013;310:1263-73. [PMID: 24065013] doi:10.1001/jama.2013.277669

Siemieniuk RAC, Harris IA, Agoritsas T, Poolman RW, Brignardello-Petersen R, Van de Velde S, et al. Arthroscopic surgery for degenerative knee arthritis and meniscal tears: a clinical practice guideline. BMJ. 2017;357:j1982. [PMID: 28490431] doi:10.1136/bmj.j1982

Thorlund JB, Juhl CB, Roos EM, Lohmander LS. Arthroscopic surgery for degenerative knee: systematic review and meta-analysis of benefits and harms. BMJ. 2015;350:h2747. [PMID: 26080045] doi:10.1136/bmj.h2747

Wang C, Schmid CH, Iversen MD, Harvey WF, Fielding RA, Driban JB, et al. Comparative effectiveness of tai chi versus physical therapy for knee osteoarthritis: a randomized trial. Ann Intern Med. 2016;165:77-86. [PMID: 27183035] doi:10.7326/M15-2143

Fibromyalgia

Adams EH, McElroy HJ, Udall M, Masters ET, Mann RM, Schaefer CP, et al. Progression of fibromyalgia: results of a 2-year observational fibromyalgia and chronic pain study in the US. J Pain Res. 2016;9:325-36. [PMID: 27330325] doi:10.2147/JPR.S100043

Bernardy K, Klose P, Busch AJ, Choy EH, Häuser W. Cognitive behavioural therapies for fibromyalgia. Cochrane Database Syst Rev. 2013:CD009796. [PMID: 24018611] doi:10.1002/14651858.CD009796.pub2

Clauw DJ. Fibromyalgia: a clinical review. JAMA. 2014;311:1547-55. [PMID: 24737367] doi:10.1001/jama.2014.3266

Macfarlane GJ, Kronisch C, Dean LE, Atzeni F, Häuser W, Fluß E, et al. EULAR revised recommendations for the management of fibromyalgia. Ann Rheum Dis. 2017;76:318-328. [PMID: 27377815] doi:10.1136/annrheumdis-2016-209724

Queiroz LP. Worldwide epidemiology of fibromyalgia. Curr Pain Headache Rep. 2013;17:356. [PMID: 23801009] doi:10.1007/s11916-013-0356-5

Wolfe F, Clauw DJ, Fitzcharles MA, Goldenberg DL, Katz RS, Mease P, et al. The American College of Rheumatology preliminary diagnostic criteria for fibromyalgia and measurement of symptom severity. Arthritis Care Res (Hoboken). 2010;62:600-10. [PMID: 20461783] doi:10.1002/acr.20140

Spondyloarthritis

Asquith M, Rosenbaum JT. The interaction between host genetics and the microbiome in the pathogenesis of spondyloarthropathies. Curr Opin Rheumatol. 2016;28:405-12. [PMID: 27152700] doi:10.1097/BOR.0000000000000299

Coates LC, Kavanaugh A, Mease PJ, Soriano ER, Laura Acosta-Felquer M, Armstrong AW, et al. Group for Research and Assessment of Psoriasis and Psoriatic Arthritis 2015 treatment recommendations for psoriatic arthritis. Arthritis Rheumatol. 2016;68:1060-71. [PMID: 26749174] doi:10.1002/art.39573

Colìa R, Corrado A, Cantatore FP. Rheumatologic and extraintestinal manifestations of inflammatory bowel diseases. Ann Med. 2016;48:577-585. [PMID: 27310096]

Gossec L, Smolen JS, Ramiro S, de Wit M, Cutolo M, Dougados M, et al. European League Against Rheumatism (EULAR) recommendations for the management of psoriatic arthritis with pharmacological therapies: 2015 update. Ann Rheum Dis. 2016;75:499-510. [PMID: 26644232] doi:10.1136/annrheumdis-2015-208337

Husni ME. Comorbidities in psoriatic arthritis. Rheum Dis Clin North Am. 2015;41:677-98. [PMID: 26476226] doi:10.1016/j.rdc.2015.07.008

Mease PJ. Biologic therapy for psoriatic arthritis. Rheum Dis Clin North Am. 2015;41:723-38. [PMID: 26476229] doi:10.1016/j.rdc.2015.07.010

Napolitano M, Caso F, Scarpa R, Megna M, Patrì A, Balato N, et al. Psoriatic arthritis and psoriasis: differential diagnosis. Clin Rheumatol. 2016;35:1893-1901. [PMID: 27156076] doi:10.1007/s10067-016-3295-9

Sieper J, Poddubnyy D. New evidence on the management of spondyloarthritis. Nat Rev Rheumatol. 2016;12:282-95. [PMID: 27052489] doi:10.1038/nrrheum.2016.42

Soriano ER. Management of psoriatic arthritis: traditional disease-modifying rheumatic agents and targeted small molecules. Rheum Dis Clin North Am. 2015;41:711-22. [PMID: 26476228] doi:10.1016/j.rdc.2015.07.012

Stolwijk C, van Onna M, Boonen A, van Tubergen A. Global prevalence of spondyloarthritis: a systematic review and meta-regression analysis. Arthritis Care Res (Hoboken). 2016;68:1320-31. [PMID: 26713432] doi:10.1002/acr.22831

Taurog JD, Chhabra A, Colbert RA. Ankylosing spondylitis and axial spondyloarthritis. N Engl J Med. 2016;374:2563-74. [PMID: 27355535] doi:10.1056/NEJMra1406182

Ward MM, Deodhar A, Akl EA, Lui A, Ermann J, Gensler LS, et al. American College of Rheumatology/Spondylitis Association of America/Spondyloarthritis Research and Treatment Network 2015 recommendations for the treatment of ankylosing spondylitis and nonradiographic axial spondyloarthritis. Arthritis Rheumatol. 2016;68:282-98. [PMID: 26401991] doi:10.1002/art.39298

Systemic Lupus Erythematosus

Abeles AM, Abeles M. The clinical utility of a positive antinuclear antibody test result. Am J Med. 2013;126:342-8. [PMID: 23395534] doi:10.1016/j.amjmed.2012.09.014

Dooley MA, Jayne D, Ginzler EM, Isenberg D, Olsen NJ, Wofsy D, et al; ALMS Group. Mycophenolate versus azathioprine as maintenance therapy for lupus nephritis. N Engl J Med. 2011;365:1886-95. [PMID: 22087680] doi:10.1056/NEJMoa1014460

Hahn BH, McMahon MA, Wilkinson A, Wallace WD, Daikh DI, Fitzgerald JD, et al; American College of Rheumatology. American College of Rheumatology guidelines for screening, treatment, and management of lupus nephritis. Arthritis Care Res (Hoboken). 2012;64:797-808. [PMID: 22556106] doi:10.1002/acr.21664

Haliloglu S, Carlioglu A, Akdeniz D, Karaaslan Y, Kosar A. Fibromyalgia in patients with other rheumatic diseases: prevalence and relationship with disease activity. Rheumatol Int. 2014;34:1275-80. [PMID: 24589726] doi:10.1007/s00296-014-2972-8

Lazzaroni MG, Dall'Ara F, Fredi M, Nalli C, Reggia R, Lojacono A, et al. A comprehensive review of the clinical approach to pregnancy and systemic lupus erythematosus. J Autoimmun. 2016;74:106-117. [PMID: 27377453] doi:10.1016/j.jaut.2016.06.016

Miner JJ, Kim AH. Cardiac manifestations of systemic lupus erythematosus. Rheum Dis Clin North Am. 2014;40:51-60. [PMID: 24268009] doi:10.1016/j.rdc.2013.10.003

Petri M, Orbai AM, Alarcón GS, Gordon C, Merrill JT, Fortin PR, et al. Derivation and validation of the Systemic Lupus International Collaborating Clinics classification criteria for systemic lupus erythematosus. Arthritis Rheum. 2012;64:2677-86. [PMID: 22553077] doi:10.1002/art.34473

Singh JA, Hossain A, Kotb A, Oliveira A, Mudano AS, Grossman J, et al. Treatments for lupus nephritis: a systematic review and network metaanalysis. J Rheumatol. 2016;43:1801-1815. [PMID: 27585688]

van Vollenhoven RF, Mosca M, Bertsias G, Isenberg D, Kuhn A, Lerstrøm K, et al. Treat-to-target in systemic lupus erythematosus: recommendations from an international task force. Ann Rheum Dis. 2014;73:958-67. [PMID: 24739325] doi:10.1136/annrheumdis-2013-205139

Sjögren Syndrome

Carsons SE, Vivino FB, Parke A, Carteron N, Sankar V, Brasington R, et al. Treatment guidelines for rheumatologic manifestations of Sjögren's syndrome: use of biologic agents, management of fatigue, and inflammatory musculoskeletal pain. Arthritis Care Res (Hoboken). 2017;69:517-527. [PMID: 27390247] doi:10.1002/acr.22968

Foulks GN, Forstot SL, Donshik PC, et al. Clinical guidelines for management of dry eye associated with Sjögren disease. Ocul Surf. 2015 Apr;13(2):118-32. [PMID: 25881996]

Shiboski CH, Shiboski SC, Seror R, Criswell LA, Labetoulle M, Lietman TM, et al; International Sjögren's Syndrome Criteria Working Group. 2016 American College of Rheumatology/European League Against Rheumatism classification criteria for primary Sjögren's syndrome: a consensus and data-driven methodology involving three international patient cohorts. Ann Rheum Dis. 2017;76:9-16. [PMID: 27789466] doi:10.1136/annrheumdis-2016-210571

Vivino FB, Carsons SE, Foulks G, Daniels TE, Parke A, Brennan MT, et al. New treatment guidelines for Sjögren's disease. Rheum Dis Clin North Am. 2016;42:531-51. [PMID: 27431353] doi:10.1016/j.rdc.2016.03.010

Inflammatory Myopathies

Basharat P, Christopher-Stine L. Immune-mediated necrotizing myopathy: update on diagnosis and management. Curr Rheumatol Rep. 2015;17:72. [PMID: 26515574] doi:10.1007/s11926-015-0548-6

Lundberg IE, Miller FW, Tjärnlund A, Bottai M. Diagnosis and classification of idiopathic inflammatory myopathies. J Intern Med. 2016;280:39-51. [PMID: 27320359] doi:10.1111/joim.12524

Mahler M, Miller FW, Fritzler MJ. Idiopathic inflammatory myopathies and the anti-synthetase syndrome: a comprehensive review. Autoimmun Rev. 2014;13:367-71. [PMID: 24424190] doi:10.1016/j.autrev.2014.01.022

Mammen AL. Necrotizing myopathies: beyond statins. Curr Opin Rheumatol. 2014;26:679-83. [PMID: 25203117] doi:10.1097/BOR.0000000000000106

Mammen AL. Statin-associated autoimmune myopathy. N Engl J Med. 2016;374:664-9. [PMID: 26886523] doi:10.1056/NEJMra1515161

Needham M, Mastaglia FL. Sporadic inclusion body myositis: a review of recent clinical advances and current approaches to diagnosis and treatment. Clin Neurophysiol. 2016;127:1764-73. [PMID: 26778717] doi:10.1016/j.clinph.2015.12.011

Qiang JK, Kim WB, Baibergenova A, Alhusayen R. Risk of malignancy in dermatomyositis and polymyositis. J Cutan Med Surg. 2017;21:131-136. [PMID: 27534779] doi:10.1177/1203475416665601

Tieu J, Lundberg IE, Limaye V. Idiopathic inflammatory myositis. Best Pract Res Clin Rheumatol. 2016;30:149-68. [PMID: 27421222] doi:10.1016/j.berh.2016.04.007

Systemic Sclerosis

Cappelli L, Wigley FM. Management of Raynaud phenomenon and digital ulcers in scleroderma. Rheum Dis Clin North Am. 2015;41:419-38. [PMID: 26210127] doi:10.1016/j.rdc.2015.04.005

Hudson M. Scleroderma renal crisis. Curr Opin Rheumatol. 2015;27:549-54. [PMID: 26352732] doi:10.1097/BOR.0000000000000221

Marder W, Littlejohn EA, Somers EC. Pregnancy and autoimmune connective tissue diseases. Best Pract Res Clin Rheumatol. 2016;30:63-80. [PMID: 27421217] doi:10.1016/j.berh.2016.05.002

McCray CJ, Mayes MD. Update on systemic sclerosis. Curr Allergy Asthma Rep. 2015;15:25. [PMID: 26139334] doi:10.1007/s11882-015-0526-0

Silver KC, Silver RM. Management of systemic-sclerosis-associated interstitial lung disease. Rheum Dis Clin North Am. 2015;41:439-57. [PMID: 26210128] doi:10.1016/j.rdc.2015.04.006

Valenzuela A, Nandagopal S, Steen VD, Chung L. Monitoring and diagnostic approaches for pulmonary arterial hypertension in patients with systemic sclerosis. Rheum Dis Clin North Am. 2015;41:489-506. [PMID: 26210131] doi:10.1016/j.rdc.2015.04.009

van den Hoogen F, Khanna D, Fransen J, Johnson SR, Baron M, Tyndall A, et al. 2013 classification criteria for systemic sclerosis: an American college of rheumatology/European league against rheumatism collaborative initiative. Ann Rheum Dis. 2013;72:1747-55. [PMID: 24092682] doi:10.1136/annrheumdis-2013-204424

Mixed Connective Tissue Disease

Mosca M, Tani C, Vagnani S, Carli L, Bombardieri S. The diagnosis and classification of undifferentiated connective tissue diseases. J Autoimmun. 2014;48-49:50-2. [PMID: 24518855] doi:10.1016/j.jaut.2014.01.019

Tani C, Carli L, Vagnani S, Talarico R, Baldini C, Mosca M, et al. The diagnosis and classification of mixed connective tissue disease. J Autoimmun. 2014;48-49:46-9. [PMID: 24461387] doi:10.1016/j.jaut.2014.01.008

Crystal Arthropathies

Abhishek A. Calcium pyrophosphate deposition disease: a review of epidemiologic findings. Curr Opin Rheumatol. 2016;28:133-9. [PMID: 26626724] doi:10.1097/BOR.0000000000000246

Hill EM, Sky K, Sit M, Collamer A, Higgs J. Does starting allopurinol prolong acute treated gout? A randomized clinical trial. J Clin Rheumatol. 2015;21:120-5. [PMID: 25807090] doi:10.1097/RHU.0000000000000235

Khanna PP, Gladue HS, Singh MK, FitzGerald JD, Bae S, Prakash S, et al. Treatment of acute gout: a systematic review. Semin Arthritis Rheum. 2014;44:31-8. [PMID: 24650777] doi:10.1016/j.semarthrit.2014.02.003

Lipsky PE, Calabrese LH, Kavanaugh A, Sundy JS, Wright D, Wolfson M, et al. Pegloticase immunogenicity: the relationship between efficacy and antibody development in patients treated for refractory chronic gout. Arthritis Res Ther. 2014;16:R60. [PMID: 24588936] doi:10.1186/ar4497

Neogi T, Jansen TL, Dalbeth N, Fransen J, Schumacher HR, Berendsen D, et al. 2015 Gout Classification Criteria: an American College of Rheumatology/European League Against Rheumatism collaborative initiative. Arthritis Rheumatol. 2015;67:2557-68. [PMID: 26352873] doi:10.1002/art.39254

Qaseem A, Harris RP, Forciea MA; Clinical Guidelines Committee of the American College of Physicians. Management of Acute and Recurrent Gout: A Clinical Practice Guideline From the American College of Physicians. Ann Intern Med. 2017;166:58-68. [PMID: 27802508]doi:10.7326/M16-0570

Richette P, Doherty M, Pascual E, Barskova V, Becce F, Castañeda-Sanabria J, et al. 2016 updated EULAR evidence-based recommendations for the management of gout. Ann Rheum Dis. 2017;76:29-42. [PMID: 27457514] doi:10.1136/annrheumdis-2016-209707

Rosenthal AK, Ryan LM. Calcium Pyrophosphate Deposition Disease. N Engl J Med. 2016;374:2575-84. [PMID: 27355536] doi:10.1056/NEJMra1511117

van Durme CM, Wechalekar MD, Buchbinder R, Schlesinger N, van der Heijde D, Landewé RB. Non-steroidal anti-inflammatory drugs for acute gout. Cochrane Database Syst Rev. 2014:CD010120. [PMID: 25225849] doi:10.1002/14651858.CD010120.pub2

Infectious Arthritis

Arvikar SL, Steere AC. Diagnosis and treatment of Lyme arthritis. Infect Dis Clin North Am. 2015;29:269-80. [PMID: 25999223] doi:10.1016/j.idc.2015.02.004

Kapadia BH, Berg RA, Daley JA, Fritz J, Bhave A, Mont MA. Periprosthetic joint infection. Lancet. 2016;387:386-394. [PMID: 26135702] doi:10.1016/S0140-6736(14)61798-0

Osmon DR, Berbari EF, Berendt AR, Lew D, Zimmerli W, Steckelberg JM, et al; Infectious Diseases Society of America. Diagnosis and management of prosthetic joint infection: clinical practice guidelines by the Infectious Diseases Society of America. Clin Infect Dis. 2013;56:e1-e25. [PMID: 23223583] doi:10.1093/cid/cis803

Sharff KA, Richards EP, Townes JM. Clinical management of septic arthritis. Curr Rheumatol Rep. 2013;15:332. [PMID: 23591823] doi:10.1007/s11926-013-0332-4

Wang DA, Tambyah PA. Septic arthritis in immunocompetent and immuno-suppressed hosts. Best Pract Res Clin Rheumatol. 2015;29:275-89. [PMID: 26362744] doi:10.1016/j.berh.2015.05.008

Systemic Vasculitis

Cacoub P, Comarmond C, Domont F, Savey L, Saadoun D. Cryoglobulinemia vasculitis. Am J Med. 2015;128:950-5. [PMID: 25837517] doi:10.1016/j.amjmed.2015.02.017

Comarmond C, Cacoub P. Granulomatosis with polyangiitis (Wegener): clinical aspects and treatment. Autoimmun Rev. 2014;13:1121-5. [PMID: 25149391] doi:10.1016/j.autrev.2014.08.017

de Souza AW, de Carvalho JF. Diagnostic and classification criteria of Takayasu arteritis. J Autoimmun. 2014;48-49:79-83. [PMID: 24461381] doi:10.1016/j.jaut.2014.01.012

De Virgilio A, Greco A, Magliulo G, Gallo A, Ruoppolo G, Conte M, et al. Polyarteritis nodosa: a contemporary overview. Autoimmun Rev. 2016;15:564-70. [PMID: 26884100] doi:10.1016/j.autrev.2016.02.015

Dejaco C, Singh YP, Perel P, Hutchings A, Camellino D, Mackie S, et al; European League Against Rheumatism. 2015 Recommendations for the management of polymyalgia rheumatica: a European League Against Rheumatism/American College of Rheumatology collaborative initiative. Ann Rheum Dis. 2015;74:1799-807. [PMID: 26359488] doi:10.1136/ann-rheumdis-2015-207492

Greco A, De Virgilio A, Rizzo MI, Gallo A, Magliulo G, Fusconi M, et al. Microscopic polyangiitis: advances in diagnostic and therapeutic approaches. Autoimmun Rev. 2015;14:837-44. [PMID: 25992801] doi:10.1016/j.autrev.2015.05.005

Greco A, Rizzo MI, De Virgilio A, Gallo A, Fusconi M, Ruoppolo G, et al. Churg-Strauss syndrome. Autoimmun Rev. 2015;14:341-8. [PMID: 25500434] doi:10.1016/j.autrev.2014.12.004

Micheletti RG, Werth VP. Small vessel vasculitis of the skin. Rheum Dis Clin North Am. 2015;41:21-32, vii. [PMID: 25399937] doi:10.1016/j.rdc.2014.09.006

Patel RM, Shulman ST. Kawasaki disease: a comprehensive review of treatment options. J Clin Pharm Ther. 2015;40:620-5. [PMID: 26547265] doi:10.1111/jcpt.12334

Rodriguez-Pla A, Monach PA. Primary angiitis of the central nervous system in adults and children. Rheum Dis Clin North Am. 2015;41:47-62, viii. [PMID: 25399939] doi:10.1016/j.rdc.2014.09.004

Stone JH, Tuckwell K, Dimonaco S, Klearman M, Aringer M, Blockmans D, et al. Trial of tocilizumab in giant-cell arteritis. N Engl J Med. 2017;377:317-328. [PMID: 28745999] doi:10.1056/NEJMoa1613849

Weyand CM, Goronzy JJ. Giant-cell arteritis and polymyalgia rheumatica [Letter]. N Engl J Med. 2014;371:1653. [PMID: 25337759] doi:10.1056/NEJMc1409206

Yates M, Watts RA, Bajema IM, Cid MC, Crestani B, Hauser T, et al. EULAR/ERA-EDTA recommendations for the management of ANCA-associated vasculitis. Ann Rheum Dis. 2016;75:1583-94. [PMID: 27338776] doi:10.1136/annrheumdis-2016-209133

Other Rheumatologic Diseases

Gerfaud-Valentin M, Jamilloux Y, Iwaz J, Sève P. Adult-onset Still's disease. Autoimmun Rev. 2014;13:708-22. [PMID: 24657513] doi:10.1016/j.autrev.2014.01.058

International Team for the Revision of the International Criteria for Behçet's Disease (ITR-ICBD). The International Criteria for Behçet's Disease (ICBD): a collaborative study of 27 countries on the sensitivity and specificity of the new criteria. J Eur Acad Dermatol Venereol. 2014;28:338-47. [PMID: 23441863] doi:10.1111/jdv.12107

Kobak S. Sarcoidosis: a rheumatologist's perspective. Ther Adv Musculoskelet Dis. 2015;7:196-205. [PMID: 26425148] doi:10.1177/1759720X15591310

Mahajan VS, Mattoo H, Deshpande V, Pillai SS, Stone JH. IgG4-related disease. Annu Rev Pathol. 2014;9:315-47. [PMID: 24111912] doi:10.1146/annurev-pathol-012513-104708

O'Regan A, Berman JS. Sarcoidosis. Ann Intern Med. 2012;156:ITC5-1, ITC5-2, ITC5-3, ITC5-4, ITC5-5, ITC5-6, ITC5-7, ITC5-8, ITC5-9, ITC5-10, ITC5-11, ITC5-12, ITC5-13, ITC5-14, ITC5-15; quiz ITC5-16. [PMID: 22547486] doi:10.7326/0003-4819-156-9-201205010-01005

Perugino CA, Wallace ZS, Meyersohn N, Oliveira G, Stone JR, Stone JH. Large vessel involvement by IgG4-related disease. Medicine (Baltimore). 2016;95:e3344. [PMID: 27428181] doi:10.1097/MD.0000000000003344

Rubartelli A. Autoinflammatory diseases. Immunol Lett. 2014;161:226-30. [PMID: 24452074] doi:10.1016/j.imlet.2013.12.013

Russo RA, Brogan PA. Monogenic autoinflammatory diseases. Rheumatology (Oxford). 2014;53:1927-39. [PMID: 24831056] doi:10.1093/rheumatology/keu170

Vitale A, Sota J, Rigante D, Lopalco G, Molinaro F, Messina M, et al. Relapsing polychondritis: an update on pathogenesis, clinical features, diagnostic tools, and therapeutic perspectives. Curr Rheumatol Rep. 2016;18:3. [PMID: 26711694] doi:10.1007/s11926-015-0549-5

Rheumatology Self-Assessment Test

This self-assessment test contains one-best-answer multiple-choice questions. Please read these directions carefully before answering the questions. Answers, critiques, and bibliographies immediately follow these multiple-choice questions. The American College of Physicians (ACP) is accredited by the Accreditation Council for Continuing Medical Education (ACCME) to provide continuing medical education for physicians.

The American College of Physicians designates MKSAP 18 Rheumatology for a maximum of 22 *AMA PRA Category 1 Credits*™. Physicians should claim only the credit commensurate with the extent of their participation in the activity.

Successful completion of the CME activity, which includes participation in the evaluation component, enables the participant to earn up to 22 medical knowledge MOC points in the American Board of Internal Medicine's Maintenance of Certification (MOC) program. It is the CME activity provider's responsibility to submit participant completion information to ACCME for the purpose of granting MOC credit.

Earn Instantaneous CME Credits or MOC Points Online

Print subscribers can enter their answers online to earn instantaneous CME credits or MOC points. You can submit your answers using online answer sheets that are provided at mksap.acponline.org, where a record of your MKSAP 18 credits will be available. To earn CME credits or to apply for MOC points, you need to answer all of the questions in a test and earn a score of at least 50% correct (number of correct answers divided by the total number of questions). Please note that if you are applying for MOC points, you must also enter your birth date and ABIM candidate number.

Take either of the following approaches:

- Use the printed answer sheet at the back of this book to record your answers. Go to mksap.acponline.org, access the appropriate online answer sheet, transcribe your answers, and submit your test for instantaneous CME credits or MOC points. There is no additional fee for this service.

- Go to mksap.acponline.org, access the appropriate online answer sheet, directly enter your answers, and submit your test for instantaneous CME credits or MOC points. There is no additional fee for this service.

Earn CME Credits or MOC Points by Mail or Fax

Pay a $20 processing fee per answer sheet and submit the printed answer sheet at the back of this book by mail or fax, as instructed on the answer sheet. Make sure you calculate your score and enter your birth date and ABIM candidate number, and fax the answer sheet to 215-351-2799 or mail the answer sheet to Member and Customer Service, American College of Physicians, 190 N. Independence Mall West, Philadelphia, PA 19106-1572, using the courtesy envelope provided in your MKSAP 18 slipcase. You will need your 10-digit order number and 8-digit ACP ID number, which are printed on your packing slip. Please allow 4 to 6 weeks for your score report to be emailed back to you. Be sure to include your email address for a response.

If you do not have a 10-digit order number and 8-digit ACP ID number, or if you need help creating a username and password to access the MKSAP 18 online answer sheets, go to mksap.acponline.org or email custserv@acponline.org.

CME credits and MOC points are available from the publication date of July 31, 2018, until July 31, 2021. You may submit your answer sheet or enter your answers online at any time during this period.

Directions

*Each of the numbered items is followed by lettered answers. Select the **ONE** lettered answer that is **BEST** in each case.*

Self-Assessment Test

Item 1

A 72-year-old man is evaluated in the emergency department after falling when his leg gave way as he tried to arise from bed. He has left hip pain, with the inability to stand and pain at rest. He was recently diagnosed with lymphoma, for which he is receiving chemotherapy. History is significant for a left hip replacement 7 years ago for osteoarthritis. His chemotherapy regimen consists of rituximab plus hyperfractionated cyclophosphamide, vincristine, doxorubicin, and dexamethasone.

On physical examination, temperature is 38.2 °C (100.8 °F); other vital signs are normal. The right upper chest is implanted with a venous access port. Warmth and tenderness around the left hip are noted. Pain in the groin is noted. There is limitation of motion in all directions on both active and passive range of motion of the left hip. There are no other joint abnormalities.

Laboratory studies show an erythrocyte sedimentation rate of 73 mm/h, a leukocyte count of 13,400/µL (13.4 × 10⁹/L), and a serum urate level of 8.2 mg/dL (0.48 mmol/L).

Left hip radiographs show periprosthetic lucency.

Which of the following is the most likely diagnosis?

(A) Gout flare
(B) Hemarthrosis
(C) Hip dislocation
(D) Prosthetic joint infection

Item 2

A 55-year-old man is hospitalized for acute respiratory failure requiring intubation and mechanical ventilation. He also has increasing leg swelling with nonhealing skin ulcers on the legs for the past 4 weeks, and pain with swelling of the bilateral wrists and finger joints for the past 6 weeks. He quit smoking 15 years ago. History is otherwise unremarkable. Prior to hospitalization he was taking no medications.

On physical examination, temperature is 37.2 °C (99.0 °F), blood pressure is 150/95 mm Hg, pulse rate is 110/min, respiration rate is 20/min (ventilator set rate, 14/min), and oxygen saturation is 92% on FIO₂ of 40%. There is blood in the endotracheal tube. Lung crackles are heard bilaterally. Swelling of the wrists, metacarpophalangeal joints, and proximal interphalangeal joints is noted. Two necrotic ulcers on the left leg and one necrotic ulcer on the right leg are present. There is 2+ pitting edema of the legs.

Laboratory studies show normal C3, C4, and rheumatoid factor; negative antinuclear antibodies; positive ANCA with a perinuclear pattern; and 3+ protein on urinalysis. Blood and sputum cultures are negative.

Chest radiograph shows diffuse bilateral infiltrates. Biopsy of a skin ulcer shows nongranulomatous, necrotizing small-vessel vasculitis with immunofluorescence negative for immune complexes.

Which of the following is the most likely diagnosis?

(A) Granulomatosis with polyangiitis
(B) IgA vasculitis
(C) Microscopic polyangiitis
(D) Rheumatoid vasculitis
(E) Thromboangiitis obliterans

Item 3

A 78-year-old woman is evaluated for a 2-year history of gout with progressively more frequent and severe attacks. She currently has pain and swelling in the right second finger. History is also significant for hypertension, chronic kidney disease, nephrolithiasis, and type 2 diabetes mellitus. Medications are lisinopril, furosemide, metformin, and the maximal dose of febuxostat; she is allergic to allopurinol.

On physical examination, vital signs are normal. The joint findings are shown.

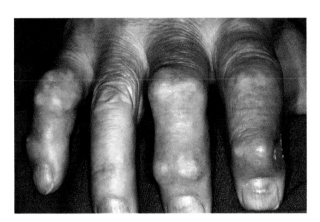

Laboratory studies show an erythrocyte sedimentation rate of 76 mm/h, a serum creatinine level of 1.5 mg/dL (132.6 µmol/L), and a serum urate level of 6.3 mg/dL (0.37 mmol/L).

Which of the following is the most appropriate treatment?

(A) Add probenecid
(B) Stop febuxostat; begin pegloticase infusions
(C) Stop lisinopril; begin losartan
(D) Continue current treatment

Item 4

A 30-year-old man is evaluated for arthritis. Three weeks ago he noticed the abrupt onset of dysuria without a discharge. Two weeks later, he developed the acute onset of warmth, pain, and swelling in the left knee. Two days later, pain and swelling developed over the left heel. He also noted the onset of stinging and redness of the right eye. He takes no medications. The dysuria and eye symptoms have since resolved.

On physical examination, vital signs are normal. A moderate effusion of the left knee is present with warmth and pain with range of motion. Diffuse swelling, warmth, erythema, and tenderness are present at the insertion of the left Achilles tendon at the calcaneus. There is no rash.

Radiographs of the left knee show a joint effusion, no bony abnormalities, and normal joint space.

Aspiration of the left knee is performed; synovial fluid analysis shows a leukocyte count of 5000/μL (5.0 × 10⁹/L) with 65% neutrophils and 35% mononuclear cells, negative Gram stain and cultures, and no crystals.

Which of the following is the most appropriate diagnostic test to perform next?

(A) *Chlamydia* nucleic acid amplification urine testing
(B) C-reactive protein
(C) HLA-B27
(D) Interferon-gamma release assay

Item 5

A 32-year-old woman is evaluated for a 15-year history of low back pain. The pain is worse with rest, improves with movement, and can awaken her during the night. Family history is notable for three paternal uncles with back problems. She takes naproxen twice daily with some relief.

On physical examination, vital signs are normal. Joint examination does not reveal any warmth, erythema, or swelling. Tenderness over the sacroiliac joints bilaterally and reduction in the range of motion of the lumbar spine are noted.

Laboratory studies are notable for an erythrocyte sedimentation rate of 27 mm/h.

A plain anteroposterior radiograph of the pelvis shows fusion of the sacroiliac joints.

Which of the following is the most appropriate diagnostic test to perform next?

(A) ANCA
(B) Anti–cyclic citrullinated peptide antibodies
(C) Antinuclear antibodies
(D) HLA-B27 antigen
(E) No additional testing

Item 6

A 43-year-old man is evaluated in the emergency department for gastrointestinal bleeding. He reports loose, dark stools of 2 weeks' duration. He has an 8-year history of diffuse cutaneous systemic sclerosis (DcSSc) complicated by Raynaud phenomenon and gastroesophageal reflux disease. He does not drink alcohol or take NSAIDs. His only medication is omeprazole.

On physical examination, temperature is normal, blood pressure is 100/60 mm Hg, pulse rate is 80/min, respiration rate is 16/min, and oxygen saturation is 94% breathing ambient air. Skin changes associated with DcSSc are noted from the hands to the elbows in the upper extremities and from the feet to the knees in the lower extremities. The abdomen is nontender to palpation. The remainder of the physical examination is normal.

Laboratory studies show a normal chemistry panel and a hematocrit level of 26%.

Upper gastrointestinal endoscopy demonstrates linear ectatic vessels resembling the stripes found on a watermelon

that arise from the pylorus. There is no evidence of a hiatal hernia or other abnormal findings.

Which of the following is the most likely diagnosis?

(A) Cameron lesions
(B) Dieulafoy lesions
(C) Gastric antral vascular ectasia
(D) Portal hypertensive gastropathy

Item 7

A 76-year-old man is evaluated for fever and a swollen, painful left knee. He was hospitalized 7 days ago for heart failure and appropriately treated. However, he developed fevers up to 38.0 °C (100.4 °F). On examination, lungs were clear to auscultation. The left knee was hot and swollen; 60 mL of turbid fluid was drained from the knee. Gram stain of the synovial fluid was negative; microscopy revealed needle-shaped intracellular crystals. Gout was diagnosed and the knee was drained again, followed by an injection of 80 mg of methylprednisolone, without improvement. Intravenous methylprednisolone, 60 mg/d for 3 days, did not improve the knee or the fevers. History is also significant for hypertension and gout. Other medications are furosemide, lisinopril, metoprolol, subcutaneous heparin, and morphine as needed.

On physical examination today, temperature is 38.0 °C (100.4 °F), blood pressure is 148/92 mm Hg, pulse rate is 116/min, and oxygen saturation is 97% on ambient air. The left knee is warm, swollen, and tender.

Blood, urine, and synovial fluid cultures are negative.

Which of the following is the most appropriate treatment for the knee?

(A) Anakinra
(B) Colchicine
(C) Ibuprofen
(D) Vancomycin

Item 8

A 55-year-old woman is evaluated for an 18-month history of increasingly severe knee pain with the inability to arise when seated on the floor. She does not have pain at rest or nocturnal pain. Medications are celecoxib and omeprazole.

On physical examination, vital signs are normal. Bony hypertrophy of both knees is present. There is no warmth, erythema, or swelling of the joints.

Plain anteroposterior knee radiographs show medial joint space narrowing, peaking of the tibial spines, and osteophytes; there are no erosions or osteopenia.

Which of the following is the most appropriate management?

(A) Glucosamine supplements
(B) Knee replacement surgery
(C) Physical therapy
(D) Prednisone

Item 9

A 25-year-old man is evaluated for the gradual onset of bilateral low back pain without radiation to the lower extremities daily, with increasing severity over the past year. The pain now awakens him during the night 2 to 3 times per week, with morning stiffness lasting more than an hour. He has improvement with exercise and no improvement at rest. He takes ibuprofen with some improvement.

On physical examination, vital signs are normal. Limited lateral bending bilaterally and a reduction in forward flexion at the lumbar spine are noted. The remainder of the examination is normal.

An anteroposterior plain radiograph of the pelvis and sacroiliac joints is unremarkable.

Which of the following is the most appropriate diagnostic test to perform next?

(A) Bone scan

(B) CT of the lumbar spine

(C) MRI of the sacroiliac joints

(D) Radiography of the hip joints

Item 10

A 75-year-old man is evaluated for a 5-year history of hand joint pain and morning stiffness lasting a few minutes. He walks about a mile every day and plays tennis 3 days a week; however, the pain has started to limit him from gripping a tennis racket. He also has noticed fatigue for the past 6 months. He reports no other constitutional symptoms, shortness of breath, or rash. History is also significant for hypertension and diet-controlled type 2 diabetes mellitus. Medications are losartan, acetaminophen as needed, and aspirin, 81 mg/d.

On physical examination, vital signs are normal. Bony enlargement of multiple proximal and distal interphalangeal joints of the hands is noted. The remainder of the physical examination is normal.

Laboratory studies show an erythrocyte sedimentation rate of 22 mm/h, a hematocrit level of 41%, and a C-reactive protein level of 0.9 mg/dL (9.0 mg/L).

Hand radiographs show joint-space narrowing and osteophytes of multiple proximal and distal interphalangeal joints, and similar changes are seen in both first carpometacarpal joints; there are no erosions.

Which of the following is the most appropriate next step in management?

(A) Anti–cyclic citrullinated peptide antibodies

(B) Antinuclear antibodies

(C) Rheumatoid factor

(D) Serum urate level

(E) No further testing

Item 11

A 47-year-old woman is evaluated for an onset over 2 to 3 weeks of low-grade, intermittent fever; blanching of the second and third right fingertips in response to cold exposure; cracking and peeling of the skin on the sides of the second digits and palms; and pain and swelling of the second and fourth proximal interphalangeal joints bilaterally. She does not take any medications.

On physical examination, temperature is 37.6 °C (99.7 °F), pulse rate is 95/min, and respiration rate is 20/min; blood pressure and oxygen saturation are normal. The tips of the digits are cool without discoloration. Erythema of the malar area, forehead, and chin is present. Pulmonary examination reveals crackles at the lung bases. There is no weakness.

Skin findings are shown.

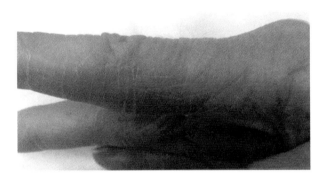

Laboratory studies:

Creatine kinase	115 U/L
Antinuclear antibodies	Titer: 1:1280
Anti–double-stranded DNA antibodies	Negative
Anti–Jo-1 antibodies	Positive
Anti–Smith antibodies	Negative

Which of the following is the most likely diagnosis?

(A) Antisynthetase syndrome

(B) Sjögren syndrome

(C) Systemic lupus erythematosus

(D) Systemic sclerosis

Item 12

A 33-year-old woman is evaluated for concerns about the development of rheumatoid arthritis (RA). She has some mild joint discomfort in the hands at the end of the day. She is a software engineer and has been smoking five cigarettes per day for the past 2 years. She takes no medications. Her identical twin sister was recently diagnosed with seropositive RA, and her maternal grandmother had RA.

On physical examination, vital signs are normal. There is no swelling or tenderness in the joints of the hands, wrists, elbows, knees, or feet.

Which of the following is the most appropriate preventive measure for this patient at risk for developing RA?

(A) Avoid food/drinks containing high-fructose corn syrup

(B) Begin hydroxychloroquine

(C) Begin probiotics

(D) Smoking cessation

Item 13

A 26-year-old man is hospitalized for a 1-week history of dry cough and progressive shortness of breath. He has a 2-year history of systemic lupus erythematosus (SLE); disease manifestations have been pleuropericarditis, polyarthritis, leukopenia, and nephritis. He currently reports no fever, sputum production, or hemoptysis, as well as no other SLE manifestations. His disease has been difficult to control and has needed multiple tapering doses of prednisone. He currently takes 15 mg/d of prednisone; other medications are hydroxychloroquine and azathioprine.

On physical examination, temperature is 36.4 °C (97.6 °F), blood pressure is 150/100 mm Hg, pulse rate is 98/min, respiration rate is 30/min, and oxygen saturation is 84% breathing ambient air. Diffuse crackles are heard on auscultation of the chest. Diffuse tenderness and swelling of multiple small joints of the hands are present. The remainder of the physical examination is normal.

Laboratory studies:

Erythrocyte sedimentation rate	68 mm/h
Hematocrit	42%
Leukocyte count	5500/µL (5.5 × 10⁹/L) with normal differential
Complements (C3 and C4)	Low
C-reactive protein	Normal
Creatinine	0.6 mg/dL (53 µmol/L)
Procalcitonin	Normal

Chest radiograph and CT scan of the chest show diffuse infiltrates in both lungs with ground glass opacities in multiple lobes. Bronchoalveolar lavage shows only increased leukocytes with lymphocytic predominance. Cultures are pending.

Which of the following is the most likely diagnosis?

(A) Acute lupus pneumonitis

(B) Acute pulmonary hypertension

(C) Community-acquired pneumonia

(D) Diffuse alveolar hemorrhage

(E) Shrinking lung syndrome

Item 14

A 45-year-old woman is evaluated for a 4-month history of diarrhea and a 4.5-kg (10-lb) weight loss. She reports explosive episodes of loose stools that follow most meals. There is a feeling of bloating and pain with the episodes. She has a 10-year history of diffuse cutaneous systemic sclerosis (DcSSc) complicated by Raynaud phenomenon with occasional digital ulceration and gastroesophageal reflux disease. Her only medication is omeprazole.

On physical examination, vital signs are normal. BMI is 21. Skin changes associated with DcSSc involve the arms, forearms, and hands. The abdominal examination reveals active and loud bowel sounds but is otherwise unremarkable.

Which of the following is the most likely diagnosis?

(A) Carcinoid syndrome

(B) Chronic mesenteric ischemia

(C) Irritable bowel syndrome

(D) Small intestinal bacterial overgrowth

Item 15

A 50-year-old man is evaluated for a left lower extremity ulcer. He has a 15-year history of worsening arthritis for which he has never been evaluated. He takes ibuprofen as needed.

On physical examination, vital signs are normal. The spleen tip is palpable. There is swelling of multiple small joints at the hands, knees, and metatarsophalangeal (MTP) joints. There is ulnar deviation and subluxation of the metacarpophalangeal joints. Subcutaneous nodules are present at the elbows bilaterally. There is a 2- × 2-cm shallow ulcer at the medial left lower extremity just above the ankle.

Laboratory studies:

Hematocrit	33%
Leukocyte count	2100/µL (2.1 × 10⁹/L), with 900 neutrophils
Platelet count	276,000/µL (276 × 10⁹/L)
Urinalysis	Normal

Which of the following is the most likely diagnosis?

(A) AA amyloidosis

(B) Felty syndrome

(C) Sarcoidosis

(D) Systemic lupus erythematosus

Item 16

A 49-year-old man is evaluated a 3-month history of right knee swelling without significant pain. He does a lot of physical activity as a park ranger in Michigan but does not recall trauma. He likes to walk for exercise and does not have significant pain when he walks. He has only minimal discomfort in the knee and stiffness when he squats. He reports no swelling or pain in other joints and no fever, rash, or other symptoms. He takes no medications.

On physical examination, vital signs are normal. Examination of the right knee shows a large effusion without erythema, but with minimal warmth and tenderness; full range of active motion is noted. The remainder of the musculoskeletal and physical examination is normal.

Knee radiographs confirm a large joint effusion in the right knee; no other abnormalities are seen.

Which of the following tests is most likely to confirm the diagnosis?

(A) HLA-B27 haplotype testing

(B) MRI of the right knee

(C) Serologic testing for *Borrelia burgdorferi*

(D) Synovial fluid analysis for crystals

Item 17

A 55-year-old man is evaluated in the emergency department for a 1-month history of low back pain and lower extremity swelling during the past 2 weeks. History is

CONT. significant for a goiter that was surgically removed 5 years ago; pathology revealed extensive fibrosis. He takes levothyroxine.

On physical examination, temperature is normal, blood pressure is 165/90 mm Hg, pulse rate is 88/min, and respiration rate is 18/min. A surgical scar over the anterior neck is noted. There is 2+ lower extremity edema to the mid calf bilaterally. The remainder of the examination is normal.

Laboratory studies show a hematocrit level of 34%, a serum creatinine level of 2.1 mg/dL (185.6 µmol/L), and a normal urinalysis.

Abdominal ultrasound shows bilateral hydronephrosis. Noncontrast CT of the abdomen and pelvis shows a soft-tissue mass surrounding the infrarenal aorta without any significant lymphadenopathy; the ureters are encased within the mass.

Which of the following is the most likely diagnosis?

(A) Germ cell tumor

(B) IgG4-associated retroperitoneal fibrosis

(C) Lymphoma

(D) Malignant peritoneal mesothelioma

Item 18

A 42-year-old woman is evaluated during a follow-up visit for Raynaud phenomenon of 6 months' duration. She also has gastroesophageal reflux disease. Her only medication is ranitidine.

On physical examination, vital signs are normal. There is no sclerodactyly or digital pitting at the fingertips. The remainder of the physical examination is normal.

Laboratory studies are significant for positive antinuclear antibodies (titer: 1:640) in a centromere pattern, with a strongly positive anticentromere B antibody level.

The nailfold capillaries are shown.

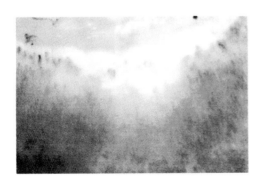

Which of the following is the most likely diagnosis?

(A) Dermatomyositis

(B) Limited cutaneous systemic sclerosis

(C) Mixed connective tissue disease

(D) Systemic lupus erythematosus

Item 19

A 65-year-old man is evaluated for a 1-month history of progressive malaise, myalgia, a 3.6-kg (8.0-lb) weight loss,

and numbness and weakness of the right foot; left testicular pain for 1 week; and a painful rash on his legs for 2 days. He was diagnosed 2 months ago with hypertension, for which he takes hydrochlorothiazide.

On physical examination, temperature is 37.2 °C (99.0 °F), and blood pressure is 165/90 mm Hg. The left testicle is tender. Small necrotic ulcers are noted on the legs. Numbness of the right lateral ankle and calf is noted, as well as weakness of right foot plantar flexion.

Laboratory studies:

Erythrocyte sedimentation rate	100 mm/h
Hemoglobin	10 g/dL (100 g/L)
Leukocyte count	13,000/µL (13 × 10⁹/L)
Platelet count	430,000/µL (430 × 10⁹/L)
Creatinine	1.7 mg/dL (150.3 µmol/L)
ANCA	Negative
Urinalysis	Normal

Renal angiogram shows microaneurysms of the renal arteries. A deep skin biopsy (deep dermis and subcutis) shows panmural inflammation with necrosis of a medium-sized artery.

Which of the following is the most likely diagnosis?

(A) Giant cell arteritis

(B) IgA vasculitis

(C) Microscopic polyangiitis

(D) Polyarteritis nodosa

Item 20

An 85-year-old woman is evaluated for left knee pain of moderate intensity that occurs with ambulation and at night. Acetaminophen provides no relief. History is significant for coronary artery disease, hypertension, and stage 3 chronic kidney disease. Medications are aspirin, lisinopril, metoprolol, and vitamin D.

On physical examination, blood pressure is 152/88 mm Hg; other vital signs are normal. The left knee demonstrates crepitus and decreased passive range of motion; a small effusion is present, and there is no warmth or tenderness.

Joint aspiration of the left knee shows a leukocyte count of 1100/µL (1.1 × 10⁹/L).

Which of the following is the most appropriate treatment for long-term symptom control?

(A) Intra-articular glucocorticoid injections

(B) Low-dose prednisone

(C) Naproxen

(D) Oxycodone

(E) Topical diclofenac

Item 21

A 79-year-old man is evaluated for a 2-month history of progressive malaise and weakness, aching bilateral shoulders and hips, and stiffness for 2 hours in the morning and after immobility. He recently noted aching in his jaw when chewing. He also reports new left-sided headaches. Last week he had an episode of diplopia lasting 1 minute. He has hypertension, for which he takes hydrochlorothiazide.

On physical examination, vital signs are normal. Tenderness and slight swelling over the left temple are present. Painful and limited range of motion of both hips and shoulders is noted. The remainder of the examination is unremarkable.

Laboratory studies show an erythrocyte sedimentation rate of 85 mm/h.

Which of the following is the most appropriate initial management?

(A) CT of the head
(B) Low-dose aspirin
(C) Methotrexate
(D) Prednisone
(E) Temporal artery biopsy

Item 22

A 67-year-old man is evaluated for a 1-year history of weakness, with increased tripping on curbs and difficulty with handwriting, which is not as neat as in the past. He reports no muscle cramping. He takes no medications.

On physical examination, vital signs are normal. There is no rash. There is symmetric weakness of the forearm and thigh muscles. Reduced grip strength and reduced wrist and finger flexion are noted. Reflexes are normal. There is atrophy of the muscles of the forearms and interosseous muscles of the right hand greater than the left. There are no fasciculations.

Laboratory studies show a serum creatine kinase level of 1150 U/L and a normal thyroid-stimulating hormone level; antinuclear and anti–Jo-1 antibody testing is negative.

Electromyogram and nerve conduction studies show myopathic changes in the proximal and distal muscles of the extremities, as well as some neurogenic changes.

Which of the following is the most likely diagnosis?

(A) Amyotrophic lateral sclerosis
(B) Inclusion body myositis
(C) Mitochondrial myopathy
(D) Polymyositis

Item 23

A 66-year-old woman is evaluated after developing five dental caries over the past year. She cannot eat crackers without accompanying water. She has lost two teeth due to caries. She also reports scratchy and itchy eyes for 2 years and intermittent joint pain, particularly of the small hand joints, for 1 year. She takes ibuprofen as needed for the joint pain, which provides relief.

On physical examination, vital signs are normal. Two molars are missing, and there is no salivary pooling below the tongue. Bilateral parotid and lacrimal enlargement is present. Mild tenderness without swelling of the second through fourth metacarpophalangeal joints bilaterally is noted.

Laboratory studies show positive rheumatoid factor, high-titer antinuclear antibodies, and high-titer anti-Ro/SSA antibodies.

A Schirmer test for ocular wetting is diminished at 3 mm. Chest radiograph is normal. Radiographs of the hands show no erosions.

Which of the following is the most appropriate treatment at this time?

(A) Artificial tears and sugar-free candies
(B) Methotrexate
(C) Pilocarpine
(D) Rituximab
(E) Topical ophthalmic NSAID drops

Item 24

A 45-year-old woman is evaluated for a 2-day history of deep boring pain in the right eye. She also describes eye redness and photophobia but no recent trauma to the eye. She has a 10-year history of rheumatoid arthritis, treated with etanercept.

On physical examination, vital signs are normal. Diffuse right eye redness is noted, and there is pain on extra-ocular movement testing. Gentle pressure over the eye with the lid closed results in pain. There is no scleromalacia in either eye. There is diminished visual acuity of the right eye. Limited range of motion of the right wrist is noted. There is no swelling of the joints of the upper or lower extremities.

Which of the following is the most likely diagnosis?

(A) Conjunctivitis
(B) Episcleritis
(C) Scleritis
(D) Subconjunctival hemorrhage

Item 25

A 26-year-old woman is evaluated in the emergency department for an acute onset of fatigue, chills, and joint pain in the fingers of the left hand, left wrist, and right ankle during the past 3 days. There is no travel history. She is currently taking ibuprofen for her symptoms; she also takes an oral contraceptive pill.

On physical examination, temperature is 39.0 °C (102.2 °F), blood pressure is 114/72 mm Hg, and pulse rate is 106/min. Fusiform enlargement of the second and fourth digits of the left hand with pain on extension is noted. Tenosynovitis over the dorsum of the left wrist and at the right ankle is present.

A painless lesion on the palm is shown (see top of next page).

Which of the following is the most likely diagnosis?

(A) Chikungunya infection
(B) Disseminated gonococcal infection
(C) Reactive arthritis
(D) Sarcoidosis

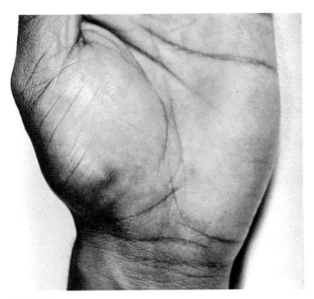

ITEM 25

On physical examination, temperature is 37.5 °C (99.5 °F), blood pressure is normal but systolic pressure is 16 mm Hg less on the right arm than the left arm, pulse rate is 90/min, respiration rate is 20/min, and oxygen saturation is 93% breathing ambient air. There is no rash. There is no temporal tenderness. A bruit is heard over the right supraclavicular fossa. The right radial pulse is reduced. A diastolic decrescendo murmur is heard in the upper right sternal border. Bibasilar crackles are heard. Painful range of motion is noted in the shoulders and hips. No joint swelling is present.

Transthoracic echocardiogram shows aortic valve regurgitation with normal leaflets, dilated aortic root, and dilated left ventricle.

Which of the following is the most likely diagnosis?

(A) Kawasaki disease
(B) Polyarteritis nodosa
(C) Subcranial giant cell arteritis
(D) Takayasu arteritis

Item 26

A 32-year-old woman is evaluated for a recent episode of transient left monocular blindness. She noted dimness of vision in the left eye that came on suddenly and persisted for 15 minutes and then resolved completely. She had no accompanying headache or other symptoms. She has an 8-year history of systemic lupus erythematosus, which initially manifested as photosensitivity, discoid rash, and arthritis. She has responded well to treatment and has been doing well without active disease for the past year. History is significant for recurrent first trimester pregnancy loss attributed to positive antiphospholipid and anticardiolipin antibodies. Medications are hydroxychloroquine, prednisone, aspirin, and a daily multivitamin.

On physical examination, vital signs are normal. Cardiac rhythm is normal. A 2/6 holosystolic murmur is heard at the apex with radiation toward the axilla. Temporal and carotid artery pulsations are normal; there is no scalp tenderness or vascular bruits. The remainder of the physical examination, including ophthalmologic examination, is normal.

Which of the following is the most likely cause of her visual symptom?

(A) Bacterial endocarditis
(B) Carotid artery stenosis
(C) Giant cell arteritis
(D) Libman–Sacks endocarditis

Item 27

A 73-year-old woman is hospitalized for symptoms of heart failure, with progression occurring over the past 2 weeks. She also reports a 6-week history of arm aching that is worse with lifting and reaching, hip aching, morning stiffness, fever, and malaise. She reports no headache or jaw claudication.

Item 28

A 43-year-old woman is evaluated for a 3-day history of left knee pain and swelling. Similar episodes have occurred in either knee as well as the left wrist during the past 2 years. She also reports a sense of generalized weakness, and has experienced constipation and vague abdominal discomfort during the past year. Because of her constipation, her thyroid-stimulating hormone level was recently measured and found to be normal. She takes no medications.

On physical examination, vital signs are normal. The left knee is warm with a moderate- to large-sized effusion, and decreased range of motion is noted. Proximal muscle strength is normal.

Radiographs show a thin white line at the chondral surfaces of both knees and at the pubic symphysis.

Joint aspiration of the left knee shows a leukocyte count of 35,000/μL (35×10^9/L), with 90% neutrophils; polarizing microscopy shows numerous positively birefringent rhomboid crystals within neutrophils.

Which of the following laboratory studies will most likely identify the cause of this patient's symptoms?

(A) Anti–cyclic citrullinated peptide antibodies
(B) Serum calcium
(C) Serum creatine kinase
(D) Serum urate

Item 29

A 66-year-old man is hospitalized for progressive dyspnea for the past 10 days. He was diagnosed with granulomatosis with polyangiitis 5 years ago; at that time, cyclophosphamide was initiated, with resolution of all symptoms. He was subsequently switched to maintenance azathioprine therapy. Today he was started on intravenous methylprednisolone.

On physical examination, temperature is 37.8 °C (100.0 °F), blood pressure is 140/85 mm Hg, pulse rate is 100/min, respiration rate is 25/min, and oxygen saturation

CONT.

is 90% on 2 L of oxygen by nasal cannula. Bilateral crackles are heard in the lower lung fields.

Laboratory studies:

Erythrocyte sedimentation rate	90 mm/h
Hemoglobin	12 g/dL (120 g/L)
Leukocyte count with differential	Normal
Platelet count	450,000 (450 × 10⁹/L)
ANCA	Positive with a cytoplasmic pattern and a titer of 1:160; positive proteinase 3 antibodies
Urinalysis	Normal

Chest radiograph shows hazy opacification and a few nodules in the mid and lower lung zones. Sputum and bronchoalveolar lavage, Gram stain, and cultures are negative. Blood cultures are negative.

In addition to discontinuing azathioprine, which of the following is the most appropriate treatment?

(A) Cyclophosphamide
(B) Etanercept
(C) Methotrexate
(D) Rituximab

Item 30

A 47-year-old woman is evaluated for a 6-month history of disequilibrium. She often feels "dizzy" and "off-balance," which has led to several falls. She does not experience vertigo. She has a 10-year history of fibromyalgia, and has experienced a 60% improvement in pain and function with graded aerobic exercise, duloxetine, and pregabalin.

On a focused physical examination, vital signs are normal. Neurologic examination, including strength testing, sensory examination (light touch, proprioception), tandem walking, and Romberg testing, is normal.

Laboratory studies show normal serum folate, thyroid-stimulating hormone, and vitamin B₁₂ levels; hemoglobin A₁c level is 5.0%.

Which of the following is the most appropriate next step in management?

(A) Discontinue duloxetine
(B) Discontinue pregabalin
(C) Measure methylmalonic acid and homocysteine levels
(D) Order an MRI of the brain
(E) Schedule vestibular rehabilitation

Item 31

A 75-year-old woman is evaluated for a 2-week history of gradually increasing pain in both shoulders and hips; the pain radiates down both arms to the elbows and down both hamstrings to the knees. She reports no headache, jaw claudication, or vision changes. She was diagnosed with polymyalgia rheumatica 3 months ago. She started prednisone, 15 mg/d, with immediate and complete relief of symptoms;

prednisone was weaned from 15 to 10 mg/d 2 months ago, then to 8 mg/d (current dose) 1 month ago. She remained asymptomatic until 2 weeks ago. She says that her current symptoms are just as bad as when she was first diagnosed.

On physical examination, vital signs are normal; blood pressure is identical in both arms. There is no temporal tenderness or induration. Painful range of motion of both shoulders and hips is noted.

Which of the following is the most appropriate management?

(A) Prednisone, 10 mg/d
(B) Prednisone, 30 mg/d
(C) Prednisone, 60 mg/d
(D) Prednisone, 20 mg/d, and methotrexate

Item 32

A 50-year-old woman is hospitalized for right arm weakness and altered mental status. Over the past 4 months, she has had gradual onset of headaches that have progressively worsened, and her family reports that the patient has had cognitive problems over the past 1 to 2 weeks. Today she developed right arm weakness. She has no other pertinent history and takes no medications.

On physical examination, the patient is not oriented to place or date. Vital signs are normal. The patient has 4+/5 strength of the right upper extremity and achieves 16 of 30 points on the Mini-Mental State Examination; the remainder of the neurologic examination is normal.

Laboratory studies show a normal erythrocyte sedimentation rate, complete blood count with differential, and comprehensive metabolic panel; a negative ANCA; and a negative urinalysis.

Cerebrospinal fluid analysis shows a leukocyte count of 12/μL (12 × 10⁹/L; all lymphocytes) and a protein level of 70 mg/dL (700 mg/L); Gram stain and cultures are negative.

MRI of the brain shows diffuse nonspecific white matter changes and a low attenuation area in the right frontal lobe. Cerebral angiogram demonstrates multiple areas of vessel dilation and stenosis. Brain biopsy shows granulomatous vessel inflammation.

In addition to high-dose glucocorticoids, which of the following is the most appropriate management?

(A) Adalimumab
(B) Cyclophosphamide
(C) Methotrexate
(D) Rituximab

Item 33

A 27-year-old woman is evaluated for a sudden onset of joint pain and significant stiffness in her fingers, wrists, knees, and ankles for the past 3 days. She had a brief fever with muscle aches a few days ago and a faint, pink rash on her arms and legs at the same time. She reports no other symptoms. She takes no medications. She works at a daycare.

On physical examination, temperature is 37.2 °C (99.0 °F); other vital signs are normal. There are no rashes, hair loss, or oral ulcers. There is mild warmth and tenderness of the first through fifth proximal interphalangeal and metacarpophalangeal joints bilaterally as well as the wrists. Warmth and tenderness of the knees and ankles are also noted, with pain on range of motion.

Which of the following will most likely confirm the diagnosis?

(A) Antinuclear antibodies
(B) HIV testing
(C) Parvovirus B19 testing
(D) Rheumatoid factor

Item 34

A 36-year-old woman is evaluated for a 2-month history of morning stiffness in the hands, wrists, knees, and feet lasting 90 minutes. She recently noted difficulty making a fist in the morning and feels like she is walking on pebbles when she first gets out of bed. She feels better after a hot shower and activity. Her only medication is ibuprofen, which is helpful.

On physical examination, vital signs are normal. There is tenderness and swelling of the second, third, and fifth metacarpophalangeal joints bilaterally, the second through fourth proximal interphalangeal joints of both hands, the right wrist, the left knee, and the second through fifth metatarsophalangeal joints bilaterally. The remainder of the examination is normal.

Which of the following is the most appropriate diagnostic test to perform next?

(A) Anti-cyclic citrullinated peptide antibodies
(B) HLA-B27
(C) Parvovirus IgG antibodies
(D) Serum urate
(E) Thyroid-stimulating hormone

Item 35

A 73-year-old woman is evaluated for a 10-year history of osteoarthritis affecting multiple joints over the years, including the distal joints of her fingers, bases of the thumbs, knees, and cervical and lower lumbar spines. She has chronic daily pain in at least one joint. She has tried nonpharmacologic measures, and she had minimal benefit from intra-articular glucocorticoid and hyaluronic acid injections to her knees. She was recently diagnosed with peptic ulcer disease. History is also significant for coronary artery disease, diabetes mellitus, and hypertension. Medications are enalapril, carvedilol, metformin, atorvastatin, pantoprazole, and low-dose aspirin.

On physical examination, vital signs are normal. Heberden nodes and squaring of the bilateral carpometacarpal joints are present. Crepitus and limited extension of the cervical spine are noted. Bilateral knee varus deformity and bony enlargement are present, with crepitus on range of motion.

Which of the following is the most appropriate treatment?

(A) Duloxetine
(B) Gabapentin
(C) Ibuprofen
(D) Topical capsaicin

Item 36

A 35-year-old woman is hospitalized for left-sided pleuritic chest pain and dyspnea that began 1 day ago. Four weeks ago, she began to experience fever once or twice a day, pharyngitis, intermittent rash on the trunk and proximal extremities that occurs with the fever, severe joint pain, and myalgia. She gave birth 10 weeks ago to a healthy female infant.

On physical examination, temperature is 39.0 °C (102.2 °F), pulse rate is 90/min, and respiration rate is 22/min. Enlarged cervical lymph nodes, hepatomegaly, and splenomegaly are present. A pleural friction rub is heard. A pink maculopapular rash is present on the trunk. Tenderness and swelling of the wrists, knees, and ankles are noted.

Laboratory studies:

Erythrocyte sedimentation rate	90 mm/h
Hemoglobin	10 g/dL (100 g/L)
Leukocyte count	20,000/µL (20×10^9/L), 90% neutrophils
Alanine aminotransferase	80 U/L
Aspartate aminotransferase	70 U/L
Ferritin	6000 ng/mL (6000 µg/L)
Urinalysis	Normal

Chest radiograph shows a small left-sided pleural effusion.

Which of the following is the most likely diagnosis?

(A) Adult-onset Still disease
(B) Cryoglobulinemic vasculitis
(C) Lymphoma
(D) Microscopic polyangiitis
(E) Systemic lupus erythematosus

Item 37

A 49-year-old woman is evaluated for recently worsening joint symptoms. She has a 13-year history of Crohn disease characterized by four to six stools daily and mild crampy abdominal pain. She also has a 1-year history of arthritis. She currently has pain in the left knee, right ankle, and two joints of the right foot; diffuse swelling involving the left third toe; and 30 minutes of morning stiffness. She has been treated with various NSAIDs, which seem to worsen her bowel disease. She has tried, in succession, azathioprine, mesalamine, and methotrexate without notable improvement in her symptoms. She currently is taking methotrexate.

On physical examination, vital signs are normal. The left knee has a small effusion. Dactylitis of the left third toe is present. The right ankle and the right second and third metatarsophalangeal joints are tender to palpation.

Which of the following is the most appropriate long-term treatment?

(A) Adalimumab
(B) Intra-articular glucocorticoid injections
(C) Prednisone
(D) Rituximab

Item 38

A 64-year-old man is evaluated for a 9-month history of a swollen and painful right knee without trauma or injury. The knee has been drained twice; synovial fluid leukocyte counts were between 15,000/µL to 20,000/µL (15-20 × 10^9/L), predominantly lymphocytes. All stains and cultures have been negative. He also reports a low-grade fever in the evening. He has no history of skin rash or tick bites. He had a positive tuberculin skin test 20 years ago and was treated with isoniazid for an unknown duration. He takes no medications.

On physical examination, vital signs are normal. The right knee is tender and has a moderate effusion, with reduced passive range of motion. The remainder of the physical examination is normal.

Laboratory studies show an erythrocyte sedimentation rate of 48 mm/h and negative Lyme disease serologies.

Chest radiograph shows three small calcified granulomas in the left upper lobe. Plain radiograph of the right knee shows joint space narrowing, osteopenia, and small sinus tracts.

Which of the following is the most appropriate diagnostic test to perform next?

(A) Angiotensin-converting enzyme level
(B) CT of the chest
(C) HLA-B27 testing
(D) Synovial biopsy

Item 39

A 59-year-old woman is evaluated for a 5-year history of bilateral hand pain and stiffness of several hand joints, with enlargement and crookedness developing at some of the hand joints over the past few years. The stiffness is present in the morning and lasts about 30 minutes. One area of enlargement, at the right fourth distal interphalangeal (DIP) joint, has occasionally become abruptly swollen, red, and tender, and is currently inflamed. Family history is significant for deformed and painful, arthritic hand joints in her mother.

On physical examination, vital signs are normal. There are no rashes or nail changes. Grossly deformed digits on both hands with bony enlargement and deviation at the right second, left second and third, and bilateral fourth DIP joints are noted. A tender, erythematous bony nodule is present over the right fourth DIP joint. Significant squaring of the right carpometacarpal joint is also present. The remainder of the musculoskeletal examination is normal.

Laboratory studies show normal erythrocyte sedimentation rate, C-reactive protein, serum urate, rheumatoid factor, and anti–cyclic citrullinated peptide antibodies.

A hand radiograph is shown (see top of next column).

Which of the following is the most likely diagnosis?

(A) Erosive osteoarthritis
(B) Gout
(C) Psoriatic arthritis
(D) Rheumatoid arthritis

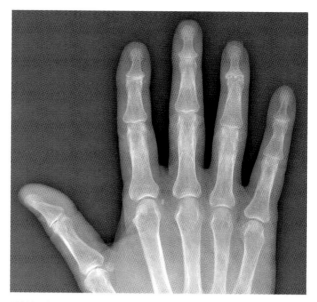

ITEM 39

Item 40

A 21-year-old woman is evaluated for a 2-week history of worsening rash and arthritis as well as intermittent low-grade fever. She has a 5-year history of systemic lupus erythematosus (SLE). She has been doing well without active disease for the past 3 years and has been compliant with hydroxychloroquine.

On physical examination, temperature is 37.8 °C (100.0 °F), and blood pressure is 150/86 mm Hg; other vital signs are normal. A malar rash is present. Diffuse tenderness and swelling of multiple small joints of the hands are present. New dependent edema is present.

Laboratory studies show low C3 and C4 complement levels, a serum creatinine level of 1.8 mg/dL (159.1 µmol/L), a urine protein-creatinine ratio of 3200 mg/g, and active urine sediment on microscopic examination.

Which of the following laboratory studies should be done next?

(A) Anti–double-stranded DNA antibodies
(B) Antinuclear antibodies
(C) Anti–Ro/SSA and anti-La/SSB antibodies
(D) Anti-Smith antibodies
(E) Anti–U1-ribonucleoprotein antibodies

Item 41

A 64-year-old woman is evaluated for worsening leg weakness. She was evaluated 2 weeks ago for a 3-week history of lower extremity weakness; laboratory studies showed a serum creatine kinase level of 23,000 U/L. History is notable for hypercholesterolemia treated with lovastatin, which was discontinued at the initial visit.

On physical examination, vital signs are normal. There is no rash. Examination shows 3/5 strength of the quadriceps and hamstrings (4/5 strength 2 weeks ago); 4/5 strength in the deltoids, biceps, and triceps; and 5/5

CONT. strength of the neck flexors, neck extensors, and distal upper and lower extremities. The remainder of the examination is normal.

Current laboratory studies show an erythrocyte sedimentation rate of 25 mm/h and a serum creatine kinase level of 20,876 U/L.

In addition to a muscle biopsy, which of the following is most likely to establish the diagnosis?

(A) Anti-cyclic citrullinated peptide antibodies
(B) Anti-cytosolic 5′-nucleotidase 1A antibodies
(C) Anti-histidyl tRNA synthetase antibodies
(D) Anti-HMG Co-A reductase antibodies

Item 42

A 32-year-old woman is evaluated for a 2-year history of dry eyes and dry mouth. She wakes up in the morning with a feeling like something is in her eyes. She cannot eat dry foods without consuming large amounts of water. She has noticed a change in the shape of her face; it has gotten more round. She previously saw an ophthalmologist who found abnormal ocular surface staining consistent with dry eyes. She uses artificial tears as needed.

On physical examination, vital signs are normal. There is no pooled saliva under the tongue. Bilateral parotid and lacrimal enlargement is present. The remainder of the examination is normal.

Antinuclear antibodies, anti-Ro/SSA antibodies, and rheumatoid factor are negative. Screening for HIV and hepatitis B and C is negative. Serum IgG levels are normal.

Chest radiograph is normal.

Which of the following is the most appropriate diagnostic test to perform next?

(A) CT of the chest
(B) Lip biopsy
(C) Parotid biopsy
(D) Schirmer test
(E) Sialography

Item 43

A 67-year-old woman is evaluated for a 3-year history of severe rheumatoid arthritis. She had an inadequate response to methotrexate and low-dose prednisone. She responded well to the addition of infliximab, but eventually the drug lost effect and she required a change in biologic therapy. She has done well with tocilizumab and methotrexate over the past year. She notes several months of prominent fatigue. History is also significant for type 2 diabetes mellitus, hypertension, and hyperlipidemia. Current medications are methotrexate, folic acid, tocilizumab, basal insulin, lisinopril, metoprolol, atorvastatin, ibuprofen, and omeprazole.

On physical examination, vital signs are normal. Joint examination reveals no swollen or tender joints. The remainder of the physical examination is normal.

Laboratory studies:

Hemoglobin	9.3 g/dL (93 g/L)
Leukocyte count	5600/μL (5.6 × 10⁹/L)
Mean corpuscular volume	111 fL
Platelet count	330,000/μL (330 × 10⁹/L)

Which of the following is the most likely cause of the anemia?

(A) Inflammation
(B) Iron deficiency
(C) Methotrexate
(D) Tocilizumab

Item 44

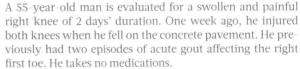

A 55-year-old man is evaluated for a swollen and painful right knee of 2 days' duration. One week ago, he injured both knees when he fell on the concrete pavement. He previously had two episodes of acute gout affecting the right first toe. He takes no medications.

On physical examination, temperature is 38.1 °C (100.6 °F); other vital signs are normal. There are superficial scrapes on the front of both knees. The right knee is swollen and tender and has a moderate effusion with redness; restriction of both passive and active range of motion due to pain is noted. The remainder of the examination is normal.

Plain radiograph of the right knee shows mild joint-space narrowing, an effusion, and soft-tissue swelling.

Which of the following is most likely to establish the diagnosis?

(A) Aspiration of the right knee
(B) Blood cultures
(C) Erythrocyte sedimentation rate
(D) MRI of the right knee

Item 45

A 65-year-old woman is evaluated during a follow-up visit for giant cell arteritis. Prior to confirmation of the diagnosis she was started on 60 mg of prednisone daily and low-dose aspirin. The diagnosis was subsequently confirmed with a temporal artery biopsy. She is otherwise healthy and takes no additional medications.

On physical examination, vital signs are normal. There is a healing incision over the right temporal artery.

Dual-energy x-ray absorptiometry (DEXA) was performed 6 months ago. Based upon the results of the Fracture Risk Assessment Tool, the patient was classified as medium risk (10%-20%) for a major osteoporotic fracture in the next 10 years.

Which of the following is the most appropriate next step in management?

(A) Begin alendronate
(B) Begin teriparatide
(C) Repeat DEXA
(D) No additional testing or therapy

Item 46

A 48-year-old woman is evaluated for 3 months of progressive exertional dyspnea. She was diagnosed with limited cutaneous systemic sclerosis 4 years ago. She also has Raynaud phenomenon and gastroesophageal reflux disease. Medications are nifedipine and omeprazole.

On physical examination, vital signs are normal. Oxygen saturation is 95% at rest, breathing ambient air. Scattered telangiectasias are present on the face, nose, and hands. Sclerodactyly at the fingers and tightness of the skin at the neck are noted. There is increased intensity of the pulmonic sound and a widened split S_2 on cardiac examination. Lungs are clear to auscultation.

Electrocardiogram and chest radiograph are normal.

Which of the following is the most likely cause of her symptom?

(A) Interstitial lung disease
(B) Myocardial fibrosis
(C) Pulmonary arterial hypertension
(D) Venous thromboembolic disease

Item 47

A 67-year-old man is evaluated for a 5-year history of right knee pain, with morning stiffness lasting 20 minutes.

On physical examination, vital signs are normal. Limitation of flexion and extension of the right knee is noted, with bony enlargement and tenderness to palpation along the medial and lateral joint lines. Crepitus is noted upon range of motion of the right knee. Bony enlargement of a few proximal interphalangeal and distal interphalangeal joints on both hands is present.

Which of the following is the most appropriate initial imaging study?

(A) CT
(B) MRI
(C) Radiography
(D) Ultrasonography

Item 48

A 50-year-old woman is evaluated for a 1-month history of pain around the lower part of the inner left knee. The pain is aggravated by ascending stairs and rising from a seated position. She has a history of knee osteoarthritis, for which she takes acetaminophen. Her new pain is different in location and intensity compared with her prior pain. She has no other pertinent personal or family history.

On physical examination, vital signs are normal. Tenderness to palpation and slight swelling over the proximal medial tibia about 6 cm below the anteromedial joint margin of the knee are noted. Examination of the knee shows no crepitus, minimal pain along the medial joint line, and no pain on valgus stress; anterior and posterior drawer signs are negative.

Which of the following is the most likely diagnosis?

(A) Medial collateral ligament tear
(B) Meniscal tear

(C) Pes anserine bursitis
(D) Quadriceps tendonitis

Item 49

A 48-year-old woman is evaluated for a 2-month history of increased dyspnea, wheezing, and nonproductive cough. She also reports intermittent pain and swelling in the wrists and knees for the past 6 months. She was diagnosed with scleritis of the left eye 1 month ago that improved with glucocorticoid drops. She also had two episodes of right pinna pain, redness, and swelling. Medications are prednisolone acetate ophthalmic and ibuprofen as needed for joint pain.

On physical examination, vital signs are normal. There is no rash. Sclerae are normal. Hearing is normal. The trachea is tender. On lung auscultation, wheezing is heard in both lung fields with no crackles or rubs. Swelling of the wrists and knees is present.

The ear findings are shown.

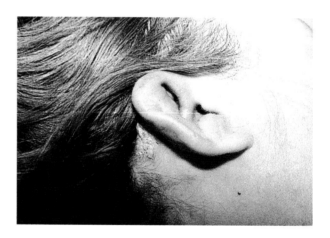

Laboratory studies show an erythrocyte sedimentation rate of 60 mm/h and a normal complete blood count with differential except for a hemoglobin level of 11 g/dL (110 g/L).

Chest radiograph is normal. CT of the chest reveals bronchial thickening with strictures; there is air trapping distal to the strictures.

Which of the following is the most likely diagnosis?

(A) Cogan syndrome
(B) Polyarteritis nodosa
(C) Relapsing polychondritis
(D) Systemic lupus erythematosus

Item 50

A 28-year-old woman requests a referral to an obstetrician. She has been attempting to conceive, and her menstrual period is now 3 weeks late. Her home pregnancy test was positive. She has a 2-year history of seropositive rheumatoid arthritis. Her only medication is hydroxychloroquine; methotrexate was stopped 4 months ago in anticipation of conception.

On physical examination, vital signs are normal. Swelling of the second and third metacarpophalangeal joints of the right hand is noted.

Pregnancy test is positive.

Which of the following is the most appropriate treatment at this time?

(A) Add etanercept

(B) Add leflunomide

(C) Discontinue hydroxychloroquine

(D) No change in therapy

Item 51

A 68-year-old man is evaluated in the emergency department for a 4-week history of severe lower left leg pain, swelling, and redness. The pain is localized to the shin and ankle. He was previously diagnosed with cellulitis, but no improvement was seen with sequential courses of cephalexin and clindamycin. History is also significant for gout and atrial fibrillation. Medications are allopurinol, colchicine, and apixaban.

On physical examination, vital signs are normal. The left lower shin is erythematous, warm, and tender to palpation; the erythema is not sharply demarcated. The left ankle is swollen, warm, and tender. There is no ulceration or skin breakdown over lower legs or feet. Solid masses at the extensor surfaces of both elbows are present.

Laboratory studies show an erythrocyte sedimentation rate of 90 mm/h and a serum urate level of 6.8 mg/dL (0.40 mmol/L). Blood cultures performed 1 week ago were negative.

Plain radiographs of the left shin and ankle show no changes suggestive of osteomyelitis.

Aspiration of the left ankle yields no fluid.

Which of the following is the most appropriate next step in management?

(A) Indomethacin

(B) Intravenous clindamycin

(C) MRI of the lower leg

(D) Prednisone

(E) Surgical debridement

Item 52

A 47-year-old woman is evaluated during a follow-up visit for a 2-year history of symptoms diagnosed 4 months ago as fibromyalgia. She reports ongoing widespread pain, fatigue, and difficulty concentrating. She does not have trouble falling asleep, but her sleep is nonrestorative. She was seen 3 months ago, and was given duloxetine and instructed to exercise. The medication produced a modest benefit, but she continues to have difficulty working as a housekeeper. She can only exercise to a limited extent without experiencing disabling pain for the next several days. On a 9-point pain scale, her pain was formerly an 8; after initiation of duloxetine, it decreased to a 5.

On physical examination, vital signs are normal. There is tenderness between the shoulder blades and at the occiput, trapezius, elbows, and hips bilaterally. There is no joint swelling.

Which of the following is the most appropriate treatment?

(A) Add meloxicam

(B) Add pregabalin

(C) Discontinue duloxetine; start gabapentin

(D) Discontinue duloxetine; start sertraline

Item 53

A 44-year-old woman is evaluated for recent-onset dyspnea on exertion and a nonproductive cough. She has a 1-year history of diffuse cutaneous systemic sclerosis. She takes no medications.

On physical examination, vital signs are normal. Oxygen saturation is 96% breathing ambient air. Skin thickening is noted on the face, neck, anterior chest, upper extremities to the mid forearm bilaterally, and lower extremities to the mid calf bilaterally. Heart examination is normal. There are fine crackles at the bases of both lungs on auscultation.

Anti–Scl-70 antibodies are strongly positive.

Pulmonary function tests:

	Today	6 Months Ago
FVC	85% of predicted	96% of predicted
D$_{LCO}$	65% of predicted	75% of predicted

High-resolution CT scan of the chest shows lower lobe ground-glass opacities in a pattern consistent with nonspecific interstitial pneumonitis.

Which of the following is the most appropriate treatment?

(A) Cyclophosphamide

(B) High-dose glucocorticoids

(C) Methotrexate

(D) Mycophenolate mofetil

Item 54

A 30-year-old woman is evaluated for a 3-month history of pain and swelling of the proximal interphalangeal (PIP) joints. She has difficulty performing tasks such as gripping or typing. Naproxen provides minimal relief.

On physical examination, vital signs are normal. There are no rashes or oral ulcers. Swelling and tenderness of the PIP joints bilaterally are noted. Pain occurs with flexion of the fingers. There is blanching coloration of the fingers and cyanosis at the fingertips. Nailfold examination shows a few dilated capillary loops. There are no cardiopulmonary friction rubs. The remainder of the examination is normal.

Laboratory studies performed 1 month ago showed the following: a positive antinuclear antibody titer of 1:320 with a speckled pattern; negative anti–double-stranded DNA antibodies, anti-Smith antibodies, anti-U1-ribonucleoprotein antibodies, anti-Ro/SSA antibodies, anti-La/SSB antibodies, anti–cyclic citrullinated peptide antibodies, and rheumatoid factor; and normal complete blood count with differential, serum creatinine, and urinalysis.

Radiographs of the hands are normal.

Which of the following is the most appropriate management?

(A) Add hydroxychloroquine
(B) Discontinue naproxen; begin ibuprofen
(C) Obtain plain radiography of the feet
(D) Repeat anti–double-stranded DNA antibodies
(E) Repeat antinuclear antibodies

Item 55

A 78-year-old woman is evaluated for knee pain that occurs when walking, ascending and descending stairs, and getting up from a seated position. She was diagnosed with bilateral knee osteoarthritis 10 years ago. She has tried acetaminophen, up to 3000 mg/d in divided doses, without significant relief.

Previous examinations have documented bony hypertrophy and crepitus on range of motion of the knees with weakness of the quadriceps.

She is scheduled to begin physical therapy. Topical diclofenac is prescribed.

The patient should be warned about which of the following possible side effects?

(A) Eye and mucous membrane irritation
(B) Localized lipoatrophy
(C) Localized skin hypopigmentation
(D) Localized skin rash

Item 56

A 78-year-old woman is evaluated for a 2-week history of pain and swelling in the left wrist. In the past year, she experienced two similar episodes, one in the left knee and one in the left wrist, each resolving after 3 weeks.

On physical examination, the patient appears well. Vital signs are normal. The left wrist is swollen, warm, and tender, with decreased range of motion.

Laboratory studies show an erythrocyte sedimentation rate of 53 mm/h and a serum urate level of 3.8 mg/dL (0.22 mmol/L).

A plain radiograph of the left wrist is shown.

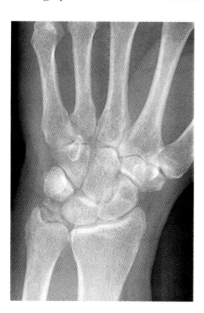

Which of the following is the most likely diagnosis?

(A) Acute calcium pyrophosphate crystal arthritis
(B) Gout
(C) Infectious arthritis
(D) Palindromic rheumatism

Item 57

A 48-year-old man is evaluated for a 3-week history of slowly progressive dyspnea on exertion, left-sided chest pain, and fever. He has a 20-year history of anti-cyclic citrullinated peptide antibody–positive rheumatoid arthritis. Prior to starting a tumor necrosis factor α inhibitor, his tuberculin skin test was nonreactive. Medications are methotrexate, etanercept, and folic acid. Despite these medications, he has morning stiffness for 1 hour and has swelling of the joints in his hands, wrists, and feet.

On physical examination, temperature is 37.8 °C (100 °F), blood pressure is 148/84 mm Hg, pulse rate is 100/min, and respiration rate is 24/min. Breath sounds are absent at the right base, with dullness on percussion. Joint changes typical of rheumatoid arthritis are present, along with swelling and tenderness of eight joints. The remainder of the examination is normal.

Chest radiograph shows a moderate right-sided pleural effusion.

Pleural fluid analysis following a thoracentesis shows a leukocyte count of 3500/μL (3.5×10^9/L) with 4% neutrophils, 87% lymphocytes, and 9% monocytes; a pleural fluid glucose level of 6.0 mg/dL (0.3 mmol/L); a pH of 7.2; and a pleural fluid lactate dehydrogenase level of 900 U/L. A pleural fluid adenosine deaminase measurement is low, at 30 U/L.

Which of the following is the most likely cause of the pleural effusion?

(A) Malignancy
(B) Parapneumonic effusion
(C) Rheumatoid pleuritis
(D) Tuberculosis

Item 58

A 36-year-old woman is hospitalized for acute kidney injury and hypertension. She has an 18-month history of diffuse cutaneous systemic sclerosis. She was well and taking no medications prior to hospitalization.

On physical examination, temperature is 36.6 °C (97.8 °F), blood pressure is 240/130 mm Hg, pulse rate is 100/min, and respiration rate is 18/min. Cardiac examination reveals a prominent S_4. Pulmonary auscultation reveals bibasilar crackles. Cutaneous examination reveals sclerodactyly of both hands as well as skin induration of the forearms and anterior chest.

Laboratory studies:

Hemoglobin	8.0 g/dL (80 g/L)
Platelet count	90,000/μL (90×10^9/L)
Creatinine	4.9 mg/dL (433.1 μmol/L)
Urinalysis	2+ protein; a few hyaline casts

Peripheral blood smear shows schistocytes and decreased platelets.

Which of the following is the most likely diagnosis?

(A) Disseminated intravascular coagulation
(B) Hemolytic uremic syndrome
(C) Scleroderma renal crisis
(D) Thrombotic thrombocytopenic purpura

Item 59

A 31-year-old man is evaluated in the emergency department for fever and red, painful eyes. He reports a 1-month history of intermittent painful oral and genital ulcers, knee pain, and fever, and 1 week of bilateral eye redness, pain, and photophobia.

On physical examination, temperature is 38.3 °C (101.0 °F), and pulse rate is 100/min. Slit lamp examination reveals white cells in the anterior chambers of both eyes. There are aphthous ulcers on the tongue and one aphthous ulcer on the scrotum. Swelling and warmth are noted in both knees. The heart, lung, abdominal, and neurologic examinations are normal.

Which of the following is the most likely diagnosis?

(A) Behçet syndrome
(B) Crohn disease
(C) Sarcoidosis
(D) Systemic lupus erythematosus

Item 60

An 82-year-old woman is evaluated for a 3-year history of chronic discomfort and stiffness in the hands, wrists, and shoulders. Some of these joints intermittently become acutely swollen and warm. She currently has 3 days of severe left wrist pain and swelling. She previously had been diagnosed with seronegative rheumatoid arthritis; there was no improvement with sulfasalazine or intravenous infliximab, both of which were discontinued. Short courses of prednisone have alleviated the acute attacks of arthritis. History is also significant for hypertension and stage 3 chronic kidney disease. Medications are hydrochlorothiazide, metoprolol, and losartan.

On physical examination, vital signs are normal. Decreased range of motion of both wrists and a few metacarpophalangeal (MCP) joints is noted, and shoulder abduction is limited to 90 degrees passively. The left wrist is swollen and tender. There are no subcutaneous nodules at the elbows, hands, or heels.

Laboratory studies:

Erythrocyte sedimentation rate	51 mm/h
Urate	4.3 mg/dL (0.25 mmol/L)
Rheumatoid factor	15 U/mL (15 kU/L)
Anti–cyclic citrullinated peptide antibodies	Negative

Radiographs show osteoarthritic changes at the second through fourth MCP joints bilaterally, both wrists, and glenohumeral joints. Chondrocalcinosis is seen in the knees

and both wrists. There are no periarticular erosions in the wrists or hands.

Which of the following is the most appropriate treatment?

(A) Adalimumab
(B) Allopurinol
(C) Low-dose prednisone
(D) Methotrexate
(E) NSAID therapy

Item 61

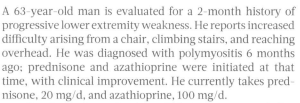

A 63-year-old man is evaluated for a 2-month history of progressive lower extremity weakness. He reports increased difficulty arising from a chair, climbing stairs, and reaching overhead. He was diagnosed with polymyositis 6 months ago; prednisone and azathioprine were initiated at that time, with clinical improvement. He currently takes prednisone, 20 mg/d, and azathioprine, 100 mg/d.

On physical examination, vital signs are normal. The patient cannot arise from the chair without using his arms to push off and can squat only by using his hands to hold on to the chair. He has cushingoid features and scattered ecchymoses on the forearms. There is no rash.

Laboratory studies show a serum creatine kinase level of 160 U/L.

Which of the following is the most appropriate management?

(A) Order electromyography
(B) Order muscle biopsy
(C) Reduce azathioprine dose
(D) Reduce prednisone dose

Item 62

A 26-year-old woman is evaluated for a 4-week history of progressive dyspnea on exertion. She has experienced malaise and myalgia for the past 6 months, noting that her arms ache when she does physical activity with them. She was previously healthy. She reports no rashes, headache or jaw claudication, gastrointestinal symptoms, or neurologic symptoms.

On physical examination, blood pressure is 120/60 mm Hg in the right arm and 95/50 in the left arm, pulse rate is 80/min, and respiration rate is 18/min. There is no rash. A reduced radial pulse in the left upper extremity is noted. A grade 2/6 decrescendo diastolic murmur at the left sternal border is heard. The lungs are clear. There is no synovitis. Strength is normal.

Laboratory studies:

Complete blood count	Normal, except for anemia
Erythrocyte sedimentation rate	90 mm/h
Hemoglobin	10 g/dL (100 g/L)
Creatinine	Normal
Antinuclear antibodies	Negative
Urinalysis	Negative

Transthoracic echocardiogram shows mild to moderate aortic valve regurgitation, dilated aortic root, normal valve leaflets, left ventricle dilation, and normal left ventricular ejection fraction.

Which of the following is the most likely diagnosis?

(A) Giant cell arteritis
(B) IgA vasculitis
(C) Kawasaki disease
(D) Polyarteritis nodosa
(E) Takayasu arteritis

Item 63

A 25-year-old woman is evaluated for a 2-month history of joint pain and swelling involving the hands, knees, and feet.

On physical examination, vital signs are normal. Swelling is noted at the second and third metacarpophalangeal joints of both hands, the left wrist, both knees, and the second through fifth metatarsophalangeal joints of both feet.

Laboratory studies are positive for rheumatoid factor and anti-cyclic citrullinated peptide antibodies.

Radiographs of the hands and feet are normal.

In addition to methotrexate and short-term prednisone, which of the following should be initiated?

(A) Folic acid
(B) Niacin
(C) Thiamine
(D) Vitamin C

Item 64

A 55-year-old man is evaluated for a 3-week history of progressive joint pain, swelling of the ankles, and occasional dry cough. He also reports a 2-day history of low-grade fever and painful red lumps on his shins. He has no other significant history and takes no medications.

On physical examination, temperature is 37.8 °C (100.0 °F); other vital signs are normal. The chest is clear to auscultation. Swelling and warmth of the ankles are noted. There are three raised, erythematous, and indurated subcutaneous nodules on the right anterior shin and one on the left anterior shin.

Laboratory studies show a normal complete blood count and an erythrocyte sedimentation rate of 70 mm/h.

Chest radiograph shows bilateral hilar adenopathy but is otherwise normal.

Which of the following is the most appropriate management?

(A) Biopsy of the hilar node
(B) Biopsy of a shin lesion
(C) Rheumatoid factor testing
(D) Synovial fluid cultures
(E) No further testing

Item 65

A 30-year-old woman is evaluated in the emergency department for worsening abdominal pain over past 2 days as well as a rash starting in the feet and spreading up to the thighs and buttocks. She feels generally achy in the joints and muscles. She reports no diarrhea, vomiting, or nausea. She was previously healthy. She takes no medications.

On physical examination, vital signs are normal. A palpable purpuric rash is noted on the feet, legs, and buttocks. There is peri-umbilical tenderness to palpation.

Stool is positive for occult blood.

Laboratory studies:

Complete blood count with differential	Normal
Erythrocyte sedimentation rate	70 mm/h
Antinuclear antibodies	Negative
ANCA	Negative
Urinalysis	Normal

CT of the abdomen shows a short segment of small bowel thickening and edema.

Which of the following is the most appropriate test to establish the diagnosis?

(A) Kidney biopsy
(B) Mesenteric angiography
(C) Serum IgA levels
(D) Skin biopsy with immunofluorescence

Item 66

A 53-year-old man is evaluated for a 5-year history of recurrent gout attacks involving the base of the great toes, mid feet, and ankles. Episodes are becoming more frequent and severe. History is also significant for hypertension and stage 3 chronic kidney disease. Medications are lisinopril and metoprolol. The patient is of Thai descent.

On physical examination, vital signs are normal. There are no tophi or swollen joints.

Laboratory studies show a serum urate level of 9.2 mg/dL (0.54 mmol/L).

Which of the following is the most appropriate next step in management?

(A) Begin allopurinol
(B) Begin probenecid
(C) Measure antinuclear antibodies
(D) Order HLA-B*5801 allele testing

Item 67

A 45-year-old man is evaluated for a 3-month history of swollen and painful hands and toes of both feet, without trauma or injury. He also has morning stiffness of the small joints of the hands and feet lasting 2 hours. He takes no medications.

On physical examination, vital signs are normal. Diffuse tenderness and swelling are noted in the third and fourth toes of the right foot, fourth toe of the left foot, and third and fourth digits of the left hand. The remainder of the joint examination is normal.

The appearance of the hand digits is shown (see top of next page).

Plain radiographs of the feet show joint-space narrowing and soft-tissue swelling of the digits without erosions.

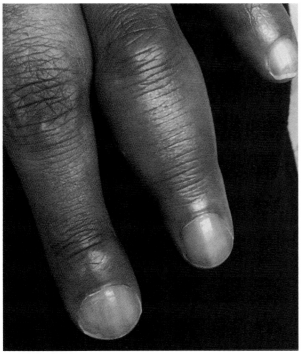

ITEM 67

Which of the following disorders is most likely to be associated with this patient's presentation?

(A) Infectious arthritis
(B) Rheumatoid arthritis
(C) Spondyloarthritis
(D) Systemic lupus erythematosus

Item 68

A 54-year-old man is evaluated for a 5-month history of mid lower back pain. The pain radiates from the center of his back to his flanks and abdomen. He has intermittent numbness in the areas of the pain. He also reports a 2.3-kg (5-lb) weight loss over the past 3 months. He emigrated from India to the United States 20 years ago and travels to India yearly. He has tried ibuprofen for the pain without relief and takes no other medications.

On physical examination, temperature is 38.2 °C (100.8 °F); other vital signs are normal. Examination of the spine reveals kyphosis, tenderness to palpation, and paraspinal muscle tightness around T10. Decreased sensation to light touch along the T10 dermatome is noted.

Chest radiograph shows calcified granuloma in the right upper lobe. Thoracic spine radiograph shows marked kyphosis and erosive changes and collapse of the anterior portions of the T10 and T11 vertebral bodies, destruction of the T10-11 disk space, and surrounding fusiform paravertebral swelling.

Which of the following is the most likely diagnosis?

(A) Herniated intervertebral disk
(B) Multiple myeloma
(C) Osteoporosis
(D) Tuberculous vertebral osteomyelitis

Item 69

A 43-year-old man is evaluated for knee, hip, shoulder, and arm stiffness, worsening over the past year. He also has pain in the arms, legs, neck, and torso, both on and between the joints. He states that his discomfort is continuous. He also reports chronic fatigue, lack of sleep, a band-like headache, and difficulty concentrating. He also has intermittent constipation and diarrhea. He takes acetaminophen and ibuprofen as needed for pain without much benefit.

On physical examination, the patient appears tired and anxious, with no acute distress. Vital signs are normal. He has minimal tenderness on palpation of multiple muscle groups. Full range of motion of all joints without crepitus is noted. There is no joint swelling or rash.

Laboratory studies, including complete blood count, erythrocyte sedimentation rate, serum creatine kinase, and thyroid-stimulating hormone, are within normal limits.

Which of the following is the most likely diagnosis?

(A) Fibromyalgia
(B) Hypothyroidism
(C) Osteoarthritis
(D) Rheumatoid arthritis

Item 70

A 25-year-old woman is hospitalized for a 4-week history of swelling of the legs, weight gain, and shortness of breath on exertion. She was diagnosed with systemic lupus erythematosus 1 year ago when she presented with polyarthritis, rash, and alopecia. She was initially treated with hydroxychloroquine and prednisone with a good response.

On physical examination, blood pressure is 142/96 mm Hg; other vital signs are normal. There is pitting edema of the lower extremities extending to the knees. The remainder of the physical examination is normal.

Laboratory studies:

Erythrocyte sedimentation rate	68 mm/h
Hematocrit	38%
Complements (C3 and C4)	Low
Creatinine	1.0 mg/dL (88.4 µmol/L)
Anti-Smith antibodies	Positive
Anti–double-stranded DNA antibodies	Positive
Urinalysis	3+ protein; no erythrocytes; no leukocytes; no casts
Urine protein	6000 mg/24 h

The patient is started on prednisone, along with diuretics and an ACE inhibitor.

Kidney biopsy results show class V (membranous) lupus nephritis with absent chronicity and mild activity.

Which of the following is the most appropriate treatment of the kidney disease?

(A) Adalimumab
(B) Belimumab
(C) Cyclophosphamide
(D) Methotrexate
(E) Mycophenolate mofetil

Item 71

A 45-year-old woman is evaluated for increased pain and swelling in her left knee and right ankle. She has a 5-year history of psoriatic arthritis and psoriasis treated with methotrexate, which previously improved her joint and skin symptoms. She also takes folic acid.

On physical examination, vital signs are normal. There is an erythematous, flaky patch on the left elbow. Nail pitting is present. The left knee has a moderate effusion and is warm without erythema, with discomfort on range of motion. The right ankle is swollen anteriorly, with discomfort on range of motion in flexion and extension.

Laboratory studies show an erythrocyte sedimentation rate of 30 mm/h.

Plain radiographs of the left knee show mild medial and lateral joint space narrowing.

Aspiration of the left knee shows a leukocyte count of 7500/µL (7.5 × 10⁹/L), with 50% neutrophils.

Which of the following is the most efficacious medication to add to this patient's treatment regimen?

(A) Abatacept
(B) Hydroxychloroquine
(C) Infliximab
(D) Rituximab

Item 72

A 24-year-old man is evaluated for increasing left buttock pain that worsens over the course of the day. It is improved by exercise and does not improve with rest. The pain had a gradual onset 1 year ago without a clear precipitant. At that time, radiographs were unremarkable, and physical therapy provided no benefit. He has stopped exercising because of the increasing discomfort. Family history includes ankylosing spondylitis in his father. The patient takes no medications.

On physical examination, vital signs are normal. Normal range of motion of the lumbar spine is noted. There is no reduction in lateral bending and no limitation of cervical spine motion in any plane. There are no warm, erythematous, or swollen joints.

Laboratory studies show the presence of HLA-B27; normal complete blood count and C-reactive protein; and negative rheumatoid factor and anti-cyclic citrullinated peptide antibodies.

Radiographs of the lumbar spine are normal.

Which of the following is the most appropriate treatment?

(A) Diclofenac
(B) Etanercept
(C) Methotrexate
(D) Sulfasalazine

Item 73

A 58-year-old man is evaluated for a 3-year history of left knee stiffness, which was intermittent but has become more persistent in the past 4 months. He reports no daily pain but has knee stiffness for 10 minutes in the morning and when he sits for an extended period of time. He reports no swelling and no knee buckling or locking. History is significant for gastroesophageal reflux disease and peptic ulcer disease diagnosed 6 months ago now treated with omeprazole. He prefers not to take medications for his knee symptoms.

On physical examination, vital signs are normal. BMI is 24. Crepitus and medial joint line tenderness to palpation are noted. There is no redness, effusion, or signs of knee instability.

Left knee radiograph shows mild medial joint space narrowing and spiking of the tibial spines.

Which of the following is the most appropriate management?

(A) Ibuprofen
(B) Intra-articular glucocorticoids
(C) Left knee MRI
(D) Physical therapy

Item 74

A 21-year-old woman is evaluated for an 8-week history of fatigue and low-grade fever. Last week she developed a facial rash. She takes a multivitamin.

On physical examination, vital signs are normal. The remainder of the examination is normal.

The appearance of the face is shown.

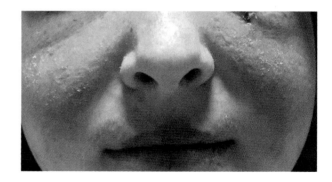

Which of the following is the most likely diagnosis for the rash?

(A) Acute cutaneous lupus erythematosus
(B) Erysipelas
(C) Rosacea
(D) Seborrheic dermatitis
(E) Subacute cutaneous lupus erythematosus

Item 75

A 53-year-old woman is evaluated for intermittent sensory loss in the hands and an occasional shock-like sensation from the neck down the back with neck flexion. She has not noted any weakness. She has a 15-year history of

CONT.

rheumatoid arthritis. Medications are methotrexate, etanercept, and folic acid.

On physical examination, vital signs are normal. Ulnar deviation of the metacarpophalangeal joints on both hands is present without active synovitis. Neck flexion triggers her symptoms. There is no muscle atrophy at the hands. Tinel and Phalen signs at the wrist are negative. Reflexes, strength, and sensation of the upper and lower extremities are normal.

Which of the following is the most appropriate diagnostic test to perform next?

(A) Electrodiagnostic studies of the upper extremities
(B) Flexion/extension radiography of the cervical spine
(C) Serum vitamin B$_{12}$ level
(D) Thyroid-stimulating hormone level

 ## Item 76

A 36-year-old woman is brought to the emergency department by her family for mental status changes. For the past 2 days, the family has noticed forgetfulness, confusion, and alteration of personality. She has a 5-year history of systemic lupus erythematosus (SLE), which has been quiescent. One week ago, she developed fatigue, a diffuse erythematous rash, and polyarthritis. There is no history of focal deficits, seizures, or neck stiffness. She does not have a fever. History is also significant for hypertension. Medications are losartan, hydroxychloroquine, prednisone, 5 mg/d, and a daily multivitamin.

On physical examination, the patient is alert, awake, and follows commands but is not oriented to place and time. She is afebrile, and vital signs are normal. Neurologic examination other than mental status is normal, with no motor or sensory deficits. There is no neck stiffness. The remainder of the examination is normal.

Laboratory studies:

Erythrocyte sedimentation rate	42 mm/h
Complements (C3 and C4)	Low
C-reactive protein	0.2 mg/dL (2.0 mg/L)
Creatinine	1.4 mg/dL (123.8 µmol/L)
Antinuclear antibodies	Titer: 1:320
Cerebrospinal fluid analysis	Normal cell count and glucose; protein, 85 mg/dL (850 mg/L)

CT scan of the brain is normal. MRI with MR angiogram of the brain shows multiple small punctate white matter changes in periventricular areas. There is no evidence of vasculitis or blood vessel narrowing.

Which of the following is the most likely diagnosis?

(A) Acute bacterial meningitis
(B) Neuropsychiatric systemic lupus erythematosus
(C) Status epilepticus
(D) Steroid-induced psychosis

Item 77

An 18-year-old man is seen for a physical examination required to join the ice hockey team at his university. He was diagnosed with Kawasaki disease at age 5 years; he

does not recall how or if he was treated for the disease. He has medical records from his pediatrician who has provided ongoing care until now.

Physical examination, including vital signs, is normal.

Which of the following disease complications is most important in determining the nature of his sports evaluation and prognosis?

(A) Bundle branch block
(B) Coronary artery aneurysm
(C) Myocarditis
(D) Pericarditis

Item 78

A 38-year-old woman seeks advice regarding preventative measures for developing osteoarthritis. One year ago, she started an exercise regimen of running approximately 20 miles per week. She has no joint pain when running. History is significant for polycystic ovary syndrome. Family history is notable for both parents having knee replacements for osteoarthritis. Her only medication is an oral contraceptive.

On physical examination, vital signs are normal. BMI is 31. Musculoskeletal examination is normal.

Which of the following is the most appropriate preventive measure for this patient?

(A) Begin chondroitin sulfate supplements
(B) Begin vitamin D
(C) Recommend weight loss
(D) Stop running

Item 79

A 32-year-old woman is evaluated in the emergency department for a 2-day history of headache and vomiting. She was diagnosed with Raynaud phenomenon 1 year ago and gastroesophageal reflux disease 6 months ago. Her only medication is omeprazole.

On physical examination, temperature is 38.0 °C (100.4 °F), blood pressure is 240/140 mm Hg, pulse rate is 88/min, respiration rate is 16/min, and oxygen saturation is 96% breathing ambient air. Skin findings are digital pitting at the ends of the fingers, thickening of the skin over the fingers and dorsum of the hands, and thickening with poikilodermic changes over the skin of the anterior chest.

Laboratory studies:

Hematocrit	32%
Platelet count	75,000/µL (75 × 10^9/L)
Creatinine	1.5 mg/dL (132.6 µmol/L)
Urinalysis	2+ protein; no blood

Peripheral blood smear shows diminished platelet numbers and schistocytes.

Which of the following is the most appropriate treatment?

(A) Captopril
(B) Cyclophosphamide
(C) Methylprednisolone
(D) Nitroprusside

Item 80

A 32-year-old woman is evaluated during a follow-up visit for a 3-month history of arthralgia affecting the hands, wrists, knees, and feet. At her initial visit 3 weeks ago, joint examination demonstrated nine tender and six swollen joints; prednisone, 10 mg/d, was initiated at that time. She now reports some benefit from the prednisone for morning stiffness and joint pain. Family history is notable for her mother with seropositive erosive rheumatoid arthritis.

Laboratory studies from 3 weeks ago showed an erythrocyte sedimentation rate of 38 mm/h, and high levels of rheumatoid factor and anti–cyclic citrullinated peptide antibodies.

On physical examination today, vital signs are normal. The second and third proximal interphalangeal joints on the right hand and the second metacarpophalangeal joint on the left hand are tender and swollen. Her clinical disease activity index score is 12, indicating moderate disease activity.

Radiographs of the hands and feet are normal.

Which of the following is the most appropriate treatment at this time?

(A) Increase prednisone
(B) Initiate ibuprofen
(C) Initiate methotrexate
(D) Initiate mycophenolate mofetil

Item 81

A 34-year-old woman is evaluated for a 6-month history of gradually increasing pain in the left groin with some radiation to the left buttock, particularly with stair climbing. She has a 2-year history of lupus nephritis. Medications are hydroxychloroquine, mycophenolate mofetil, and prednisone.

On physical examination, vital signs are normal. Musculoskeletal examination reveals weakness of the left hip flexors. Decreased passive range of motion of the left hip in both external and internal rotation with pain is noted.

Which of the following is the most appropriate initial test to evaluate the patient's hip pain?

(A) Dual-energy x-ray absorptiometry
(B) MRI of the left hip
(C) Plain radiography of the left hip
(D) Ultrasonography

Item 82

A 65-year-old man is evaluated in the emergency department for left knee pain and swelling of 10 days' duration. He reports no other joint pain. He has a 15-year history of rheumatoid arthritis, which has been well controlled with methotrexate and adalimumab. He began taking over-the-counter naproxen 8 days ago, without improvement.

On physical examination, temperature is 38.1 °C (100.6 °F), blood pressure is 106/68 mm Hg, and pulse rate is 97/min. The left knee is erythematous, warm, and tender to touch, with a large effusion; range of motion is limited, especially flexion. Examination of the other joints is normal.

Laboratory studies show an erythrocyte sedimentation rate of 53 mm/h and a leukocyte count of 12,000/µL (12 × 10⁹/L).

Which of the following is the most appropriate next step in management?

(A) Perform arthrocentesis
(B) Start colchicine
(C) Start prednisone
(D) Start sulfasalazine

Item 83

A 52-year-old man is evaluated for an episodic rash on the legs for the past month; diffuse arthralgia and Raynaud phenomenon for 2 months; and burning pain and tingling of the feet for 3 months. He has a remote history of intravenous drug use. He takes no medications.

On physical examination, vital signs are normal. Cyanosis of the fingertips is noted. There is no sclerodactyly, dilated capillary loops of fingernail beds, or digital pitting. Palpable purpura is present on the lower legs. Reduced sensation to pinprick of the soles of the feet is noted. The remainder of the examination is normal.

Laboratory studies:

Erythrocyte sedimentation rate	70 mm/h
C3	Normal
C4	Low
Rheumatoid factor	Positive
Antinuclear antibodies	Negative
Cryoglobulins	Positive
Urinalysis	1+ blood; 2+ protein

Chest radiograph is normal. Skin biopsy shows leukocytoclastic vasculitis.

Which of the following is the most appropriate test to perform next?

(A) Anticentromere antibodies
(B) Anti–cyclic citrullinated peptide antibodies
(C) Anti–Jo-1 antibodies
(D) Anti–U1-ribonucleoprotein antibodies
(E) Hepatitis C antibodies

Item 84

A 30-year-old man is evaluated for a 7-year history of intermittent pain and swelling in multiple fingers and toes, along with 1 hour of morning stiffness. History is notable for an episode of swelling of the left second toe 2 years ago. He has been treated with multiple NSAIDs over the years, with ibuprofen being the most efficacious.

On physical examination, vital signs are normal. Mild soft-tissue swelling of the fourth and fifth distal interphalangeal (DIP) joints bilaterally is present. Tenderness is present with metacarpophalangeal joint squeeze on the left. There is no rash.

The patient's nail findings are shown (see top of next page).

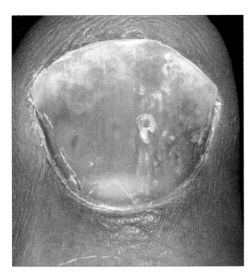

ITEM 84

Laboratory studies show a serum urate level of 6.7 mg/dL (0.40 mmol/L); rheumatoid factor and anti-cyclic citrullinated peptide antibodies are negative.

Plain radiographs of the hands show pencil-in-cup deformities of the DIP joints of the third and fourth digits bilaterally; there is no periarticular osteopenia.

Which of the following is the most likely diagnosis?

(A) Gouty arthritis
(B) Psoriatic arthritis
(C) Reactive arthritis
(D) Rheumatoid arthritis

Item 85

A 32-year-old woman is evaluated for an 8-week history of fatigue and low-grade fever. She also reports swelling and tenderness of the hand joints, along with morning stiffness lasting 2 hours. Over the past 2 weeks, she has been taking naproxen with relief. Last week, she developed swelling of the legs and gained 4.5 kg (10 lb).

On physical examination, blood pressure is 152/96 mm Hg; other vital signs are normal. A malar rash is present. Active tenderness and swelling of multiple joints of the hands are noted. There is pitting edema of the lower extremities. The remainder of the physical examination is normal.

Laboratory studies:

Erythrocyte sedimentation rate	88 mm/h
Hematocrit	38%
Complements (C3, C4)	Low
Creatinine	1.1 mg/dL (97.2 µmol/L)
Antinuclear antibodies	Titer: 1:320
Anti-Smith antibodies	Positive
Anti–double-stranded DNA antibodies	Positive
Urinalysis	3+ protein; no erythrocytes; no leukocytes; no casts
Urine protein	4000 mg/24 h

Which of the following tests is most appropriate to perform next to assess this patient's kidney disease?

(A) Antiphospholipid antibodies
(B) CT of the abdomen and pelvis
(C) Kidney biopsy
(D) Renal arteriography
(E) Serum and urine protein electrophoresis

Item 86

A 71-year-old woman is evaluated for a 3-year history of rheumatoid arthritis. She reports burning and tingling sensations in her feet and legs that are worse at night, without exacerbation with position or activity. She has not noted back pain, lower extremity weakness, or bowel or bladder dysfunction. Medications are methotrexate, hydroxychloroquine, low-dose prednisone, and folic acid. Her rheumatoid arthritis was moderately active 6 months ago, at which time leflunomide was added with good response.

On physical examination, vital signs are normal. Decreased sensation to light touch and vibration is limited to the feet. Joint examination reveals one tender and two swollen metacarpophalangeal joints. Strength testing is intact throughout, and reflexes are intact. There are no skin rashes or lesions.

Laboratory studies show normal complete blood count, serum creatinine, blood glucose, and hemoglobin A_{1c} values.

Which of the following is the most appropriate next step in management?

(A) Begin gabapentin
(B) Increase prednisone
(C) Stop leflunomide
(D) Stop methotrexate

Item 87

An 83-year-old woman is evaluated for a 15-year history of gout. Attacks were initially limited to the first metatarsophalangeal joints and occurred once or twice a year. She now has recurrent attacks, occurring every 3 months. Her feet, ankles, knees, wrists, elbows, and hands have been affected. Attacks last for 1 to 2 weeks and have been treated with NSAIDs. History is also significant for recurrent nephrolithiasis, stage 3 chronic kidney disease, and hypertension. Medications are allopurinol, 400 mg/d; colchicine, 0.6 mg/d; and lisinopril. She tolerates her medications well.

On physical examination, vital signs are normal. There are palpable masses at the olecranon processes and white nodules on a few distal and proximal interphalangeal joints of both hands.

Laboratory studies show a serum creatinine level of 1.0 mg/dL (88.4 µmol/L) and a serum urate level of 5.8 mg/dL (0.34 mmol/L).

Which of the following is the most appropriate next step in management?

(A) Add probenecid
(B) Discontinue allopurinol; begin pegloticase infusions
(C) Increase allopurinol
(D) Increase colchicine

Item 88

A 40-year-old woman is evaluated for a 12-year history of inflammatory arthritis, puffy fingers, Raynaud phenomenon, serositis, and gastroesophageal reflux disease.

On physical examination, vital signs are normal. The fingers are puffy, and cyanosis of the fingertips is noted. Cardiac examination is normal. The lungs are clear. There is no friction rub heard on examination.

Laboratory studies show positive anti-U1-ribonucleoprotein antibodies.

Which of the following complications of this patient's disease is a major cause of early mortality?

(A) Central nervous system vasculitis

(B) Pericarditis

(C) Pulmonary arterial hypertension

(D) Rapidly progressive glomerulonephritis

Item 89

A 75-year-old woman is evaluated for a 15-year history of right knee pain, which recently has become more constant, with morning stiffness lasting 15 minutes. She participates in a home exercise program. Her knee pain persists despite treatment with acetaminophen. She could not tolerate topical capsaicin or diclofenac. History is also significant for atrial fibrillation and hypertension. Medications are dabigatran and diltiazem. She would like to improve her knee pain, because she is going on vacation in 2 weeks and will be walking a lot.

On physical examination, vital signs are normal. Examination of the right knee reveals crepitus upon movement, bony hypertrophy presenting as varus deformity, and no effusion or warmth.

Weight-bearing knee radiographs show moderate medial joint space narrowing, osteophytes at the medial femoral and tibial joint margins, and subchondral sclerosis at the medial tibia.

Which of the following is the most appropriate treatment?

(A) Alendronate

(B) Arthroscopic debridement and lavage

(C) Intra-articular glucocorticoid injection

(D) Pregabalin

(E) Tramadol

Item 90

A 26-year-old woman is evaluated for a rash on her scalp and polyarthritis associated with systemic lupus erythematosus (SLE). She was diagnosed with SLE 8 years ago with an initial presentation of photosensitivity, malar and discoid rashes, pleuropericarditis, and arthritis. She was initially treated with hydroxychloroquine, azathioprine, and glucocorticoids with a good response, but she has had intermittent flare-ups of arthritis and rash. She developed lupus nephritis 3 years ago and had a 6-month course of cyclophosphamide followed by mycophenolate mofetil (MMF). She is currently on MMF, hydroxychloroquine, and prednisone but continues to have joint and skin disease.

Methotrexate and leflunomide were tried, but she was not able to tolerate them. Her kidney disease is well controlled without any active nephritis.

On physical examination, vital signs are normal. Several hyperkeratotic, dyspigmented, discoid plaques are present on the scalp. Multiple joints of the hands are tender and swollen. The remainder of the examination is normal.

Laboratory studies:

Erythrocyte sedimentation rate	56 mm/h
Hematocrit	38%
Complements (C3, C4)	Low
Creatinine	1.5 mg/dL (132.6 µmol/L)
Anti-double-stranded DNA antibodies	Elevated
Urinalysis	Normal

Chest radiograph is normal.

Which of the following is the most appropriate therapeutic option to consider in this patient?

(A) Abatacept

(B) Adalimumab

(C) Belimumab

(D) Secukinumab

Item 91

A 74-year-old man is evaluated for pain and stiffness in the mid and lower spine that has progressively worsened over the past 10 years. The pain is worse with physical activity. He notes recent difficulty when bending to pick something up from the floor. He takes no medications.

On physical examination, vital signs are normal. No rash or nail changes are seen. Limited range of motion and pain on motion of thoracic and lumbar spine are noted. There is no peripheral joint swelling or tenderness and no sacroiliac tenderness. The FABER test of the hip is normal.

Laboratory studies show a normal erythrocyte sedimentation rate.

Thoracolumbar spine radiographs reveal bridging ossification on the right side along the anterolateral aspects of the vertebral bodies of T9-L2. Radiographs of the sacroiliac joints are normal.

Which of the following is the most likely diagnosis?

(A) Ankylosing spondylitis

(B) Calcium pyrophosphate deposition disease

(C) Diffuse idiopathic skeletal hyperostosis

(D) Psoriatic arthritis

Item 92

A 78-year-old man is evaluated in the emergency department. Five days ago he was diagnosed with community-acquired pneumonia at an urgent care center for which he was prescribed clarithromycin. Yesterday he developed generalized weakness and diarrhea. History is also significant for hypertension and gout. He has a history of allopurinol-induced drug rash. Current medications are lisinopril, colchicine, clarithromycin, and febuxostat.

CONT.

On physical examination, temperature is 36.9 °C (98.4 °F), blood pressure is 104/60 mm Hg, pulse rate is 112/min, respiration rate is 18/min, and oxygen saturation is 98% breathing ambient air. There is no rash. The oropharynx appears dry. The chest is clear to auscultation. Tophi are noted at the olecranon processes. There are no swollen or tender joints. Neurologic examination is normal.

Laboratory studies:

Absolute neutrophil count	1300/µL (1.3 × 10⁹/L)
Hemoglobin	9.8 g/dL (98 g/L)
Leukocyte count	2700/µL (2.7 × 10⁹/L)
Platelet count	96,000/µL (96 × 10⁹/L)
Reticulocyte count (corrected)	1.2%
Creatine kinase	8433 U/L
Creatinine	1.7 mg/dL (150.1 µmol/L)
Urinalysis	4+ blood; 0-1 erythrocytes/hpf; 0-2 leukocytes/hpf

There are no schistocytes seen on peripheral blood smear.

Which of the following is the most appropriate next step in management?

(A) Begin high-dose glucocorticoids

(B) Begin plasma exchange

(C) Stop colchicine and clarithromycin

(D) Stop febuxostat

Item 93

A 33-year-old woman is evaluated for a 4-week history of recurrent worsening joint pain and a new rash on the chest and upper back. She reports sun exposure from spending time at the beach. She has no other symptoms. She has no other medical problems and takes no medications.

On physical examination, vital signs are normal. Diffuse tenderness of multiple small joints of the hands is noted. The remainder of the examination is normal.

The appearance of the rash is shown.

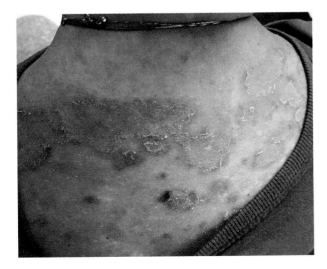

Which of the following is the most likely diagnosis for the rash?

(A) Acute cutaneous lupus erythematosus

(B) Dermatomyositis

(C) Discoid lupus erythematous

(D) Subacute cutaneous lupus erythematous

Item 94

A 49-year-old man is evaluated for a 10-year history of intermittent low back pain with 30 to 60 minutes of morning stiffness, both of which improve with exercise. The back pain can awaken him from sleep. He also reports occasional pain in the neck, shoulder blades, and buttocks on one side or the other. History is notable for anterior uveitis diagnosed more than 30 years ago, the symptoms of which recurred every 3 to 4 years but have been subsequently controlled by topical glucocorticoids. Current medications are as-needed NSAIDs and ophthalmic glucocorticoid drops.

On physical examination, vital signs are normal. Lumbar spine range of motion is restricted for forward flexion. There are no warm, erythematous, or swollen joints. There is no spinal or sacroiliac tenderness. Conjunctivae are without injection.

Which of the following is the most appropriate test to perform next?

(A) Bone scan

(B) CT of the sacroiliac joints

(C) MRI of the lumbar spine

(D) Radiography of the sacroiliac joints

Item 95

A 48-year-old man is evaluated during a routine follow-up visit for gout diagnosed 2 months ago, at which time he started allopurinol and colchicine. Since then, he has had three acute attacks separately involving the left wrist, right knee, and left foot. He has no current joint pain. He also reports having diarrhea two to three times daily over the past 6 weeks. History is also significant for type 2 diabetes mellitus, for which he takes insulin.

On physical examination, vital signs are normal. Musculoskeletal examination is normal.

Laboratory studies show a serum creatinine level of 0.8 mg/dL (70.7 µmol/L) and a serum urate level of 5.5 mg/dL (0.32 mmol/L).

Which of the following is the most appropriate next step to decrease the frequency of gout attacks?

(A) Add prednisone

(B) Add probenecid

(C) Discontinue colchicine; begin meloxicam

(D) Increase allopurinol

(E) Increase colchicine

Item 96

A 28-year-old woman is evaluated for a 3-week history of isolated left groin pain. The pain is worse with weight bearing. She has a 10-year history of systemic lupus erythematosus (SLE) and lupus nephritis. She has also received high-dose glucocorticoids multiple times in the past 10 years. She is currently doing well without any active SLE manifestations. Medications are hydroxychloroquine and low-dose prednisone.

On physical examination, vital signs are normal. The left groin has slight discomfort with hip movement and weight bearing but is nontender. There is no active synovitis. The remainder of the examination is normal.

Pelvic and hip radiographs are normal.

Which of the following is the most appropriate test to perform next in this patient?

(A) CT of the hip
(B) MRI of the hip
(C) Radionuclide bone scan
(D) Single photon emission CT

Answers and Critiques

Item 1 Answer: D

Educational Objective: Diagnose prosthetic joint infection.

Prosthetic joint infection is the most likely diagnosis. This patient has a prosthetic hip and is currently undergoing chemotherapy. Malignancy and immunosuppression are risk factors for prosthetic joint infection, and this patient also has a central venous catheter that increases his risk for bacteremia. The elevated leukocyte count and erythrocyte sedimentation rate, along with periprosthetic lucency on radiographs, are all suggestive of prosthetic joint infection. Prosthetic joint infections are divided into early onset (<3 months after placement), delayed (3 to 24 months postsurgery), and late onset (>24 months after placement). Early and delayed infections are usually related to surgical contamination at the time of the implantation, whereas late infections result from hematogenous seeding of the joint. Early and late prosthetic joint infections typically present with pain, warmth, effusion, and fever. *Staphylococcus aureus* is a leading causative agent in prosthetic joint infections; treatment involves prompt intravenous antibiotics and sometimes removal of the prosthesis.

Gout flare may also cause joint pain and loss of mobility, as well as fever, elevated leukocyte count, and inflammatory markers. However, this patient has no prior history of gout, and the hip is an uncommon place for a gout flare, especially an initial flare. Most initial gout flares affect the foot and/or ankle joints.

Hemarthrosis causes bleeding into a joint and is characterized by pain, swelling, warmth, and impaired mobility. It is diagnosed by synovial fluid aspiration. This patient does not have a history or findings suggestive of a bleeding diathesis to put him at risk for a traumatic hemarthrosis.

A patient with hip dislocation may present in a similar manner as one with prosthetic joint infection, namely pain and difficulty moving the joint; however, a dislocation would be evident on radiographs.

KEY POINT

- Both early and late prosthetic joint infections are typically characterized by pain, warmth, effusion, and fever; treatment involves prompt intravenous antibiotics and possible removal of the prosthesis.

Bibliography

Osmon DR, Berbari EF, Berendt AR, Lew D, Zimmerli W, Steckelberg JM, et al; Infectious Diseases Society of America. Diagnosis and management of prosthetic joint infection: clinical practice guidelines by the Infectious Diseases Society of America. Clin Infect Dis. 2013;56:e1-e25. [PMID: 23223583] doi:10.1093/cid/cis803

Item 2 Answer: C

Educational Objective: Diagnose microscopic polyangiitis.

The most likely diagnosis is microscopic polyangiitis (MPA), which characteristically affects the lungs and kidneys, along with other organ systems. Diagnosis is suspected based upon typical clinical findings and positive ANCA. The diagnostic gold standard is a biopsy demonstrating nongranulomatous necrotizing pauci-immune vasculitis of small vessels or pauci-immune necrotizing crescentic glomerulonephritis in the kidney. This patient has pulmonary hemorrhage, pauci-immune small-vessel necrotizing vasculitis of the skin, proteinuria, inflammatory arthritis, and a positive p-ANCA (directed against myeloperoxidase)—all consistent with the diagnosis of MPA.

Granulomatosis with polyangiitis (GPA) can cause the same lung, skin, joint, and kidney findings but is usually associated with a positive c-ANCA (directed against proteinase-3). Furthermore, GPA causes granulomatous inflammation; absence of granulomas distinguishes MPA from GPA.

IgA vasculitis (Henoch-Schönlein purpura) can affect lungs, skin, joints, and kidneys but it is an immune complex–mediated vasculitis with deposition of IgA containing immune complexes identified on biopsy, which is not present in this patient.

Rheumatoid vasculitis usually occurs in long-standing disease with positive rheumatoid factor and is immune complex mediated, none of which is present in this patient.

Thromboangiitis obliterans is a smoking-related vasculopathy affecting small to medium vessels with inflammation and thrombosis of vessels in upper and lower limbs, leading to reduced pulses and gangrenous ulcers. This diagnosis is unlikely because this patient no longer smokes, and has involvement of internal organs in addition to the legs.

KEY POINT

- The diagnostic gold standard of microscopic polyangiitis is a biopsy demonstrating nongranulomatous necrotizing pauci-immune vasculitis of small vessels or pauci-immune necrotizing crescentic glomerulonephritis in the kidney.

Bibliography

Kallenberg CG. The diagnosis and classification of microscopic polyangiitis. J Autoimmun. 2014;48-49:90-3. [PMID: 24461388] doi:10.1016/j.jaut.2014.01.023

Item 3 Answer: B

Educational Objective: Treat severe tophaceous gout.

In addition to stopping febuxostat, the most appropriate treatment is pegloticase infusions. This patient has severe recurrent and tophaceous gout that has been resistant to standard therapies, including febuxostat. Pegloticase is an intravenously administered porcine-derived uricase (infused every 2 weeks), which reduces serum urate to nearly zero within hours of administration. If anti-drug antibodies do not form, tophi may resolve over the course of months. Other urate-lowering therapies should be discontinued with initiation of pegloticase because they can mask the development of antibodies that manifest as rising serum urate levels. Patients starting pegloticase should be placed on prophylaxis to prevent acute gout attacks; colchicine, prednisone, or NSAIDs are appropriate. In this case, glucocorticoids and NSAIDs should be avoided because of the concomitant type 2 diabetes mellitus and chronic kidney disease; therefore, low-dose colchicine is the appropriate prophylactic agent.

It is important to note that two recently published guidelines differ regarding the role of pharmacologic urate-lowering therapy in patients with gout. The 2016 American College of Physicians guideline (http://annals.org/aim/article/2578528/management-acute-recurrent-gout-clinical-practice-guideline-from-american-college) notes a lack of evidence supporting a specific target level for urate lowering; this guideline stresses discussing the risks and benefits of urate-lowering therapy with patients and suggests a "treat to avoid symptoms" approach without specifically considering the serum urate levels. The 2016 European League Against Rheumatism (EULAR) recommendations support a "treat-to-target" approach (consistent with the 2012 ACR gout guidelines), reducing the serum urate level to less than 6.0 mg/dL (0.35 mmol/L) in patients without tophi and less than 5.0 mg/dL (0.30 mmol/L) in patients with tophi. The patient's serum urate level is 6.3 mg/dL (0.37 mmol/L) on febuxostat therapy, and she continues to have symptoms; therefore, escalation of treatment is appropriate according to both the ACP and EULAR guidelines.

Probenecid is not appropriate for those with an estimated glomerular filtration rate of less than 60 mL/min/1.73 m^2 or with a history of kidney stones; this patient has both.

Losartan has a modest uricosuric effect, but not significant enough that it would be recommended in a patient with severe tophaceous gout, especially one who remains symptomatic with an elevated serum urate level despite febuxostat therapy.

KEY POINT

- Pegloticase may be considered for patients with severe recurrent and/or tophaceous gout that is intolerant or resistant to standard therapies.

Bibliography

Sundy JS, Baraf HS, Yood RA, Edwards NL, Gutierrez-Urena SR, Treadwell EL, et al. Efficacy and tolerability of pegloticase for the treatment of chronic gout in patients refractory to conventional treatment: two randomized controlled trials. JAMA. 2011;306:711-20. [PMID: 21846852] doi:10.1001/jama.2011.1169

Item 4   Answer: A

Educational Objective: Diagnose reactive arthritis.

The most appropriate diagnostic test to perform next is nucleic acid amplification urine testing for chlamydia. *Chlamydia*

trachomatis is the most common agent causing urethritis that is associated with reactive arthritis. This patient has the triad of conjunctivitis, urethritis, and arthritis seen in a subset of patients with chlamydial reactive arthritis. Typically, affected men experience dysuria and note a urethral discharge, although less frequently than in arthritis related to gonococcal infection. Gonococcal arthritis, however, is not associated with conjunctivitis and is often accompanied by vesicopustular skin lesions and tenosynovitis. Reactive arthritis typically occurs 3 to 6 weeks after the infectious trigger, with a latency range of 2 weeks to 6 months. In a significant minority of cases, the triggering infection may go unrecognized. Although infection has usually resolved by the time of arthritis onset in patients with reactive arthritis, nucleic acid amplification urine testing for *C. trachomatis* should be performed because some individuals may have asymptomatic persistent infection or carriage of this organism.

C-reactive protein would not be of value in establishing the diagnosis. The patient has an acute inflammatory process in the joints based on his history, physical examination, and synovial fluid analysis. C-reactive protein would not lend further diagnostic information.

HLA-B27 antigen may be present in those with reactive arthritis, but it has little diagnostic specificity in this disorder. The presence of HLA-B27 antigen would neither rule in nor rule out reactive arthritis.

The interferon-gamma release assay can indicate prior exposure to tuberculosis. The clinical picture in this scenario is not that of tuberculous arthritis, which tends to be monoarticular, most frequently affects the hip, has a course that is subacute with progressive pain and loss of function over weeks to months, and is not often associated with features of inflammatory synovitis on physical examination (warmth, erythema).

KEY POINT

- Nucleic acid amplification urine testing is the appropriate diagnostic test for suspected chlamydial reactive arthritis.

Bibliography

Carter JD, Hudson AP. Recent advances and future directions in understanding and treating Chlamydia-induced reactive arthritis. Expert Rev Clin Immunol. 2017;13:197-206. [PMID: 27627462] doi:10.1080/1744666X.2017.1233816

Item 5   Answer: E

Educational Objective: Diagnose ankylosing spondylitis.

No additional tests are necessary. Different criteria have been proposed for the diagnosis of ankylosing spondylitis. Common requirements include the presence of inflammatory back pain for 3 or more months in a person younger than age 45 years, limited lumbar spine motion, elevated inflammatory markers, and evidence of bilateral sacroiliitis on imaging. The patient has a long history of inflammatory back pain (improves with exercise, worsens with sleep or inactivity), loss of range of motion of the lumbar spine, and radiographs showing fusion of the sacroiliac joints, one of the typical features of ankylosing spondylitis. It is important to establish the diagnosis of ankylosing spondylitis to assess the risk of further joint fusion and deformity in this patient.

ANCA is present in some forms of medium-vessel vasculitis. In the absence of cutaneous or internal organ manifestations suggestive of vasculitis (sinus, pulmonary, kidney, cutaneous, and ophthalmologic abnormalities), it is not appropriate as the next step in this patient's evaluation.

Anti–cyclic citrullinated peptide antibodies have specificity for the diagnosis of rheumatoid arthritis and are appropriately ordered when patients present with bilaterally symmetric inflammatory arthritis of the small joints of the hands. These antibodies will not establish the diagnosis of ankylosing spondylitis.

Testing for antinuclear antibodies should be carried out when there is suspicion for the presence of systemic lupus erythematosus. This patient does not have rash, sun sensitivity, alopecia, oral ulcers, pleuropericarditis, kidney disease, or laboratory abnormalities that would raise suspicion for lupus.

The presence of HLA–B27 antigen is not a diagnostic criterion for ankylosing spondylitis. However, such testing may be particularly helpful in patients with inflammatory back pain and other manifestations of ankylosing spondylitis but without evidence of sacroiliitis on imaging.

KEY POINT

- A diagnosis of ankylosing spondylitis can be made in a patient younger than age 45 years with symptoms of inflammatory back pain for 3 months or more and bilateral sacroiliitis on imaging.

Bibliography

Taurog JD, Chhabra A, Colbert RA. Ankylosing spondylitis and axial spondyloarthritis. N Engl J Med. 2016;374:2563-74. [PMID: 27355535] doi:10.1056/NEJMra1406182

Item 6   Answer: C

Educational Objective: Diagnose gastric antral vascular ectasia associated with diffuse cutaneous systemic sclerosis.

The most likely diagnosis is gastric antral vascular ectasia (GAVE) associated with systemic sclerosis. GAVE is the proliferation of blood vessels typically in the antrum of the stomach; on endoscopy, it has the appearance of watermelon stripes (watermelon stomach). Approximately 60% of patients with GAVE have an underlying autoimmune disease; the remainder have portal hypertension secondary to hepatic cirrhosis. GAVE can be a source of both acute and chronic gastrointestinal bleeding. First-line therapy is argon plasma coagulation or laser coagulation.

Cameron lesions are erosions found on the crest of gastric folds within a large hiatal hernia and are thought to be caused by mechanical trauma as the hiatal hernia slides up and down. Up to 5% of patients with known hiatal hernias

may have Cameron lesions. There is no evidence of a hiatal hernia, making this diagnosis unlikely.

Dieulafoy lesions are submucosal arterioles that intermittently protrude through the mucosa and cause hemorrhage. Dieulafoy lesions are of unknown etiology and account for about 2% of all causes of acute upper gastrointestinal bleeding and are located in the proximal stomach along the lesser curvature. When bleeding they appear as an isolated pumping arteriole in the absence of a mass or ulcer. The patient's findings do not match those of Dieulafoy lesions.

Portal hypertensive gastropathy (PHG) commonly occurs with advanced cirrhosis and has a characteristic mosaic appearance on endoscopy, most often seen in the body and fundus. It can be confused with GAVE. This patient has no history of cirrhosis or findings to suggest chronic liver disease, making PHG an unlikely diagnosis.

KEY POINT

- Patients with diffuse cutaneous systemic sclerosis are at risk for acute and chronic gastrointestinal bleeding secondary to gastric antral vascular ectasia.

Bibliography

Fuccio L, Mussetto A, Laterza L, Eusebi LH, Bazzoli F. Diagnosis and management of gastric antral vascular ectasia. World J Gastrointest Endosc. 2013;5:6-13. [PMID: 23330048] doi:10.4253/wjge.v5.i1.6

Item 7   Answer: A

Educational Objective: Treat refractory acute gout.

Anakinra is the most appropriate treatment for this patient's knee. He has a persistent fever due to a severe acute gouty attack. Synovial fluid analysis permits definitive diagnosis and can rule out other conditions. Under polarized light, monosodium urate crystals are needle shaped and negatively birefringent. Whereas extracellular crystals confirm a chronic gout diagnosis, crystals within neutrophils define active, gout-induced inflammation. Even in the setting of acute gout, Gram stain and cultures must be obtained to exclude infection because acute gout and joint infection occasionally coexist. This patient has not responded favorably to glucocorticoid therapy, which characterizes some severe acute episodes. In a case such as this, an interleukin-1 inhibitor such as anakinra should be provided as a reliable (although expensive) off-label treatment.

Colchicine is unlikely to be effective for an established attack of greater than 12 to 24 hours' duration. It is also unlikely to be useful when intravenous and intra-articular glucocorticoids have been ineffective.

The absence of a response to intra-articular or intravenous glucocorticoids necessitates an alternative treatment; however, NSAIDs would not be as effective as the two previously provided failed alternatives. Additionally, NSAIDs have numerous side effects that might be even more likely to occur during critical illness, and they are relatively contraindicated in a patient with heart failure.

CONT.

Blood, urine, and synovial fluid cultures have all been negative, the pneumonia is resolving, and there is no clinical evidence of infection. Vancomycin for methicillin-resistant staphylococcus is unnecessary.

KEY POINT

- For patients with severe and refractory gouty attacks or with contraindications to other treatments, off-label use of interleukin-1 inhibitors (anakinra or canakinumab) can be considered.

Bibliography

Thueringer JT, Doll NK, Gertner E. Anakinra for the treatment of acute severe gout in critically ill patients. Semin Arthritis Rheum. 2015;45:81-5. [PMID: 25795473] doi:10.1016/j.semarthrit.2015.02.006

Item 8   Answer: C

Educational Objective: Treat osteoarthritis with physical therapy.

Physical therapy is appropriate for this patient whose history, physical examination, and radiographic findings are consistent with the diagnosis of osteoarthritis (OA). Physical therapy is an effective intervention for the management of pain and reduced functioning due to OA, with numerous guidelines supporting exercise as an appropriate intervention for all patients with OA. Evidence is most robust for knee OA. Many patients become sedentary due to their symptoms, and physical therapy is often a useful starting point to transition patients to participation in a regular exercise program. Physical therapy can be prescribed at any point in the course of the disease instead of medication, as a supplement to medication that does not adequately reduce pain, or prior to surgery to increase strength and potentially influence surgical outcomes.

Glucosamine supplements are the most widely used over-the-counter products worldwide for OA. Many randomized controlled trials have found that pain, function, and radiographic progression improve overall at a level equivalent to the effects of placebo in patients taking glucosamine.

Knee replacement surgery is effective for treatment of pain and disability but is not appropriate in a patient who has not been through a trial of physical therapy, particularly a patient who is not regularly exercising. Assessment of the ability to carry out activities of daily living, as well as occupational and recreational activities, will be important in the decision to seek surgery, and a physical therapist can be particularly helpful to the primary care provider in carrying out this assessment. Considerations for surgical referral include the presence of pain at rest or pain that awakens the patient in the middle of the night, both of which are less likely to respond to analgesics, exercise, or physical modalities.

Prednisone is an oral glucocorticoid that can be used as an adjunctive medication in the treatment of some forms of inflammatory arthritis. However, insufficient evidence exists to support the use of oral glucocorticoids in the treatment of OA.

KEY POINT

- Physical therapy can be prescribed at any point in the course of osteoarthritis instead of medication, as a supplement to medication that does not adequately reduce pain, or prior to surgery to increase strength and potentially influence surgical outcomes.

Bibliography

Hochberg MC, Altman RD, April KT, Benkhalti M, Guyatt G, McGowan J, et al; American College of Rheumatology. American College of Rheumatology 2012 recommendations for the use of nonpharmacologic and pharmacologic therapies in osteoarthritis of the hand, hip, and knee. Arthritis Care Res (Hoboken). 2012;64:465-74. [PMID: 22563589]

Item 9   Answer: C

Educational Objective: Diagnose ankylosing spondylitis using MRI.

The most appropriate diagnostic test to perform next is MRI of the sacroiliac joints. This patient has symptoms suggestive of back pain due to inflammation, including young age of onset, gradual onset, pain during the night, morning stiffness, improvement with motion, no history of trauma, and no improvement with rest. A single anteroposterior pelvis plain radiograph to view the sacroiliac joints is an appropriate first diagnostic step in this setting, which may reveal joint space widening (early) or narrowing (late), erosions, sclerosis, and ankylosis, and can establish the diagnosis of ankylosing spondylitis. However, plain radiographs may be normal early in the course of disease, as seen in this patient. MRI of the sacroiliac joints can then be utilized, which is more sensitive for detecting early spine and sacroiliac joint inflammation. The finding of bone marrow edema on STIR or T2-weighted images with fat suppression is not specific for ankylosing spondylitis but does suggest active inflammation, particularly if found in characteristic periarticular and subchondral locations. MRI can also identify soft-tissue evidence of inflammation in the entheses, bursae, and tendons, as well as subtle structural abnormalities.

Bone scan is sensitive for the detection of osteoblast activity and is the study of choice for detecting bone metastases from various forms of cancer. However, bone scan is not used in the diagnosis of any form of inflammatory arthritis because it lacks specificity.

CT of the lumbar spine can be useful in the diagnosis of ankylosing spondylitis when radiography of the sacroiliac joints is normal. However, it is not routinely used in the evaluation of patients for arthritis due to the high dose of radiation required.

Hip pathology frequently results in anterior groin pain and would be unlikely to cause back pain. Therefore, radiography of the hip joints is not likely to aid in the diagnosis and is not indicated for this patient.

KEY POINT

- MRI is more sensitive than radiography for detecting early spine and sacroiliac joint inflammation and may be indicated in the evaluation of suspected spondyloarthritis if radiographs are normal.

Bibliography

Sieper J, Poddubnyy D. Axial spondyloarthritis. Lancet. 2017. [PMID: 28110981] doi:10.1016/S0140-6736(16)31591-4

Item 10   Answer: E

Educational Objective: Avoid serologic testing in patients with low pretest probability of connective tissue disease.

No further testing is currently needed in this 75-year-old man with no clinical findings suggestive of a connective tissue disease. His symptoms of hand joint pain are noninflammatory (pain with use, no warmth or swelling, and only minimal morning stiffness), and the distribution and findings are consistent with a diagnosis of osteoarthritis. Furthermore, the radiographs confirm these findings and do not show changes consistent with an inflammatory rheumatologic disorder (such as erosive joint disease seen in rheumatoid arthritis and psoriatic arthritis, or tophi seen in gout). Therefore, no further testing is indicated.

Positive antinuclear antibodies (ANA) in a patient with nonspecific symptoms are difficult to interpret. As with all tests, the positive predictive value of ANA rests upon the pretest probability of disease. In the presence of 0 or 1 clinical manifestations of systemic lupus erythematosus (SLE), a positive ANA is associated with a very low posttest probability of SLE. The American College of Rheumatology's Choosing Wisely list currently recommends against testing ANA and ANA subserologies without a clinical suspicion of immune-mediated disease. The clinical suspicion for a connective tissue disorder such as SLE or rheumatoid arthritis is low in this patient, and ANA, rheumatoid factor, or anti–cyclic citrullinated peptide antibodies should not be tested.

Osteoarthritis, psoriatic arthritis, and gout can involve distal interphalangeal joints. However, this patient does not have the rash seen in psoriatic arthritis or symptoms of crystal-induced arthritis such as recurrent acute attacks and/or tophaceous deposits. Serum urate levels are helpful in a patient with symptoms suggestive of gout but are unlikely to helpful here.

KEY POINT

- The positive predictive value of antinuclear antibody (ANA) tests is determined by the pretest probability of disease; in the presence of 0 or 1 clinical manifestations of systemic lupus erythematosus (SLE), a positive ANA is associated with a very low posttest probability of SLE.

Bibliography

Yazdany J, Schmajuk G, Robbins M, Daikh D, Beall A, Yelin E, et al; American College of Rheumatology Core Membership Group. Choosing wisely: the American College of Rheumatology's top 5 list of things physicians and patients should question. Arthritis Care Res (Hoboken). 2013;65:329-39. [PMID: 23436818] doi:10.1002/acr.21930

Item 11   Answer: A

Educational Objective: Diagnose antisynthetase syndrome.

The most likely diagnosis is antisynthetase syndrome, which is characterized by interstitial lung disease, myositis, Raynaud phenomenon, nonerosive inflammatory arthritis, constitutional findings such as low-grade fever, and mechanic's hands. Mechanic's hands is a dermatologic manifestation unique to antisynthetase syndrome and is characterized by hyperkeratotic skin along the ulnar aspect of the thumb and radial aspects of the digits, most commonly on the index and middle fingers, and involvement of the palms. Unlike eczema, there is no pruritus, vesicles, or hand dominance. Antisynthetase syndrome can occur in patients with dermatomyositis or polymyositis; about one third of patients with dermatomyositis belong to this subset characterized by a relatively abrupt onset and features. Antinuclear antibodies (ANA) are often positive in patients with antisynthetase syndrome, but anti–aminoacyl-tRNA synthetases antibodies, including the subset anti–Jo-1 antibodies, are more specific for the diagnosis.

In patients with Sjögren syndrome, constitutional findings and inflammatory arthritis are common, but Raynaud phenomenon is less so. Rash and mechanic's hands are not characteristics. Furthermore, dry eyes and dry mouth are the most common presenting symptoms, along with positive anti-Ro/SSA and anti-La/SSB antibodies.

Fever, Raynaud phenomenon, rash, inflammatory arthritis, and positive ANA are seen in systemic lupus erythematosus. However, an abrupt onset rarely occurs, mechanic's hands are not a feature, and anti–Jo-1 antibodies are not characteristic.

In patients with systemic sclerosis, fever and inflammatory arthritis are far less likely. Furthermore, although Raynaud phenomenon is very common in systemic sclerosis, the findings of either localized or diffuse skin tightening and thickening, including sclerodactyly, are absent in this patient. Mechanic's hands is not a feature of systemic sclerosis, and anti–Jo-1 antibodies are not characteristic.

KEY POINT

- Antisynthetase syndrome is characterized by interstitial lung disease, myositis, Raynaud phenomenon, nonerosive inflammatory arthritis, constitutional findings such as low-grade fever, and mechanic's hands; anti-aminoacyl-tRNA synthetases antibodies, such as anti-Jo-1, are highly suggestive of the diagnosis.

Bibliography

Lega JC, Fabien N, Reynaud Q, Durieu I, Durupt S, Dutertre M, et al. The clinical phenotype associated with myositis-specific and associated autoantibodies: a meta-analysis revisiting the so-called antisynthetase syndrome. Autoimmun Rev. 2014;13:883-91. [PMID: 24704867] doi:10.1016/j.autrev.2014.03.004

Item 12   Answer: D

Educational Objective: Prevent rheumatoid arthritis with smoking cessation.

The most preventive measure for this patient at risk for developing rheumatoid arthritis (RA) is smoking cessation. Smoking has been definitively identified as a risk factor for the development of RA, especially in genetically susceptible individuals. This woman has a strong family history of RA, including an identical twin sister who was recently diagnosed. Smoking increases the risk for RA 2 to 21 times depending on the presence of one or two copies of the shared epitope in the HLA makeup of the individual. Data suggest that if she stops smoking now, the risk for developing RA will decline each year that she does not smoke and will eventually be 30% lower than if she continued to smoke, but will not reach the level of someone who has never smoked for up to 20 years. There is additional evidence that if she stops smoking now and does develop RA, future mortality will be favorably affected, as will her disease activity. Smoking stimulates the production of enzymes that modify arginine to citrulline, and the modified proteins containing citrulline are targets for the immune system in susceptible individuals. This patient's hand symptoms seem more mechanical in nature (that is, end of the day) rather than inflammatory (prolonged morning stiffness).

High-fructose corn syrup has been identified as a possible risk factor for hyperuricemia and gout but not RA.

The use of hydroxychloroquine to prevent the development of RA in susceptible individuals is unproven. A clinical trial will soon evaluate the impact of hydroxychloroquine in patients positive for anti-cyclic citrullinated peptide antibodies, but it is premature to recommend this intervention without supporting evidence.

To date, probiotics have not been shown to modify risk for RA.

KEY POINT

- Smoking is a risk factor for the development of rheumatoid arthritis, especially in genetically susceptible individuals; all patients should be counseled to quit smoking.

Bibliography

Di Giuseppe D, Orsini N, Alfredsson L, Askling J, Wolk A. Cigarette smoking and smoking cessation in relation to risk of rheumatoid arthritis in women. Arthritis Res Ther. 2013;15:R56. [PMID: 23607815] doi:10.1186/ar4218

Item 13   Answer: A

Educational Objective: Diagnose acute lupus pneumonitis.

Acute lupus pneumonitis is the most likely diagnosis in this patient who has difficult-to-control systemic lupus erythematosus (SLE) requiring aggressive therapy with prednisone and azathioprine. Lupus pneumonitis is a rare but severe presentation of SLE characterized by shortness of breath, hypoxia, and diffuse pulmonary infiltrates. Other major entities in the differential diagnosis include infection and diffuse alveolar hemorrhage. He has clear evidence of active SLE with polyarthritis, a high erythrocyte sedimentation rate, hypocomplementemia, and diffuse pulmonary infiltrates on radiologic studies, as well as lymphocytic predominance on bronchoalveolar lavage. These findings are very suggestive of lupus pneumonitis. It usually requires rapid and aggressive therapy with glucocorticoids and/or immunosuppressive agents.

Pulmonary hypertension does not present with diffuse infiltrates with ground glass opacities, as seen in this patient, and it cannot explain the bronchoalveolar lavage findings.

This patient has no fever or sputum production, and testing shows a normal leukocyte count and differential, normal C-reactive protein (CRP), and normal procalcitonin, making infection less likely. CRP is a marker of inflammation, and levels are significantly increased in bacterial pneumonia but frequently normal or only slightly elevated in SLE flares. Procalcitonin is produced by cells as a response to bacterial toxins, which result in serum procalcitonin elevations in bacterial infections.

The patient reports no hemoptysis, and lack of anemia and absence of erythrocytes on bronchoalveolar lavage exclude a diagnosis of diffuse alveolar hemorrhage.

Shrinking lung syndrome presents with chronic insidious shortness of breath with low lung volumes possibly related to diaphragmatic dysfunction. This patient's acute presentation and diffuse infiltrates on imaging is not consistent with this syndrome.

KEY POINT

- Lupus pneumonitis is a rare but severe presentation of systemic lupus erythematosus characterized by shortness of breath, hypoxia, and diffuse pulmonary infiltrates.

Bibliography

Mittoo S, Fell CD. Pulmonary manifestations of systemic lupus erythematosus. Semin Respir Crit Care Med. 2014;35:249-54. [PMID: 24668539] doi:10.1055/s-0034-1371537

Item 14   Answer: D

Educational Objective: Diagnose small intestinal bacterial overgrowth associated with systemic sclerosis.

The most likely diagnosis is small intestinal bacterial overgrowth (SIBO) associated with systemic sclerosis (SSc). More than 70% of patients with SSc have clinical gastrointestinal involvement. Gastrointestinal motility is compromised in 40% to 90% of patients with systemic sclerosis, especially those with diffuse disease. Because of the decrease in motility of the small bowel, bacterial overgrowth occurs and leads to the symptoms described in this patient history, including diarrhea, bloating, and pain, and can lead to malabsorption. Patients with SSc can also develop chronic pancreatic insufficiency and develop symptoms similar to SIBO, which must be considered in the differential diagnosis. Diagnosis of SIBO can be confirmed with glucose hydrogen breath testing or jejunal aspirate cultures. Treatment is with rotating antibodies to try to reduce the overgrowth using agents with both aerobic and anaerobic coverage. Probiotics may have some benefit in such patients. It is important to screen such patients for nutritional deficiencies.

Carcinoid tumors are neuroendocrine tumors arising from the aerodigestive tract. Although most neuroendocrine tumors are hormonally nonfunctioning, a few produce serotonin and are responsible for the clinical manifestations of the carcinoid syndrome characterized by diarrhea and facial flushing. The diarrhea associated with the carcinoid syndrome is secretory, and symptoms are not confined to periods of food intake; nocturnal diarrhea is a clinical hallmark.

Chronic mesenteric ischemia is almost always associated with atherosclerotic disease. Symptoms consist of postprandial pain within 60 minutes after meals, which results in fear of eating and weight loss. It is not associated with postprandial bloating or explosive diarrhea.

Irritable bowel syndrome is a symptom complex characterized by abdominal pain and altered bowel habits. Diagnosis is established by fulfilling specific diagnostic criteria, including recurrent abdominal pain or discomfort at least 3 days per month in the last 3 months associated with two or more of the following: improvement with defecation; onset associated with a change in frequency of stool; and onset associated with a change in form (appearance) of stool. The presence of "red flags" such as anemia, fever, or weight loss strongly suggests the presence of an alternative diagnosis.

KEY POINT

- In patients with systemic sclerosis, gastrointestinal dysmotility can result in small intestinal bacterial overgrowth with resultant chronic diarrhea and malabsorption.

Bibliography

Gyger G, Baron M. Systemic sclerosis: gastrointestinal disease and its management. Rheum Dis Clin North Am. 2015;41:459-73. [PMID: 26210129] doi:10.1016/j.rdc.2015.04.007

Item 15   Answer: B

Educational Objective: Diagnose Felty syndrome.

The most likely diagnosis is Felty syndrome, which consists of the triad of long-standing aggressive rheumatoid arthritis (RA), neutropenia, and splenomegaly. Patients with Felty syndrome are almost always seropositive. This patient has the typical findings of long-standing RA, including involvement of multiple small joints of the hands and feet, joint subluxation, and subcutaneous nodules. Felty syndrome is associated with the risk for serious infections, lower extremity ulcers, lymphoma, and vasculitis. Treatment of Felty syndrome consists of more aggressive therapy for the underlying RA.

AA amyloid results from accumulation of the AA protein, an acute phase reactant seen in chronic inflammatory diseases. Although AA amyloidosis can be associated with hepatosplenomegaly, the most common organ involved in AA amyloidosis is the kidney and is evidenced by heavy proteinuria. Hematologic abnormalities may include anemia as the result of chronic kidney disease and thrombocytopenia secondary to splenomegaly, but neutropenia is unusual. AA amyloidosis cannot account for this patient's joint findings or lower extremity ulcer.

Sarcoidosis most commonly affects the lungs. Severe sarcoidosis can uncommonly be associated with a chronic arthritis that is typically polyarticular, involving the shoulders, hands, wrists, knees, and ankles, and often coexists with lung and cutaneous sarcoidosis. An entire digit may be affected, leading to dactylitis. Sarcoidosis can also be associated with slightly tender subcutaneous nodules of the upper extremities and (rarely) splenomegaly. Sarcoidosis does not cause leukopenia or cutaneous ulcers and is an unlikely cause of this patient's findings.

Joint involvement occurs in 90% of patients with systemic lupus erythematosus (SLE), with inflammatory polyarthralgia the most common presentation. Frank arthritis occurs in 40% of patients with SLE. Both small and large joints can be affected. Persistent periarticular inflammation can damage soft-tissue structures that support joints, resulting in reducible subluxation of the digits, swan neck deformities, and ulnar deviation (Jaccoud arthropathy). All three bone marrow cell lines can be affected in SLE. Leukopenia occurs in 50% of patients, with lymphopenia predominating. Subcutaneous nodules are not usually found in SLE. In addition, up to 90% of patients with SLE have skin (acute, subacute, or chronic lupus) or mucous membrane involvement. The presence of splenomegaly and subcutaneous nodules and absence of skin rash argue against the diagnosis of SLE. In addition, serologies would help distinguish RA from SLE.

KEY POINT

- Felty syndrome consists of the triad of long-standing aggressive rheumatoid arthritis, neutropenia, and splenomegaly and is associated with the risk for serious infections, lower extremity ulcers, lymphoma, and vasculitis.

Bibliography

Owila MB, Newman K, Akhtari M. Felty's syndrome, insights and updates. Open Rheumatol J. 2014 Dec 31; 8:129-36. [PMCID: PMC4296472] doi: 10.2174/1874312901408010129.

Item 16   Answer: C

Educational Objective: Diagnose Lyme arthritis.

The most likely diagnosis is Lyme arthritis, which can be confirmed by serologic testing for detection of *Borrelia burgdorferi*-specific antibodies using a two-tiered approach: enzyme-linked immunosorbent assay (ELISA) followed by Western blot. This patient is a park ranger in an area endemic for Lyme disease, thus the diagnosis should be strongly suspected, especially given a monoarthritis of the knee that is not overly painful, which is typical for Lyme arthritis. Lyme arthritis is a late manifestation of Lyme disease; after the first month of infection, at least 5/10 bands should be present on Western blot testing for IgG antibodies to different *B. burgdorferi* proteins. It is not uncommon for patients to be unaware of or experience manifestations of early stages of disease, such as erythema migrans or constitutional symptoms.

Positive HLA-B27 haplotype may be seen in patients who have spondyloarthritis such as ankylosing spondylitis, psoriatic arthritis, or reactive arthritis. Although these conditions commonly involve the peripheral joints, including the knees, the arthritis is usually painful and oligoarticular, not monoarticular. Additionally, inflammatory symptoms such as morning stiffness are prominent.

CONT.

MRI of the knee can be useful to diagnose meniscal, ligamentous, and other soft-tissue abnormalities, as well as synovitis and effusion. It is particularly useful to localize knee pathology in the clinical setting of trauma, which has not occurred in this patient. Degenerative meniscal tears due to knee osteoarthritis may be seen on MRI, without a clinical history of trauma, but this patient does not have clinical or radiographic symptoms/signs of osteoarthritis.

In crystal arthropathies, metabolic abnormalities promote the formation and deposition of crystals that stimulate inflammation. Symptoms are typically of an acute painful arthritis, which is not present in this patient. Synovial fluid analysis for crystals is therefore not indicated.

KEY POINT

- Chronic monoarticular arthritis with a large effusion and stiffness but minimal pain is characteristic of Lyme arthritis; diagnosis is made by serologic testing (enzyme-linked immunosorbent assay followed, if positive, by Western blot).

Bibliography

Arvikar SL, Steere AC. Diagnosis and treatment of Lyme arthritis. Infect Dis Clin North Am. 2015;29:269-80. [PMID: 25999223] doi:10.1016/j.idc.2015.02.004

 ### Item 17   Answer: B

Educational Objective: Diagnose IgG4-associated retroperitoneal fibrosis.

The most likely diagnosis is IgG4-associated retroperitoneal fibrosis. Most of the conditions that are under the banner of IgG4-related disease (IgG4-RD) are characterized by IgG4-producing plasma cell infiltration and tumefaction of the affected tissue with resultant organ enlargement, fibrosis, and dysfunction. Patients commonly present with a sentinel organ enlargement, but careful evaluation often reveals more extensive disease. Clinical signs include painless enlargement of lymph nodes or the thyroid, parotid, or submandibular glands; proptosis with orbital pseudo-tumor; back or chest pain from aortic involvement; and abdominal pain from pancreatic or biliary tree disease. This patient presents with a classic picture of retroperitoneal fibrosis with back pain and kidney failure from the periaortic mass that is large enough to encase the ureters resulting in obstructive uropathy and kidney injury. In a recent study, almost 60% of patients with retroperitoneal fibrosis were found to have IgG4-RD. Some patients present with an inflammatory aortitis as well. The patient's history of a fibrotic thyroid gland is also a feature of IgG4-RD.

Young men with germ cell tumor can present with bulky retroperitoneal or mediastinal lymphadenopathy. A testicular mass may not always be present. Similarly, involvement of retroperitoneal, mesenteric, and pelvic nodes is common in many types of non-Hodgkin lymphoma and can lead to urinary tract obstruction. It is uncommon for either of these conditions to present as a retroperitoneal

mass in the absence of lymphadenopathy, and neither germ cell tumor nor lymphoma can account for the fibrous goiter.

Mesothelioma is a highly lethal disease that most commonly involves the pleura but also the peritoneum. The most frequently noted symptoms are abdominal pain, weight loss, and increase in abdominal girth due to ascites. Malignant peritoneal mesothelioma does not present as a retroperitoneal mass and does not cause urinary obstruction or a fibrous thyroid goiter.

KEY POINT

- IgG4-related disease is characterized by IgG4-producing plasma cell infiltration and tumefaction of the affected tissue with resultant organ enlargement, fibrosis, and dysfunction.

Bibliography

Khosroshahi A, Carruthers MN, Stone JH, Shinagare S, Sainani N, Hasserjian RP, et al. Rethinking Ormond's disease: "idiopathic" retroperitoneal fibrosis in the era of IgG4-related disease. Medicine (Baltimore). 2013;92:82-91. [PMID: 23429355] doi:10.1097/MD.0b013e318289610f

Item 18   Answer: B

Educational Objective: Diagnose limited cutaneous systemic sclerosis.

The most likely diagnosis is limited cutaneous systemic sclerosis (LcSSc). This patient has Raynaud phenomenon and abnormal nailfold capillary changes that suggest that the Raynaud disease is part of the features of an underlying connective tissue disease. Raynaud phenomenon (sequential white, blue, and red color changes in the digits precipitated by cold or stress) occurs in almost all patients with systemic sclerosis (SSc). Raynaud phenomenon in LcSSc is initially transient and reversible; later, structural changes develop within small blood vessels, resulting in permanently impaired flow that produces acrocyanosis, digital pitting, and/or ulcerations. Office-based examination of the nailfold capillaries of patients with SSc using a dermatoscope or ophthalmoscope reveals both capillary destruction and dilated capillary loops, which can distinguish SSc from primary Raynaud. Early changes in nailfold capillaries in the setting of a connective tissue disease include dilatation. In the scleroderma spectrum disorders, nailfolds can demonstrate capillary dropout and then more disorganized loops as the vasculopathy progresses. Elevated antinuclear antibodies in a centromere pattern occur in 20% to 40% of patients with SSc and have a 90% specificity for the disease, and in particular for LcSSc. The presence of anticentromere antibodies also increases the risk for developing pulmonary arterial hypertension (PAH). This patient will need to be monitored for progression, including PAH screening.

Anticentromere B antibodies are not seen in patients with dermatomyositis or mixed connective tissue disease, neither of which is the likely diagnosis in this patient. The pathognomonic cutaneous features of dermatomyositis are the heliotrope rash and Gottron papules, which are absent in this patient, as is another key feature, proximal muscle weakness.

Mixed connective tissue disease (MCTD) is an overlap syndrome that includes features of systemic lupus erythematosus (SLE), SSc, and/or polymyositis in the presence of anti-U1-ribonucleoprotein antibodies. More than 50% of patients with MCTD have hand edema and synovitis at disease onset, which is not present in this patient.

Anticentromere B antibodies are rarely seen in SLE (4% or less), and this patient does not have any findings associated with this disorder. SLE should be considered in any patient who presents with unexplained multisystem disease. The most common early SLE manifestations include constitutional symptoms (fever, weight loss, or severe fatigue), arthralgia/arthritis, and skin disease, all of which are absent in this patient.

KEY POINT

- Elevated antinuclear antibodies in a centromere pattern have a 90% specificity for systemic sclerosis, and in particular for limited cutaneous systemic sclerosis.

Bibliography

Mehra S, Walker J, Patterson K, Fritzler MJ. Autoantibodies in systemic sclerosis. Autoimmun Rev. 2013;12:340-54. [PMID: 22743034] doi:10.1016/j.autrev.2012.05.011

Item 19   Answer: D

Educational Objective: Diagnose polyarteritis nodosa.

The most likely diagnosis is polyarteritis nodosa (PAN), a vasculitis affecting medium-sized arteries. This entity may occur in the setting of chronic hepatitis B virus infection, HIV infection, and hairy cell leukemia. The most common symptoms are constitutional, including fever, malaise, and weight loss, and neurologic symptoms such as mononeuritis multiplex. Skin rashes, including purpura and necrotic ulcers, occur in more than half of patients. Kidney involvement manifests as hypertension due to renal artery vasculitis with renal infarction, not glomerulonephritis. Orchitis, an uncommon manifestation, is usually unilateral and due to testicular artery involvement. Mesenteric vasculitis may cause abdominal pain, perforation, and bleeding. This patient has all of these findings except for mesenteric involvement. Diagnosis of PAN is best established by demonstrating necrotizing arteritis in biopsy specimens or finding characteristic medium-sized artery aneurysms and stenoses on imaging studies of the mesenteric or renal arteries. This patient's renal angiogram confirms the presence of vasculitis and skin biopsy confirms medium-vessel vasculitis, consistent with the diagnosis of PAN.

Giant cell arteritis causes myalgia and elevated erythrocyte sedimentation rate but involves large vessels usually in the head and neck area or great vessels of the chest, not medium-sized vessels. Furthermore, it usually does not involve nerves or kidneys.

IgA vasculitis can cause testicular involvement, mononeuritis, and rash (palpable purpura), but it affects small vessels and causes glomerulonephritis rather than renovascular involvement.

Microscopic polyangiitis (MPA) is an ANCA-associated vasculitis affecting small vessels. It can cause neurologic involvement and skin rash, but kidney involvement is due to glomerulonephritis rather than renal artery vasculitis. Furthermore, MPA is associated with a positive ANCA with perinuclear pattern, directed against myeloperoxidase. This patient does not have a positive ANCA or glomerulonephritis, making MPA an unlikely diagnosis.

KEY POINT

- Polyarteritis nodosa is a vasculitis affecting medium-sized arteries and is characterized by constitutional and neurologic symptoms, skin rashes, and kidney involvement that is renovascular rather than glomerular in origin.

Bibliography

De Virgilio A, Greco A, Magliulo G, Gallo A, Ruoppolo G, Conte M, et al. Polyarteritis nodosa: a contemporary overview. Autoimmun Rev. 2016;15:564-70. [PMID: 26884100] doi:10.1016/j.autrev.2016.02.015

Item 20   Answer: E

Educational Objective: Treat osteoarthritis in an elderly patient using a topical NSAID.

Topical diclofenac is the most appropriate treatment for long-term symptom control for this elderly patient with knee osteoarthritis (OA). Acetaminophen has not provided relief; furthermore, the efficacy of acetaminophen for OA is increasingly being questioned because recent controlled trials and meta-analyses demonstrated no benefit from the drug, even at high doses. NSAIDs are available in oral, topical, and intravenous forms. Due to efficacy and cost-effectiveness, oral preparations are usually first-line NSAID therapy in patients without contraindications to treatment. In OA, topical NSAIDs are considered to provide similar pain relief as oral medications with fewer gastrointestinal effects. Furthermore, the American College of Rheumatology currently recommends topical NSAIDs rather than oral NSAIDs for patients aged 75 years or older. However, they are associated with more skin reactions and are significantly more expensive than oral NSAIDs. This elderly woman with unilateral knee OA is an ideal candidate for topical NSAIDs—she has just one area of musculoskeletal pain and has several relative contraindications to oral NSAIDs (age, chronic kidney disease, coronary artery disease, and aspirin intake).

When a single symptomatic joint is present, injection directly into the joint may deliver medication to the affected site while minimizing the potential for systemic effects. Intra-articular injections may be used along with or in place of oral or topical analgesics. Intra-articular glucocorticoids are associated with short-term benefit with few side effects.

Glucocorticoid injection alone would not likely provide long-term benefit for this patient.

Low-dose oral prednisone is associated with modest reductions in short-term knee pain and may increase a 6-minute walk distance in older patients with moderate-to-severe knee OA. However, long-term use is associated with significant complications, including an increased risk for diabetes mellitus, osteoporosis, osteonecrosis, weight gain, fluid retention, hypertension, cardiovascular disease, striae and bruising, and glaucoma and cataracts.

Oral naproxen and other oral NSAIDs are relatively contraindicated given the patient's hypertension, chronic kidney disease, and coronary artery disease.

Traditional opiates may rarely be warranted to control pain in patients with OA who have not responded to other agents or are poor candidates for other interventions to treat painful joints, such as surgery. Opioid analgesics are inappropriate for this patient because other treatment options are available. In addition, opioids have limited effectiveness for chronic joint pain and are associated with substantial side effects in the elderly, especially increased fall risk, cognitive changes, and constipation.

KEY POINT

- Topical NSAIDs are beneficial for patients at high risk for toxicity from oral NSAIDs.

Bibliography

Rannou F, Pelletier JP, Martel-Pelletier J. Efficacy and safety of topical NSAIDs in the management of osteoarthritis: Evidence from real-life setting trials and surveys. Semin Arthritis Rheum. 2016;45:S18-21. [PMID: 26806189] doi:10.1016/j.semarthrit.2015.11.007

Item 21   Answer: D

Educational Objective: Treat giant cell arteritis.

The most appropriate treatment is prednisone, 60 mg/d. This patient has signs and symptoms of giant cell arteritis (GCA), including headache, jaw claudication, visual changes, and an elevated erythrocyte sedimentation rate, as well as symptoms of polymyalgia rheumatica (PMR). GCA is the most common primary vasculitis. Median age of onset is 70 years; GCA in patients under age 50 is rare. GCA characteristically affects the second- to fifth-order branches of the aorta. Affected arteries include the external carotids, temporal arteries, and ciliary and ophthalmic arteries. Subclavian and brachial arteries can be affected. Uncommonly, intracranial arteritis may occur. Up to 50% of patients with GCA have PMR that may occur prior to, concurrent with, or following diagnosis of GCA. It is imperative that high-dose prednisone be initiated without delay to prevent irreversible visual loss from GCA; some advocate intravenous pulse methylprednisolone for patients with significant visual changes. Prednisone should generally be administered for approximately 1 month (or until resolution of signs and symptoms), with subsequent dose reduction at a rate of about 10% every few weeks.

CT of the head would be helpful in assessing for stroke-induced vision changes, but this patient's clinical presentation is not that of stroke. Stroke cannot explain the patient's malaise, weakness, aching, and tenderness over the left temporal area.

There are insufficient data from randomized controlled trials to recommend daily low-dose aspirin to prevent GCA complications, and this therapy would be inappropriate without concomitant high-dose prednisone.

Methotrexate may be helpful as adjunctive therapy for GCA and PMR, especially for those patients who have relapses and are unable to taper glucocorticoids. It is not appropriate initial therapy for GCA, especially as it will not take effect for several weeks, and this patient requires immediate treatment to prevent vision loss.

Temporal artery biopsy is the gold standard for diagnosing GCA; at least 1 cm is required in order to reduce the false-negative rate because of skip lesions. However, glucocorticoid therapy should not be delayed in order to establish the diagnosis of GCA. If necessary, temporal artery biopsy can be obtained 1 to 2 weeks after glucocorticoids have been initiated, and will still reveal diagnostic abnormalities.

KEY POINT

- High-dose prednisone must be initiated immediately in patients with signs and symptoms that are highly suggestive of giant cell arteritis to prevent irreversible visual loss.

Bibliography

Buttgereit F, Dejaco C, Matteson EL, Dasgupta B. Polymyalgia rheumatica and giant cell arteritis: a systematic review. JAMA. 2016;315:2442-58. [PMID: 27299619] doi:10.1001/jama.2016.5444

Item 22   Answer: B

Educational Objective: Diagnose inclusion body myositis.

The most likely diagnosis is inclusion body myositis (IBM), an inflammatory myopathy that can involve both the proximal and distal muscles; although typically symmetric, muscle distribution may be asymmetric. Sporadic IBM is the most common muscle disease in elderly populations, is more common in men than women, and typically develops after age 50 years and does not appear to affect individuals younger than 45 years old. Serum creatine kinase levels are typically less than 10 to 12 times the upper limit of normal. Its insidious onset and distal muscle involvement help to distinguish IBM from the other inflammatory myopathies. The absence of rash helps to exclude dermatomyositis. Electromyogram may show myopathic, neurogenic, or mixed changes with both short and long duration motor unit potentials and spontaneous activity. Diagnosis of IBM is confirmed by muscle biopsy showing muscle fibers containing multiple rimmed vacuoles. Distinguishing IBM from polymyositis is important because IBM is usually not treated with immunosuppressive therapy and has an overall poor response to treatment.

Amyotrophic lateral sclerosis (ALS) is a progressive, neurodegenerative disease that can have an insidious onset causing muscle weakness. Upper and lower motor neuron signs may be seen, including spasticity, abnormal gait, increased reflexes, and difficulty with coordination (including manipulation of small objects), tripping, and falling. Findings may initially be proximal or distal and asymmetric. ALS can be distinguished from IBM by the presence of fasciculations, and ALS does not raise serum creatine kinase levels.

Mitochondrial myopathy can present in childhood, adolescence, or young adulthood, and a family history of mitochondrial disease is often evident. When myopathy predominates, the patient generally presents with proximal muscle weakness. However, exercise intolerance, painful and sometimes severe muscle cramping, and eye symptoms such as ptosis and diplopia are common. Serum creatine kinase levels are usually within the normal range, but serum lactate levels may be elevated.

Polymyositis occurs more frequently in women than in men and has its age of onset before 50 more often than IBM. It generally presents with proximal, rather than distal, muscle weakness, and serum creatine kinase levels can be substantially higher than those seen in IBM, often greater than 10 to 50 times normal.

KEY POINT

- Inclusion body myositis (IBM) is an inflammatory myopathy that can involve both the proximal and distal muscles with typically symmetric muscle distribution; its insidious onset and distal muscle involvement help to distinguish IBM from the other inflammatory myopathies.

Bibliography

Needham M, Mastaglia FL. Sporadic inclusion body myositis: a review of recent clinical advances and current approaches to diagnosis and treatment. Clin Neurophysiol. 2016;127:1764-73. [PMID: 26778717] doi:10.1016/j.clinph.2015.12.011

Item 23   Answer: A

Educational Objective: Treat sicca symptoms associated with Sjögren syndrome.

Artificial tears and sugar-free candies are the most appropriate treatment at this time. This patient meets diagnostic criteria for Sjögren syndrome, with objective documentation of sicca in the presence of anti-Ro/SSA antibodies, antinuclear antibodies, and rheumatoid factor. Her dental carries and missing teeth are almost certainly due to her dry mouth, as evidenced by lack of salivary pooling below the tongue. She has arthralgia but no definite arthritis and, consistent with Sjögren joint involvement, no evidence of erosive joint disease on radiograph. The immediate treatment goal of sicca is the re-establishment of wetting of the eyes and mouth. For the eyes, topical application of artificial tears is usually the first strategy, potentially followed by addition of topical cyclosporine or lifitegrast if artificial tears prove insufficient. For oral dryness, sugar-free candy or chewing gum can

help to increase saliva flow. Regular intake or rinsing with small sips of water is also recommended. Artificial saliva substitutes would be considered next if these approaches are insufficient.

Methotrexate is a nonbiologic disease-modifying antirheumatic drug occasionally used in Sjögren syndrome for arthritis. Because the patient's joint disease is unlikely to result in future bony damage and is responsive to ibuprofen, no additional arthritis management is needed at this time. There is no documented indication for methotrexate to treat sicca symptoms associated with Sjögren syndrome.

Pilocarpine is a muscarinic agonist that may stimulate saliva secretion. It is often poorly tolerated and would not be considered unless basic measures to treat oral dryness are insufficient.

Rituximab depletes B cells and has shown early promise for the management of Sjögren syndrome. Early studies suggest a possible benefit for treating sicca, but it is generally reserved for patients with systemic Sjögren complications or severe disease. At the present time, its use is not warranted in this patient.

Topical ophthalmic NSAID drops are absolutely contraindicated in Sjögren syndrome because they carry risk for severe corneal damage.

KEY POINT

- Initial management of Sjögren syndrome typically involves treatment of sicca symptoms by restoring moisture of the eyes and mouth.

Bibliography

Baer AN, Walitt B. Sjögren Syndrome and Other Causes of Sicca in Older Adults. Clin Geriatr Med. 2017;33:87-103. [PMID: 27886700] doi:10.1016/j.cger.2016.08.007

Item 24   Answer: C

Educational Objective: Diagnose scleritis in a patient with rheumatoid arthritis.

The most likely diagnosis is scleritis in this patient with rheumatoid arthritis (RA). RA is one of the most common diseases associated with scleritis. Typical features include eye pain, pain with gentle palpation of the globe, and photophobia. The deep scleral vessels are involved and may lead to scleromalacia, which is characterized by thinning of the sclera and is seen as a dark area in the white sclera. Scleromalacia may lead to perforation of the sclera called scleromalacia perforans. Scleritis can be vision-threatening and lead to blindness; it is therefore important to urgently refer the patient to an ophthalmologist for care.

Conjunctivitis also causes a red eye. Typically, the underlying vessels are visible, a discharge may be seen, and often there is mattering of the eye in the morning. The eye may feel irritated but there is no pain or loss of visual acuity. In general, conjunctivitis is a diagnosis of exclusion. The presence of pain and decreased visual acuity exclude conjunctivitis in this patient.

Episcleritis is an abrupt inflammation of the superficial vessels of the episclera, a thin membrane that lies just beneath the conjunctiva. The cause is often unclear; rarely, it is associated with systemic rheumatologic disease. Patients with episcleritis frequently present without pain or decreased visual acuity. On examination, the inflammation appears localized. White sclera can be seen between superficial dilated blood vessels. Episcleritis typically resolves spontaneously. The presence of pain, diffuse redness, and decreased visual acuity make episcleritis an unlikely diagnosis.

Subconjunctival hemorrhage is a common disorder and typically benign in origin. It is caused by painless bleeding into the superficial portion of the eye. Examination reveals a blotchy redness (from extravascular blood) that is typically confined to one area of the conjunctiva. Subconjunctival hemorrhage is painless and not associated with loss of vision. Most cases resolve within several weeks without intervention. The patient's findings are not compatible with subconjunctival hemorrhage.

KEY POINT

- Rheumatoid arthritis is one of the most common diseases associated with scleritis, which can be vision-threatening and lead to thinning of the sclera and perforation.

Bibliography

Artifoni M, Rothschild PR, Brézin A, Guillevin L, Puéchal X. Ocular inflammatory diseases associated with rheumatoid arthritis. Nat Rev Rheumatol. 2014;10:108-16. [PMID: 24323074] doi:10.1038/nrrheum.2013.185

Item 25   Answer: B

Educational Objective: Diagnose disseminated gonococcal infection.

The most likely diagnosis is disseminated gonococcal infection (DGI). This patient has the arthritis-dermatitis syndrome of DGI due to *Neisseria gonorrhoeae*. This syndrome is characterized by a triad of tenosynovitis, dermatitis (usually painless pustular or vesiculopustular lesions), and polyarthralgia without frank arthritis. Fever, chills, and malaise are common. Inflammation of multiple tendons of the wrists, fingers, ankles, and toes distinguishes this syndrome from other forms of infectious arthritis. This presentation of DGI is associated with positive blood cultures and characteristic skin lesions. Diagnosis is established by blood and synovial fluid cultures, as well as pharynx, cervix, urethra, and rectum cultures, and/or nucleic acid amplification testing. Testing patients and their sexual partners for both gonorrhea and chlamydia is critical. Initial therapy for DGI is usually with ceftriaxone plus either azithromycin or doxycycline, and is rapidly effective.

Chikungunya virus is an alphavirus endemic to Asia and Africa, where it is transmitted by mosquito vectors; however, cases are increasingly seen in the United States secondary to travel to endemic countries. In addition to fever, maculopapular rash, and headache, patients may experience synovitis and tenosynovitis of the fingers and wrists that is usually symmetric and may resemble rheumatoid arthritis. The presence of a pustular rash and lack of travel to an endemic area makes this diagnosis unlikely.

Reactive arthritis is an acute, asymmetric arthritis that typically follows chlamydial urethritis or infectious gastroenteritis within 6 weeks. It mainly affects lower extremity joints. Enthesitis, particularly at the Achilles tendon, can also occur. Patients also often have conjunctivitis, circinate balanitis, or keratoderma blenorrhagicum. A pustular or vesiculopustular rash is not part of the reactive arthritis syndrome.

Acute sarcoid arthritis presents most often as part of Löfgren syndrome, which is characterized by the triad of hilar adenopathy, acute arthritis, and erythema nodosum. The acute polyarthritis is mostly oligoarticular, with symmetric involvement most commonly involving the ankles or other lower extremity joints. This is in contrast to DGI, which is usually asymmetric and involves the upper extremity joints. Sarcoidosis may involve the skin, but lesions may be papular, nodular, plaque-like, or indurated and deep.

KEY POINT

- The arthritis-dermatitis syndrome of disseminated gonococcal infection due to *Neisseria gonorrhoeae* is characterized by a triad of tenosynovitis, dermatitis, and polyarthralgia without frank arthritis; fever, chills, and malaise are common.

Bibliography

García-Arias M, Balsa A, Mola EM. Septic arthritis. Best Pract Res Clin Rheumatol. 2011;25:407-21. [PMID: 22100289] doi:10.1016/j.berh.2011.02.001

Item 26   Answer: D

Educational Objective: Diagnose Libman-Sacks endocarditis.

Libman-Sacks endocarditis (nonbacterial thrombotic endocarditis) is the most likely cause of this patient's transient monocular blindness. She has an 8-year history of systemic lupus erythematosus (SLE) and positive antiphospholipid antibodies (anticardiolipin antibodies plus lupus anticoagulant) with recurrent pregnancy loss. She meets the criteria for antiphospholipid syndrome. Patients who have SLE with positive antiphospholipid antibodies are at a high risk for developing valvular dysfunction/thickening, and in some cases manifesting as Libman-Sacks endocarditis. A recent study confirmed this significant association between valvular heart disease and antiphospholipid antibody positivity. It was also found that the highest risk was seen in double-positive antiphospholipid antibodies/lupus anticoagulant patients, as is the case in this patient. Libman-Sacks endocarditis may affect 11% or more of patients

CONT.

with SLE and has no relationship to disease activity. The condition is associated with large verrucous lesions near the edge of the valve, most often the mitral valve. Typical lesions consist of immune complexes, mononuclear cells, and fibrin and platelet thrombi. Libman-Sacks endocarditis is usually asymptomatic but can be responsible for numerous complications, including embolic stroke, or in this case a transient ischemic attack in the territory of the ophthalmic artery, peripheral emboli, and infective endocarditis.

Bacterial endocarditis can be a source of cardiogenic emboli, but 90% of patients with infective endocarditis have fever, and often other constitutional symptoms, which are absent in this patient.

Patients with SLE are prone to develop premature atherosclerosis (and can be a cause of stroke or transient ischemia attack), but this patient has no findings of atherosclerosis involving the carotid artery; furthermore, this diagnosis cannot account for the patient's heart murmur.

Transient monocular blindness can be a manifestation of giant cell arteritis, but this diagnosis is extremely rare in individuals less than 40 years old.

KEY POINT

- Patients with systemic lupus erythematosus and positive antiphospholipid antibodies are at a high risk for developing valvular dysfunction/thickening, in some cases manifesting as Libman Sacks endocarditis.

Bibliography

Vivero F, Gonzalez-Echavarri C, Ruiz-Estevez B, Maderuelo I, Ruiz-Irastorza G. Prevalence and predictors of valvular heart disease in patients with systemic lupus erythematosus. Autoimmun Rev. 2016;15:1134-1140. [PMID: 27639157] doi:10.1016/j.autrev.2016.09.007

 Item 27   **Answer:**   **C**

Educational Objective: Diagnose subcranial giant cell arteritis.

The most likely diagnosis is giant cell arteritis (GCA), a large-vessel vasculitis that most commonly affects vessels in the head and neck area (cranial GCA), resulting in jaw claudication, headaches (from involvement of the superficial temporal artery), and visual changes (due to involvement of ophthalmic arteries). Polymyalgia rheumatica (PMR), although not a vasculitis, is an inflammatory disorder that frequently accompanies GCA. Symptoms of PMR (shoulder and hip girdle pain and stiffness) may precede, accompany, or follow the diagnosis of GCA, and may be the only symptom of silent or subclinical GCA. As in this case, GCA less commonly affects the great vessels of the chest (subcranial GCA), causing upper extremity claudication and/or aortitis, as seen in this patient. Aortitis may lead to aortic root dilation, aortic regurgitation, and heart failure, as seen in this patient; this manifestation is usually a late feature of GCA.

Kawasaki disease initially presents in childhood, affects medium-sized (coronary) vessels, and can lead to heart failure due to myocardial damage years after the inflammation from vasculitis has resolved. Kawasaki disease does not have an onset in late adulthood.

Polyarteritis nodosa is a medium-vessel vasculitis that rarely affects the heart, and when it does, involves coronary vessels, not large vessels; this patient has a large-vessel vasculitis affecting the aorta.

In Takayasu arteritis (TA), the affected arteries are primarily the aorta (ascending, descending thoracic, and abdominal aorta) and its major branches. In contrast to GCA, TA is rare (2 cases/million patient-years) and mainly affects young women (9:1 ratio) with a typical age at onset between 15 and 25 years. Histologically, the pathophysiologic processes of TA and GCA are similar, with infiltration of T cells, macrophages, and giant cells in the vessel wall. This patient's age effectively excludes TA as the cause of her symptoms.

KEY POINT

- Giant cell arteritis can affect the great vessels of the chest causing upper extremity claudication and/or aortitis; aortitis may lead to aortic root dilation, aortic regurgitation, and heart failure.

Bibliography

González-Gay MA, Pina T. Giant cell arteritis and polymyalgia rheumatica: an update. Curr Rheumatol Rep. 2015;17:6. [PMID: 25618572] doi:10.1007/s11926-014-0480-1

Item 28   **Answer:**   **B**

Educational Objective: Diagnose a secondary cause of acute calcium pyrophosphate crystal arthritis.

A serum calcium measurement is most likely to identify the cause of this patient's symptoms. This young woman has recurrent attacks of acute calcium pyrophosphate (CPP) crystal arthritis (pseudogout). Clues to the diagnosis include acute and recurrent self-limited monoarticular arthritis, chondrocalcinosis on radiograph, and, most tellingly, identification of CPP crystals under polarizing microscopy. This condition usually affects the elderly; therefore, evidence of acute CPP crystal arthritis in a young person should always prompt an investigation for secondary causes. Secondary causes include hyperparathyroidism, hypothyroidism, hypophosphatasia, hypomagnesemia, and hemochromatosis. This patient has recent-onset signs and symptoms suggestive of hypercalcemia and hyperparathyroidism, including abdominal discomfort, constipation, and weakness. Therefore, measuring the serum calcium is appropriate (and serum parathyroid hormone, if hypercalcemia is present), because this patient appears to have CPP deposition due to hyperparathyroidism.

Anti–cyclic citrullinated peptide antibodies are useful in the diagnosis of rheumatoid arthritis (RA). RA typically presents with the insidious onset of symmetric arthritis in the hands and feet along with morning stiffness. Monoarthritis is a rare presenting feature of RA, but it is usually followed by development of the symmetric arthritis.

Checking serum creatine kinase would not be a first-line test for this patient. Although muscle disease is associated with weakness, myositis would not account for many of the other manifestations, including the monoarticular arthritis, radiographic chondrocalcinosis, and synovial fluid crystals.

Serum urate would be an appropriate laboratory study to measure if gout was suspected, but the synovial fluid analysis is consistent with acute CPP crystal arthritis rather than gout, in which negatively birefringent crystals are seen. Gout also more typically affects the metatarsophalangeal joints, the mid foot, ankles, and knees, although the finger joints may be affected in postmenopausal women.

KEY POINT

- Evidence of acute calcium pyrophosphate crystal arthritis (pseudogout) in a young person should always prompt an investigation for secondary causes such as hyperparathyroidism, hypothyroidism, hypophosphatasia, hypomagnesemia, and hemochromatosis.

Bibliography

Rosenthal AK, Ryan LM. Calcium Pyrophosphate Deposition Disease. N Engl J Med. 2016;374:2575-84. [PMID: 27355536] doi:10.1056/NEJMra1511117

Item 29   Answer: D

Educational Objective: Treat relapsed granulomatosis with polyangiitis.

Rituximab is the most appropriate treatment for this patient who has experienced a relapse of granulomatosis with polyangiitis (GPA), manifesting with pulmonary inflammation and nodules despite maintenance treatment with azathioprine. GPA is a rare systemic autoimmune disease of unknown cause that leads to vasculitis and granulomatosis of small- to medium-sized blood vessels. Without treatment, most patients die within 1 year. With treatment, most patients achieve remission within 6 months. Relapses of GPA are common, occurring in more than 50% of patients within 5 years, and may occur in different organs from the initial presentation. Both rituximab and cyclophosphamide are efficacious for initial induction therapy in patients with severe GPA. The choice of which therapy to use depends upon the individual patient presentation and comorbid conditions.

The RAVE (Rituximab versus Cyclophosphamide for ANCA-Associated Vasculitis) trial demonstrated that rituximab is superior to cyclophosphamide in the subgroup of patients with relapse. In this study, remission without

prednisone at 6 months was observed in 67% of rituximab-treated patients compared with 42% of cyclophosphamide patients ($P = 0.01$; NNT = 4). Rituximab was also as effective as cyclophosphamide in the treatment of patients with kidney disease or alveolar hemorrhage. There were no significant differences between the treatment groups with respect to rates of adverse events.

In trials of etanercept treatment for GPA, patients manifested an increased risk for the development of solid malignancies, especially if they had previously been treated with cytotoxic drugs. Therefore, etanercept is not considered first-line treatment for GPA.

Methotrexate is inadequate as induction therapy for severe disease; it can be used alone either as maintenance therapy after induction, or for mild and limited disease.

KEY POINT

- Rituximab is appropriate treatment for patients who experience a relapse of granulomatosis with polyangiitis.

Bibliography

Comarmond C, Cacoub P. Granulomatosis with polyangiitis (Wegener): clinical aspects and treatment. Autoimmun Rev. 2014;13:1121-5. [PMID: 25149391] doi:10.1016/j.autrev.2014.08.017

Item 30   Answer: B

Educational Objective: Manage disequilibrium caused by pregabalin.

The most appropriate next step in management is to discontinue pregabalin. Disequilibrium is an unsteadiness, or sense of imbalance, with standing or walking. Patients may experience disequilibrium as a side effect of medication use. This patient has fibromyalgia, which is characterized by widespread pain, fatigue, disturbed sleep, and cognitive dysfunction. Education, exercise, and psychosocial support are cornerstones of treatment, although pharmacotherapy is often warranted. Pregabalin can be effective for patients with fibromyalgia, but use is often limited by side effects, including weight gain, peripheral edema, lethargy, and especially dizziness (31% of all patients in trials versus 9% on placebo). The patient has fallen several times; therefore, it is imperative to remove any possible offending agent, and pregabalin is the most likely culprit among her medications. Once the troubling side effects resolve off medication, restarting at a lower dose could be considered.

Duloxetine can cause dizziness but not nearly as frequently as pregabalin (10% of patients in controlled trials versus 6% on placebo). Because pregabalin is the more likely cause, it should be stopped first; if possible, only one variable should be changed at a time.

There is no need to measure methylmalonic acid and homocysteine levels in this patient. Although vitamin B_{12} deficiency can cause peripheral neuropathy, the normal B_{12} level and neurologic examination make this a very unlikely diagnosis.

Given the high likelihood that pregabalin is causing the dizziness as well as the normal neurologic examination, MRI of the brain is not indicated at this time. It would be most useful if a space-occupying lesion were suspected, but there are no neurologic symptoms or signs referable to the central nervous system. If the patient were to develop neurologic signs or if symptoms did not improve with discontinuation of the pregabalin, this decision would need to be reevaluated.

Vestibular rehabilitation may be appropriate as a means of adapting to long-lasting or permanent vestibular damage. It includes exercises and balance training intended to stabilize gait and decrease symptoms and falls. It is not an appropriate first step in this case, however, because drug discontinuation alone is likely to result in improvement of her symptoms.

KEY POINT

- Use of pregabalin is often limited by side effects, including weight gain, peripheral edema, lethargy, and dizziness; discontinuation may be needed to manage the side effects.

Bibliography

Derry S, Cording M, Wiffen PJ, Law S, Phillips T, Moore RA. Pregabalin for pain in fibromyalgia in adults. Cochrane Database Syst Rev. 2016;9:CD011790. [PMID: 27684492]

Item 31   Answer: A

Educational Objective: Treat relapsed polymyalgia rheumatica.

Prednisone, 10 mg/d, is the most appropriate treatment for this patient with a relapse of polymyalgia rheumatica (PMR) after her prednisone dose was weaned to 8 mg/d. Patients with PMR experience symmetric pain and stiffness in the shoulder, neck, and hip regions, typically without synovitis. PMR is a clinical diagnosis based on the characteristic symptoms in a patient older than 50 years and is supported by an elevated erythrocyte sedimentation rate and/or C-reactive protein. Recent guidelines for the management of PMR (developed by a collaborative effort of the American College of Rheumatology and the European League Against Rheumatism) recommend increasing the prednisone to the last pre-relapse dose at which the patient was doing well, followed by a gradual reduction within 4 to 8 weeks back to the relapse dose. This patient was asymptomatic on 10 mg/d, prior to reducing to her current relapse dose; therefore, an increase to 10 mg/d is appropriate. After the flare-up subsides, a slow taper of 1 mg every 4 weeks may be better tolerated then larger increments over 2- to 4-week periods.

Prednisone, 30 mg/d, would also help treat the flare-up, but this higher dose is probably unnecessary, and a lower dose should be attempted first.

Prednisone, 60 mg/d, is not a typical dose used for PMR, and in the absence of concomitant giant cell arteritis is not needed to treat a PMR flare-up.

Methotrexate can be added as a glucocorticoid-sparing agent for patients who cannot be successfully weaned off prednisone or who are experiencing significant glucocorticoid toxicity; this patient has only had one flare-up and may do well after a modest increase followed by a more gradual taper of prednisone, making the addition of methotrexate premature at this time.

KEY POINT

- A relapse of polymyalgia rheumatica should be treated with an increase in prednisone to the last pre-relapse dose at which the patient was doing well, followed by a gradual reduction within 4 to 8 weeks back to the relapse dose.

Bibliography

Dejaco C, Singh YP, Perel P, Hutchings A, Camellino D, Mackie S, et al; European League Against Rheumatism. 2015 Recommendations for the management of polymyalgia rheumatica: a European League Against Rheumatism/American College of Rheumatology collaborative initiative. Ann Rheum Dis. 2015;74:1799-807. [PMID: 26359488] doi:10.1136/annrheumdis-2015-207492

Item 32   Answer: B

Educational Objective: Treat primary angiitis of the central nervous system.

In addition to high-dose glucocorticoids, cyclophosphamide is the most appropriate treatment for this patient who has primary angiitis of the central nervous system. Patients typically present with gradual progressive neurologic symptoms such as headaches, cognitive impairment, and other neurologic deficits such as strokes. Laboratory studies, including erythrocyte sedimentation rate, are typically normal, but 90% of patients have abnormal cerebrospinal fluid with lymphocytic pleocytosis and elevated total protein. MRI, MR angiogram, or CT angiogram often demonstrates nonspecific findings; cerebral angiogram sometimes reveals beading, or alternating stenosis and dilation of vessels consistent with vasculitis. Brain biopsy is falsely negative in 50% of patients due to patchy distribution of abnormalities, but when positive will show granulomatous vasculitis. Due to the rarity of this vasculitis, treatment is based on expert opinion and retrospective studies. High-dose glucocorticoids and cyclophosphamide have been reported to be effective in inducing remission and, given the severity of this patient's presentation, is the most appropriate choice. Glucocorticoids could be weaned over 3 to 6 months or longer, depending upon patient response to treatment. Cyclophosphamide could be discontinued after 3 to 6 months, and a maintenance drug such as azathioprine or mycophenolate mofetil could be started.

Anecdotal reports indicate that rituximab and tumor necrosis factor α inhibitors (such as adalimumab) may be effective; however, until more reports and studies are available, these would not be the first choice of treatment.

Methotrexate is not indicated for this patient because it does not penetrate the central nervous system well and would not be effective.

KEY POINT

- Cyclophosphamide with high-dose glucocorticoids is appropriate treatment for primary angiitis of the central nervous system.

Bibliography

Rodriguez-Pla A, Monach PA. Primary angiitis of the central nervous system in adults and children. Rheum Dis Clin North Am. 2015;41:47-62, viii. [PMID: 25399939] doi:10.1016/j.rdc.2014.09.004

Item 33 Answer: C

Educational Objective: Diagnose parvovirus B19.

Parvovirus B19 testing will most likely confirm the diagnosis. Parvovirus B19, which causes the childhood condition known as fifth disease (erythema infectiosum), is a DNA virus with a tropism for erythrocyte precursors. Adults usually contract the virus from children; individuals at risk include daycare or school workers and parents. Infection may be asymptomatic or produce a flu-like illness. In adults, the rash may be absent or atypical. The arthritis begins acutely, with symmetric pain and stiffness of the small joints of the hands and feet, as well as wrists and knees, in a pattern often mimicking rheumatoid arthritis (RA). This arthritis typically lasts for several weeks before resolving. Circulating anti-parvovirus IgM antibodies provide evidence of active disease; IgG antibodies indicate prior infection and are found in many healthy persons. Treatment is supportive.

Antinuclear antibody testing may be appropriate if systemic lupus erythematosus (SLE) or other related autoimmune diseases are suspected. Although some features of parvovirus B19 may overlap with those of SLE (fever, arthritis, cytopenias), other features of SLE (rashes, other mucocutaneous abnormalities) are notably absent in this patient.

Although HIV testing may be part of the complete workup for this patient's arthritis, the patient's exposure to children and the resolved antecedent brief febrile illness with an evanescent rash make parvovirus B19 much more likely.

Only 50% of patients with RA have detectable rheumatoid factor at onset, increasing to 60% to 80% in established disease. Conversely, up to 20% of patients with RA lack rheumatoid factor. Although rheumatoid factor testing may be part of this patient's evaluation because she has findings resembling RA, diagnosis requires that symptoms be chronic, usually for at least 6 weeks. Additionally, RA usually does not follow a viral infection.

KEY POINT

- Parvovirus B19 infection should be suspected in patients with an acute onset of small-joint symmetric polyarthritis following a febrile illness with rash, who have exposure to children.

Bibliography

Young NS, Brown KE. Parvovirus B19. N Engl J Med. 2004;350:586-97. [PMID: 14762186]

Item 34 Answer: A

Educational Objective: Diagnose rheumatoid arthritis with anti–cyclic citrullinated peptide antibodies.

Anti–cyclic citrullinated peptide (CCP) antibody testing is appropriate. This patient has a symmetric inflammatory polyarthritis involving the small joints of the hands and feet, which is highly suggestive of rheumatoid arthritis (RA). Laboratory studies, including rheumatoid factor, anti-CCP antibodies, and inflammatory markers, can assist in confirming the diagnosis, with anti-CCP antibodies the most helpful. Anti-CCP antibodies have a sensitivity of 70%, similar to that of rheumatoid factor, but they have a much higher specificity than rheumatoid factor (95%) and are more predictive than rheumatoid factor for erosive disease, making this test very useful to diagnose RA. The dual presence of rheumatoid factor and anti-CCP antibodies makes a diagnosis of RA substantially more likely.

Spondyloarthritis disorders share an overlapping set of features, including inflammation of the axial skeleton, tendons, and entheses; tendon and enthesis calcification; and an association with HLA-B27 antigen. HLA-B27 testing can define a probability for spondyloarthritis but cannot independently confirm or exclude any specific diagnosis. This patient does not have any features besides peripheral arthritis to suggest spondyloarthritis.

Parvovirus can cause polyarthralgia/arthritis but is generally transient, lasting 3 weeks or less, and is often accompanied by a net-like rash on the extremities and low-grade fever. IgM serology would indicate a recent infection and has to be checked within 8 to 10 weeks of infection because it declines thereafter as IgG rises. An elevated IgG antibody would simply indicate a past infection with the virus. This patient's persistent joint findings lasting 8 weeks argue against parvovirus infection.

Serum urate is useful in the diagnosis of gout in patients with typical findings. Although chronic recurrent gout can be polyarticular, this patient does not have features that suggest underlying gout such as palpable tophaceous depositions, and gout is rare in women before menopause.

Hypothyroidism can cause fatigue and uncommonly cause arthralgia and joint stiffness but is not associated with the active synovitis seen in this patient. Therefore, measuring thyroid-stimulating hormone would not be indicated.

KEY POINT

- Anti–cyclic citrullinated antibody testing is beneficial in diagnosing rheumatoid arthritis.

Bibliography

Chang PY, Yang CT, Cheng CH, Yu KH. Diagnostic performance of anti-cyclic citrullinated peptide and rheumatoid factor in patients with rheumatoid arthritis. Int J Rheum Dis. 2016;19:880-6. [PMID: 25940989]

Item 35   Answer: A

Educational Objective: Treat osteoarthritis with duloxetine.

Duloxetine, a serotonin and norepinephrine reuptake inhibitor with central nervous system effects, is a good treatment option for this patient with generalized osteoarthritis (OA). Duloxetine is FDA approved for chronic musculoskeletal pain and has been shown to have analgesic efficacy for chronic low back pain and knee OA pain, implicating the role of central sensitization in OA pain modulation. This patient has already tried multiple nonpharmacologic measures, as well as intra-articular glucocorticoid and hyaluronic injections, all with insufficient symptomatic relief. Duloxetine is a reasonable choice given the patient's comorbidities and generalized musculoskeletal pain.

Gabapentin and pregabalin are more effective than placebo in the treatment of neuropathic pain conditions such as postherpetic neuralgia and diabetic neuropathy. These drugs are expensive and both are associated with dose-dependent dizziness and sedation. There is no evidence of their effectiveness specifically for chronic OA pain.

NSAIDs inhibit cyclooxygenase (COX) enzymes, blocking the generation of the lipid prostaglandin E_2 (PGE_2). PGE_2 stimulates inflammation, vasodilation, smooth muscle contraction, pain, and fever. However, PGE_2 also maintains gastric mucosa and promotes kidney sodium excretion and glomerular filtration. Other COX products include thromboxane A_2, a prothrombotic regulator of platelets, and prostacyclin, an antithrombotic and vasodilatory lipid. Because NSAIDs inhibit all of these, the consequences of COX inhibition are complex and accompanied by multiple potential side effects. Side-effect risk is increased in older patients and those with preexisting comorbidities. Therefore, ibuprofen is not an advisable choice in an elderly patient with peptic ulcer disease, hypertension, and heart disease.

Topical capsaicin may benefit localized OA (for example, knee only) but is impractical in this case given the multiple areas of involvement. Furthermore, duloxetine is more likely to be efficacious given how many treatments this patient has tried and failed.

KEY POINT

- Duloxetine is FDA approved for chronic musculoskeletal pain and has been shown to have analgesic efficacy for chronic low back pain and knee osteoarthritis pain.

Bibliography

McAlindon TE, Bannuru RR, Sullivan MC, Arden NK, Berenbaum F, Bierma-Zeinstra SM, et al. OARSI guidelines for the non-surgical management of knee osteoarthritis. Osteoarthritis Cartilage. 2014;22:363-88. [PMID: 24462672] doi:10.1016/j.joca.2014.01.003

Item 36   Answer: A

Educational Objective: Diagnose adult-onset Still disease.

The most likely diagnosis is adult-onset Still disease (AOSD), a systemic inflammatory disease of multiple organ systems. This patient displays the typical signs and symptoms of AOSD, with spiking fevers, pharyngitis, an evanescent salmon pink rash that occurs in conjunction with fever, adenopathy, hepatosplenomegaly with elevated liver enzymes, leukocytosis with neutrophil predominance, inflammatory arthritis, and myalgia. Patients with AOSD can also develop other manifestations such as serositis. Extremely high serum ferritin levels are a typical feature. AOSD may also be seen during pregnancy or in the postpartum period. The diagnosis is clinical, and other entities such as infection and malignancy must be excluded.

Cryoglobulinemic vasculitis can cause arthritis, rash, and fever and may be associated with liver abnormalities, particularly if it is related to hepatitis C virus. However, the rash of cryoglobulinemia is related to small-vessel vasculitis characterized by palpable purpura of the lower extremities. Other organs characteristically involved include peripheral nerves and the kidneys (glomerulonephritis). Cryoglobulinemia cannot explain the elevated serum ferritin level.

Lymphoma can cause arthralgia, fever, rash, lymphadenopathy, and organomegaly. Lymphoma would not explain the patient's pleural friction rub, arthritis, or elevated serum ferritin level.

Microscopic polyangiitis is a form of ANCA-associated vasculitis in which patients can develop fever, rash, arthritis, and pulmonary disease, but this patient's rash (pink, evanescent, involving the trunk) is not typical for vasculitis (palpable purpura, urticaria, livedo reticularis, nodules). In addition, kidney involvement is nearly ubiquitous in microscopic polyangiitis, and the normal urinalysis argues against this diagnosis.

Similarly, systemic lupus erythematosus (SLE) can cause the same symptoms, but the rash associated with SLE is unlike that of AOSD. The malar rash of acute cutaneous lupus erythematosus consists of bright erythematous patches over both cheeks and the nasal bridge, almost always sparing the nasolabial folds; the rash is unrelated to fever. In addition, SLE cannot explain the elevated ferritin level.

KEY POINT

- Adult-onset Still disease is characterized by spiking fever, an evanescent salmon-colored rash on the trunk and extremities that occurs in conjunction with fever, arthritis, lymphadenopathy, and leukocytosis; an extremely high serum ferritin level is characteristic.

Bibliography

Gerfaud-Valentin M, Jamilloux Y, Iwaz J, Sève P. Adult-onset Still's disease. Autoimmun Rev. 2014;13:708-22. [PMID: 24657513] doi:10.1016/j.autrev.2014.01.058

Item 37   Answer: A

Educational Objective: Treat inflammatory bowel disease–associated arthritis.

Adalimumab is the most appropriate treatment for this patient with inflammatory bowel disease–associated arthritis. Various pharmacologic agents may be useful in the treatment of both intestinal manifestations and peripheral arthritis related to Crohn disease and ulcerative colitis, including sulfasalazine, azathioprine, 6-mercaptopurine, methotrexate, glucocorticoids, and certain tumor necrosis factor (TNF)-α inhibitors. Adalimumab, certolizumab pegol, golimumab, and infliximab are more effective than other TNF-α inhibitors in treating the combination of bowel and joint manifestations. This patient with Crohn disease has developed peripheral oligoarthritis and dactylitis ("sausage digit"). She also has symptomatic bowel disease. She is most likely to improve her bowel and joint disease by the addition of a TNF-α inhibitor.

Intra-articular glucocorticoid injections can be used to treat inflammatory arthritis. However, the duration of symptom relief can be short term, practical use is limited by the size and number of joints involved, and this therapy will have no effect on the patient's dactylitis or inflammatory bowel disease.

Glucocorticoids are effective for inducing but not maintaining remission in Crohn disease. Although prednisone could be used to improve the patient's joint and bowel symptoms on a short-term basis, it is unlikely to control her bowel and joint symptoms in the long term and is increasingly likely to be associated with significant side effects the longer it is used.

Rituximab depletes B cells and is used in combination with methotrexate to treat rheumatoid arthritis in patients who have not adequately responded to a TNF-α inhibitor. Rituximab is not indicated for this patient's arthritis or bowel disease and is not recommended.

KEY POINT

- Long-term treatment options for bowel and joint symptoms associated with inflammatory bowel disease include sulfasalazine, azathioprine, 6-mercaptopurine, methotrexate, and the tumor necrosis factor α inhibitors adalimumab, certolizumab pegol, golimumab, and infliximab.

Bibliography

Peluso R, Manguso F, Vitiello M, Iervolino S, Di Minno MN. Management of arthropathy in inflammatory bowel diseases. Ther Adv Chronic Dis. 2015;6:65-77. [PMID: 25729557] doi:10.1177/2040622314563929

Item 38   Answer: D

Educational Objective: **Choose the most appropriate test to diagnose tuberculosis as the cause of chronic monoarthritis.**

The most appropriate test to perform next is a synovial biopsy. This patient has persistent inflammatory swelling of the right knee, with synovial fluid leukocyte counts between 15,000 and 20,000/µL (15-20 × 10⁹/L). The differential diagnosis in this patient with chronic inflammatory monoarthritis includes mycobacterial, fungal, or *Borrelia burgdorferi* infection and other systemic rheumatologic diseases such as sarcoidosis. Frequently in these patients, synovial fluid analysis

alone may be inadequate for diagnosis; serologies or other laboratory tests or synovial biopsy is required to establish the diagnosis. In this patient, a synovial biopsy is the most appropriate test to evaluate for all of the conditions in the differential diagnosis. The biggest concern here is *Mycobacterium tuberculosis* arthritis, given this patient's history of latent tuberculosis and a high risk due to advancing age.

Sarcoidosis is characterized by formation of noncaseating granulomas in multiple organs and tissues. These granulomas may increase angiotensin-converting enzyme levels. A history of latent tuberculosis, calcified granulomas in the upper lobe, and a chronically inflamed joint are more consistent with tuberculosis infection. In addition, the angiotensin-converting enzyme level is only 75% specific (25% of cases will be missed) and 90% specific (10% of positive results will be false positive), decreasing the usefulness of this test for sarcoidosis.

Multiple small pulmonary nodules (<5 mm) found incidentally in a patient without a known malignancy are likely to be nonmalignant. Like solitary pulmonary nodules, multiple pulmonary nodules may be further assessed with helical CT to better characterize their number, location, and morphology. However, in this patient, the previous history of tuberculosis, fever, and a chronic inflammatory monoarthritis strongly suggest tuberculosis, and a tissue diagnosis can be most easily established with synovial biopsy.

HLA-B27 testing may be useful in the evaluation of spondyloarthritis, which can present with chronic lower extremity inflammatory monoarthritis. However, this patient has no other findings of spondyloarthritis such as rash, bowel symptoms, or inflammatory back pain. Furthermore, HLA-B27 lacks specificity and is unlikely to yield the correct diagnosis.

KEY POINT

- Synovial fluid analysis can confirm inflammation but may be inadequate for diagnosis of a chronic inflammatory monoarthritis; synovial biopsy may be required.

Bibliography

Gerlag DM, Tak PP. How to perform and analyse synovial biopsies. Best Pract Res Clin Rheumatol. 2013;27:195-207. [PMID: 23731931] doi:10.1016/j.berh.2013.03.006

Item 39   Answer: A

Educational Objective: **Diagnose erosive osteoarthritis.**

Erosive osteoarthritis (OA) is the most likely diagnosis. Erosive OA is thought to be an aggressive subset of hand osteoarthritis that has periods of prominent inflammatory symptoms and characteristic erosive changes on imaging. Patients often experience pain, swelling, and joint deformities. Inflammatory damage to soft-tissue structures can result in deviation of the digits. Diagnosis is mostly based on the radiographic findings of articular surface erosions at the central portion of the joint. Erosions are often symmetric and occur mainly in the distal interphalangeal (DIP) and, to a lesser extent, proximal interphalangeal (PIP) joints. Radiographs reveal a "gull-wing" deformity, resulting from marginal sclerosis and osteophytes on the distal side of the joints, whereas the proximal side is centrally eroded or collapsed and thinned. Women are affected more frequently than men. Erythrocyte sedimentation rate (ESR), C-reactive protein (CRP), rheumatoid factor, and anti-cyclic citrullinated peptide antibodies are usually normal, as seen in this patient. Heberden nodes and squaring at the carpometacarpal joint also support a diagnosis of erosive OA in this patient.

Although gout flares may be superimposed upon sites of nodal OA, the inflamed DIP joints in this patient are less likely to represent a gouty flare given the normal ESR, CRP, and urate levels. Moreover, radiographs of patients with tophaceous gout often show marginal and juxta-articular punched-out erosions, which are not seen in this patient.

Psoriatic arthritis may be symmetric and affect the hands, including the DIP joints, but the patient reports no personal history of psoriasis, does not indicate significant morning stiffness, has no rashes or nail pitting, and does not have the marginal erosions on radiograph that would support this diagnosis.

Although the patient has symmetric hand arthritis and fits the typical demographics of a patient with rheumatoid arthritis (RA), the predominance of DIP symptoms, the lack of prolonged morning stiffness, the laboratory studies negative for inflammatory markers and/or RA autoantibodies, and the typical "gull-wing" deformity on radiograph (rather than marginal erosions) do not support RA as the diagnosis.

KEY POINT

- Diagnosis of erosive hand osteoarthritis is based essentially on radiographic findings of articular surface erosions at the central portion of the joint; erosions are often symmetric and occur mainly in the distal interphalangeal joints.

Bibliography
Kloppenburg M, Kwok WY. Hand osteoarthritis—a heterogeneous disorder. Nat Rev Rheumatol. 2011;8:22-31. [PMID: 22105244] doi:10.1038/nrrheum.2011.170

Item 40   Answer: A

Educational Objective: Diagnose a systemic lupus erythematosus flare.

Measurement of the anti-double-stranded DNA antibodies will be most helpful in evaluating this patient with a systemic lupus erythematosus (SLE) flare. She has recent inflammatory swelling of multiple joints, malar eruption, hypertension, and new-onset edema. She also has an elevated urine protein-creatinine ratio, suggesting the presence of active lupus nephritis. In this situation, the measurement of inflammatory markers and other tests associated with SLE flares can be very useful in establishing a diagnosis and directing treatment. Elevation of the erythrocyte sedimentation rate, rising

anti-double-stranded DNA antibody titer, and low complement levels reliably diagnose an SLE flare. Elevated C-reactive protein (CRP) is common in inflammatory states except in SLE, in which CRP levels do not rise during SLE flare-up (but do rise during an infectious episode). Complements are especially helpful in patients with SLE. Most inflammatory states are associated with increased complement levels except in certain immune complex-mediated diseases (SLE; cryoglobulinemic and urticarial vasculitis), where the levels decrease due to excessive consumption during active disease state. C3 and C4 are the commonly measured complements, and their levels decrease during the flare-up. An increase in the anti-double-stranded DNA antibody titer also indicates an SLE flare and has the best correlation with flare-up of lupus nephritis. A kidney biopsy to evaluate SLE kidney involvement should also be considered here.

Antinuclear antibody (ANA) testing is a useful screening tool for SLE but does not correlate with disease activity. Anti-Ro/SSA and anti-La/SSB antibodies correlate with SLE rashes and photosensitivity but do not correlate with disease activity. Anti-Smith antibodies are highly specific for the diagnosis of SLE but also do not correlate with disease activity. Anti-U1-ribonucleoprotein antibodies are found in patients with SLE and mixed connective tissue disease but do not correlate with disease activity.

KEY POINT

- Elevation of the erythrocyte sedimentation rate, rising anti-double-stranded DNA antibody titer, and low complement levels reliably diagnose a systemic lupus erythematosus flare.

Bibliography
Pisetsky DS. Anti-DNA antibodies—quintessential biomarkers of SLE. Nat Rev Rheumatol. 2016;12:102-10. [PMID: 26581343] doi:10.1038/nrrheum.2015.151

Item 41   Answer: D

Educational Objective: Diagnose immune-mediated necrotizing myopathy.

In addition to a muscle biopsy, anti-HMG Co-A reductase antibody testing is most likely to establish the diagnosis. A small number of patients taking statins develop immune-mediated necrotizing myopathy (IMNM), which can be easily confused with polymyositis. IMNM is thought to occur as a result of an immune response to HMGCR, the pharmacologic target of statins. IMNM can be a paraneoplastic phenomenon related to connective tissue disease, or drug related, most commonly statins. Statin use may initiate or worsen the syndrome. In patients taking statins, myositis may rapidly progress and persist despite drug discontinuation due to this abnormal immune response and is often associated with the production of anti-HMG Co-A reductase antibodies. The histologic finding of necrotic muscle fibers with only minimal inflammatory cells that do not invade the muscle fibers is characteristic of IMNM, and, given the patient's history of exposure to statins,

CONT.

a muscle biopsy and determination of anti-HMG CO-A reductase antibodies will most likely establish the diagnosis. The condition may respond to immunosuppressive therapy.

Anti–cyclic citrullinated peptide antibodies are not seen in inflammatory myopathies; they have a relatively high specificity (>90%) for rheumatoid arthritis and may be useful in the differential diagnosis of early polyarticular inflammatory arthritis.

Anti-cytosolic 5′-nucleotidase 1A antibodies have been identified in about half of patients with inclusion body myositis. Strong reactivity for these antibodies has relatively high specificity for inclusion body myositis compared with other muscle diseases.

Anti-histidyl-tRNA synthetase antibodies, particularly the subset anti-Jo-1 antibodies, are associated with the presence of interstitial lung disease in patients with inflammatory myopathies and, in particular, with antisynthetase syndrome of interstitial lung disease, Raynaud phenomenon, inflammatory arthritis, and mechanic's hands.

KEY POINT

- In patients with immune-mediated necrotizing myopathy, myositis may persist despite statin discontinuation and is often associated with the production of anti-HMG Co-A reductase antibodies.

Bibliography

Musset L, Allenbach Y, Benveniste O, Boyer O, Bossuyt X, Bentow C, et al. Anti-HMGCR antibodies as a biomarker for immune-mediated necrotizing myopathies: a history of statins and experience from a large international multi-center study. Autoimmun Rev. 2016;15:983-93. [PMID: 27491568] doi:10.1016/j.autrev.2016.07.023

Item 42   Answer: B

Educational Objective: Diagnose Sjögren syndrome.

The most appropriate diagnostic test to perform next is a lip biopsy. This patient has parotid and lacrimal enlargement and sicca. The differential diagnosis of sicca with parotid/lacrimal enlargement includes Sjögren syndrome, sarcoidosis, IgG4-related disease, HIV-associated diffuse lymphocytic infiltrate syndrome, and others. The American College of Rheumatology/European League Against Rheumatism has proposed diagnostic criteria for Sjögren syndrome. The most heavily weighted criteria include focal lymphocytic sialadenitis in labial salivary gland biopsy and the presence of anti-Ro/SSA antibodies. The presence of both will establish the diagnosis. Alternatively, the diagnosis can be established with one of the two major criteria and an abnormal ocular staining score of ≥5, abnormal Schirmer test, or abnormal whole saliva flow test. In addition, entities in the differential diagnosis should be excluded. The patient meets the criteria for keratoconjunctivitis sicca, but because of the absence of anti-Ro/SSA antibodies, additional support is needed. A lip biopsy to assess minor salivary gland pathology is relatively noninvasive; it can provide evidence sufficient to meet the proposed diagnostic criteria and might assist in ruling out other entities in the differential diagnosis.

CT of the chest might identify findings to support an alternative diagnosis. For example, findings of hilar lymphadenopathy or pulmonary nodules might support a diagnosis of sarcoidosis. However, the yield would be low given the normal chest radiograph.

Like lip biopsy, parotid biopsy can provide evidence of Sjögren syndrome; however, it is more invasive and risks seventh cranial nerve damage. Its use is currently limited to special situations.

A Schirmer test could conveniently confirm dry eyes, but dry eyes have already been confirmed by a more rigorous and reproducible ophthalmologic examination.

Sialography can assess the extent of mouth dryness, but the diagnosis of sicca has already been sufficiently confirmed.

KEY POINT

- A lip biopsy should be considered in a patient with sicca and suspected Sjögren syndrome when initial serologic evaluation is uninformative.

Bibliography

Giovelli RA, Santos MC, Serrano ÉV, Valim V. Clinical characteristics and biopsy accuracy in suspected cases of Sjögren's syndrome referred to labial salivary gland biopsy. BMC Musculoskelet Disord. 2015;16:30. [PMID: 25887888] doi:10.1186/s12891-015-0482-9

Item 43   Answer: C

Educational Objective: Diagnose methotrexate-induced anemia.

The most likely diagnosis is methotrexate-induced anemia. Methotrexate can cause stomatitis, hepatic inflammation and fibrosis, and myelotoxicity, including megaloblastic anemia and pancytopenia. Folic acid supplementation is mandatory in all patients receiving methotrexate and can prevent the development of stomatitis and hepatotoxicity (as measured by elevated aminotransferase levels). Hematologic toxicity, however, can occur even with folic acid supplementation. In this patient, a rise in mean corpuscular volume (MCV) indicates a likely megaloblastic anemia, and methotrexate is the likely cause. Guidelines from the American College of Rheumatology recommend periodic monitoring of the complete blood count every 4 weeks during the first 3 months of therapy, every 8 to 12 weeks from 3 to 6 months, and every 8 to 12 weeks thereafter.

Inflammatory anemia (anemia of chronic disease) is a common manifestation of rheumatoid arthritis and is usually a mild, normocytic anemia. Most patients experience symptoms related to their underlying disease rather than the anemia. Inflammatory anemia would not present with this degree of anemia or macrocytosis.

Typical features of iron deficiency are identical to those of any symptomatic anemia but may be subtle owing to an insidious onset of the condition. Headache and pica (craving for typically undesirable items such as ice, dirt, clay, paper, and laundry starch) are frequently associated symptoms;

other less common symptoms include restless legs syndrome and hair loss. The hallmark of iron deficiency is a microcytic hypochromic anemia. However, this is usually only seen in advanced iron deficiency, and anemia tends to precede morphologic changes in the cells. The presence of macrocytosis makes iron deficiency unlikely.

Tocilizumab is not associated with a macrocytic anemia. Through its anti-inflammatory properties, it may decrease the likelihood of inflammatory-induced anemia in patients with rheumatoid arthritis.

KEY POINT

- Methotrexate use can result in a megaloblastic anemia or pancytopenia; periodic monitoring of the complete blood count is recommended.

Bibliography

Shea B, Swinden MV, Ghogomu ET, Ortiz Z, Katchamart W, Rader T, et al. Folic acid and folinic acid for reducing side effects in patients receiving methotrexate for rheumatoid arthritis. J Rheumatol. 2014;41:1049-60. [PMID: 24737913] doi:10.3899/jrheum.130738

Item 44 Answer: A

Educational Objective: Evaluate acute monoarthritis with joint aspiration.

Aspiration of the right knee is the most appropriate test to establish the diagnosis. This patient has isolated inflammatory swelling of the right knee. Synovial fluid aspiration is essential when evaluating for infection and crystal-related disease and can distinguish between inflammatory and noninflammatory conditions. The most useful tests of synovial fluid for infection are leukocyte count, stains, and cultures, as well as evaluation of synovial fluid for crystals under polarized light. Synovial fluid leukocyte counts less than 200/μL (0.2 × 10⁹/L) are considered normal, between 200/μL and 2000/μL (0.2-2.0 × 10⁹/L) are associated with noninflammatory conditions, and greater than 2000/μL (2.0 × 10⁹/L) are associated with inflammatory states. The higher the count is, the more inflammatory the fluid and the greater the suspicion for crystal-related or infectious disease. There is no absolute cutoff value that distinguishes infection from crystal-related disease, because some infections may have lower counts than expected and crystal-related disease may have counts greater than 100,000/μL (100 × 10⁹/L). Thus, the proper application of synovial fluid leukocyte counts requires conservative interpretation. Generally, counts greater than 50,000/μL (50 × 10⁹/L) should be managed as infectious until explicitly proven otherwise; if there is clinical suspicion for infection, fluid should be sent for stains and cultures even in the setting of counts less than 50,000/μL (50 × 10⁹/L). Synovial fluid analysis can also confirm or rule out hemarthrosis, which can have a similar clinical presentation as in this case.

Blood cultures are appropriate in this patient but are only positive in 30% to 40% of patients with infectious arthritis and do not replace the need for arthrocentesis, which is the test most likely to establish the diagnosis.

The erythrocyte sedimentation rate (ESR) commonly indicates the presence of inflammation, and elevations are used to identify and monitor disease activity in rheumatologic diseases. However, obtaining an ESR will not provide additional information not already gleaned from the physical examination and will not establish a specific diagnosis.

MRI can detect soft-tissue abnormalities, inflammation, and fluid collections but is not the most appropriate next step to establish the cause of this patient's acute monoarthritis because it cannot distinguish between infection and acute gout.

KEY POINT

- Joint aspiration and synovial fluid analysis for Gram stain, cultures, and crystals are indicated to help diagnose the underlying cause of acute monoarthritis.

Bibliography

Becker JA, Daily JP, Pohlgeers KM. Acute monoarthritis: diagnosis in adults. Am Fam Physician. 2016;94:810-816. [PMID: 27929277]

Item 45 Answer: A

Educational Objective: Prevent glucocorticoid-induced osteoporosis.

This patient at risk for glucocorticoid-induced osteoporosis should begin alendronate. One of the many risks and side effects of chronic glucocorticoid therapy is osteoporosis. The Fracture Risk Assessment Tool (FRAX) calculator defines the 10-year fracture risk for patients with T-scores in the –1.0 to –2.5 range. The FRAX calculator (www.shef.ac.uk/FRAX) incorporates multiple risk factors, including sex, fracture history, femoral neck bone mineral density, glucocorticoid use, smoking, BMI, age, and alcohol intake to determine projected fracture risk. The American College of Rheumatology recommends that patients over the age of 40 years at moderate or high risk for osteoporotic fractures who are to be on at least 2.5 mg of prednisone daily for 3 months or more should begin prophylactic bisphosphonate therapy with alendronate, risedronate, or zoledronic acid. In patients on chronic glucocorticoid therapy, prophylactic bisphosphonate therapy significantly increases bone mineral density compared with placebo, and these patients also have fewer new vertebral fractures.

In patients at high risk for major osteoporotic fracture (10-year risk greater than 20% or a T score ≤–2.5 or a history of a fragility fracture) taking any dose of glucocorticoids for at least 1 month should receive prophylactic treatment (although these patients should be treated regardless of glucocorticoid therapy). Alendronate, risedronate, zoledronic acid, or teriparatide are therapeutic options. This patient is not in the high-risk category, and teriparatide is therefore not a recommended option.

Dual-energy x-ray absorptiometry (DEXA) is useful at the outset of chronic glucocorticoid therapy to risk-stratify patients and to provide baseline values. Although there is no consensus on the optimal frequency of monitoring bone mineral density with DEXA, there is no role for repeating the study in less than 1 year.

Because of her prolonged need for prednisone and risk for osteoporotic fracture, no additional therapy would be inappropriate management for this patient.

KEY POINT

- Patients at moderate or high 10-year risk for a major osteoporotic fracture taking at least 2.5 mg of prednisone daily for 3 months or more should begin prophylactic bisphosphonate therapy.

Bibliography

Buckley L, Guyatt G, Fink HA, Cannon M, Grossman J, Hansen KE, et al. 2017 American College of Rheumatology Guideline for the Prevention and Treatment of Glucocorticoid-Induced Osteoporosis. Arthritis Care Res (Hoboken). 2017;69:1095-1110. [PMID: 28585410] doi:10.1002/acr.23279

Item 46   Answer: C

Educational Objective: Diagnose pulmonary arterial hypertension in a patient with limited cutaneous systemic sclerosis.

The most likely cause of her symptom is pulmonary arterial hypertension. Pulmonary vascular disease occurs in up to 40% of patients with systemic sclerosis. Vascular disease leading to pulmonary arterial hypertension may occur secondary to interstitial lung disease (typically in patients with diffuse cutaneous systemic sclerosis) or as an isolated process (typically in limited cutaneous systemic sclerosis). Patients are usually asymptomatic in early disease but later develop dyspnea on exertion and diminished exercise tolerance. Severe disease can lead to right-sided heart failure. This patient with limited cutaneous systemic sclerosis and progressive dyspnea has a normal chest radiograph and a normal pulmonary examination, but an increased pulmonic sound and a widened split of S_2 on cardiac examination compatible with pulmonary hypertension. Taken together, the most likely cause of the patient's progressive dyspnea is pulmonary arterial hypertension. Initial evaluation of this patient should proceed with pulmonary function tests and echocardiography.

Interstitial lung disease (ILD) usually develops subacutely with progressive fibrosis. Patients with diffuse cutaneous systemic sclerosis and anti–Scl-70 antibodies are at higher risk for developing ILD. The most common symptom of ILD is slowly progressive dyspnea, at first on exertion, but later at rest. Other symptoms include nonproductive cough, decreased exercise tolerance, and chest pain. Auscultation reveals "Velcro"-like inspiratory crackles, most prominent at the lung bases. This patient's symptom complex limited to exertional dyspnea and normal pulmonary examination and chest radiograph make this diagnosis less likely.

Cardiac involvement in systemic sclerosis may be due to cardiac fibrosis or coronary artery disease or secondarily due to systemic or pulmonary hypertension. Intrinsic cardiac fibrosis is uncommon and usually asymptomatic.

Conduction disturbances and arrhythmias are common and probably relate to fibrosis of the conduction system. This uncommon complication is not the most likely cause of progressive exertional dyspnea in this patient.

There is an increased risk for venous thromboembolism in patients with systemic sclerosis, and risk is greatest during the first year after diagnosis. This patient's 3-month history of progressive exertional dyspnea is unlikely due to acute venous thromboembolic disease.

KEY POINT

- Patients with systemic sclerosis, especially those with limited disease, are at risk for pulmonary arterial hypertension.

Bibliography

Thakkar V, Lau EM. Connective tissue disease-related pulmonary arterial hypertension. Best Pract Res Clin Rheumatol. 2016;30:22-38. [PMID: 27421214] doi:10.1016/j.berh.2016.03.004

Item 47   Answer: C

Educational Objective: Select the most appropriate imaging study for probable osteoarthritis.

Radiography is the most appropriate initial imaging study. Radiography is used to assess inflammatory arthritis and osteoarthritis (OA). Radiography does not visualize soft tissues nearly as well as bone, and due to the two-dimensional nature of the images, not all bone findings are visible on every view. Radiography may not detect early or mild erosive arthritic changes. Despite these limitations, serial radiography can be useful for monitoring arthritis disease progression. Radiography is relatively inexpensive and readily available. Despite low levels of ionizing radiation, radiography is considered safe except for pregnant women. In this case, the most likely diagnosis is OA of the right knee. Weight-bearing views should be obtained to more accurately assess the knee joint on radiographs. Typical radiographic OA features are osteophytes, joint-space narrowing, subchondral sclerosis, and cysts. Erosions are uncommon unless the erosive OA subtype is present, which usually is more aggressive and inflammatory on clinical evaluation.

In contrast to radiography, CT permits multiple views and orientations from a single study. CT is more sensitive for detecting bony abnormalities, such as bone erosions, than radiography or MRI. CT is more expensive than radiography and exposes the patient to more radiation.

MRI is useful in detecting soft-tissue abnormalities, inflammation, and fluid collections, but is less effective than CT in demonstrating bony abnormalities and erosive changes. MRI is more sensitive than radiography in detecting early spine and sacroiliac joint inflammation. MRI is more expensive than radiography and CT and is generally ordered when assessment of soft-tissue imaging is required. Radiography is a better choice than MRI to detect typical changes of OA.

Ultrasonography can detect soft-tissue abnormalities such as synovitis, tendinitis, bursitis, and joint fluid, and Doppler can assess for increased tissue blood flow consistent with synovitis. Ultrasonography can diagnose and monitor disease, and can be used to guide arthrocentesis. Ultrasonography is relatively inexpensive, and there is no ionizing radiation. Because inflammatory disease or joint aspiration is not anticipated and radiography will be better able to detect bony changes of OA, ultrasonography is not indicated.

KEY POINT

- Radiography is typically used as the initial imaging modality to assess inflammatory arthritis and osteoarthritis.

Bibliography

Jacobson JA, Girish G, Jiang Y, Sabb BJ. Radiographic evaluation of arthritis: degenerative joint disease and variations. Radiology. 2008;248:737-47. [PMID: 18710973] doi:10.1148/radiol.2483062112

Item 48   Answer: C

Educational Objective: Diagnose pes anserine bursitis.

The most likely diagnosis is pes anserine bursitis, an inflammatory condition affecting the bursa at the insertion of the conjoined medial knee tendons into the anteromedial proximal tibia. This condition has been known to affect athletes but can also occur in those with concurrent knee osteoarthritis (usually in obese women) even without a history of trauma or overuse. The diagnosis of pes anserine bursitis is clinical, based on a history of increased medial knee pain worsened with climbing or descending stairs or rising from a seated position. Patients may also note morning pain and stiffness lasting more than 1 hour, and pain may worsen at night. Physical examination showing severe point tenderness at the insertion of the anserine tendon about 3 to 6 cm (2 in) below the medial joint line, often with local edema, supports the diagnosis. Relief with injection of a local anesthetic is also supportive.

A medial collateral ligament (MCL) tear may cause medial knee pain, which can also extend to where the MCL inserts on the anteromedial proximal tibia; however, an MCL injury is very painful and may cause difficulty ambulating. MCL injury is suspected when there is pain and/or laxity on valgus stress of the knee.

A meniscal tear could cause medial knee pain, but the pain is usually around the joint line; patients may also have unusual sensations in the knee such as clicking, locking, catching, or a sensation that the joint gives way. There are several provocative maneuvers on physical examination that may suggest a meniscal tear.

Quadriceps tendonitis occurs as a result of stress placed upon the quadriceps tendon, usually from sports-related activities. Pain can be felt at the lower part of the thigh, just above the patella. There may also be swelling around the quadriceps tendon.

KEY POINT

- Pes anserine bursitis is an inflammatory condition affecting the bursa at the insertion of the conjoined medial knee tendons into the anteromedial proximal tibia and should be considered when there is localized pain inferomedial to the knee joint.

Bibliography

Alvarez-Nemegyei J, Canoso JJ. Evidence-based soft tissue rheumatology IV: anserine bursitis. J Clin Rheumatol. 2004;10:205-6. [PMID: 17043509]

Item 49   Answer: C

Educational Objective: Diagnose relapsing polychondritis.

The most likely diagnosis is relapsing polychondritis (RP). RP is characterized by inflammation and damage of cartilaginous tissues; tissues most commonly affected include the cartilaginous portions of the external and middle ear, nose, tracheobronchial tree, and joints. Auricular involvement affects the helix but spares the earlobes. Nasal chondritis can result in collapse of the nasal bridge (saddle nose deformity), which can also be seen in trauma, granulomatosis with polyangiitis, cocaine use, congenital syphilis, and leprosy. Airway stenosis from tracheal ring involvement and aortitis/large-vessel vasculitis may occur and be life-threatening. RP is diagnosed by its typical clinical manifestations. Laboratory tests are nonspecific; acute phase reactants are elevated in 80%, and mild anemia is present in 44%. Patients with RP should undergo imaging (CT or MRI) to evaluate the large airways for inflammation/stenosis. This patient has a history of recurrent inflammation of the cartilage of the right ear, inflammatory eye disease, inflammatory arthritis, and bronchial strictures due to inflammation of bronchial cartilage, consistent with a diagnosis of RP.

Cogan syndrome (interstitial keratitis, with cochlear and vestibular dysfunction) is an unlikely diagnosis because the patient has neither vestibular nor cochlear findings.

Polyarteritis nodosa, a medium-vessel vasculitis, affects the mesenteric and renal arteries. Patients usually present with abdominal symptoms, neurologic involvement, and skin findings. Polyarteritis nodosa does not involve the eye or cartilage of the ear, nose, or airways, making this an unlikely diagnosis.

Besides the inflammatory arthritis, this patient has no typical symptoms or signs of systemic lupus erythematosus (SLE). In addition, SLE does not typically cause inflammation and destruction of cartilaginous structures.

KEY POINT

- Relapsing polychondritis is characterized by inflammation and damage of cartilaginous tissues; tissues most commonly affected include the cartilaginous portions of the external and middle ear, nose, tracheobronchial tree, and joints.

Answers and Critiques

Bibliography

Vitale A, Sota J, Rigante D, Lopalco G, Molinaro F, Messina M, et al. Relapsing polychondritis: an update on pathogenesis, clinical features, diagnostic tools, and therapeutic perspectives. Curr Rheumatol Rep. 2016;18:3. [PMID: 26711694] doi:10.1007/s11926-015-0549-5

Item 50   Answer: D

Educational Objective: Treat rheumatoid arthritis during pregnancy.

No change in therapy is needed for this pregnant patient with rheumatoid arthritis (RA). For women with established RA, two thirds will go into remission or achieve low disease activity during pregnancy; however, one third will not improve or will get worse. Improvement may depend on an HLA-DQ mismatch between mother and child and/or other factors such as microchimerism (sharing of maternal cells with the fetus and vice versa). The benefit begins in the first trimester and continues throughout the pregnancy. Disease activity typically returns, often with a flare, after delivery. Medication management of a patient with RA is a major issue, and pregnancy plans should be discussed with any woman of childbearing age who will be placed on therapy. Hydroxychloroquine is an antimalarial medication that appears to inhibit antigen processing. It can be used to treat RA and other forms of inflammatory arthritis. Although its efficacy in arthritis is modest, its excellent side-effect profile makes it a useful adjunctive therapy. Hydroxychloroquine crosses the placenta; however, there does not appear to be fetal toxicity with doses used for the treatment of RA. This patient currently has minimal disease activity and is likely to improve during pregnancy; therefore, she requires no change in therapy.

Limited case studies suggest that use of tumor necrosis factor α inhibitors during pregnancy may be safe, but a relationship to rare birth defects has been raised. Different agents may have different potential to cross the placenta. Decisions regarding the use of any biologic agent in pregnancy should incorporate risk-benefit analysis. Etanercept could be used only if this patient has a significant flare of disease during pregnancy but is not needed at the current time.

Leflunomide is contraindicated in this patient; this medication is extremely teratogenic and must not be used before/during pregnancy. Pregnancy must be avoided until the drug is no longer detectable in the serum; cholestyramine may be used to hasten the elimination of leflunomide from the body.

Methotrexate was discontinued prior to attempted conception, which is highly appropriate. Methotrexate is highly teratogenic and abortifacient, and it must be discontinued at least 3 months before pregnancy.

KEY POINT

- Methotrexate and leflunomide are contraindicated in pregnant patients because these medications are highly teratogenic and must not be used before/during pregnancy; hydroxychloroquine can be safely used during pregnancy.

Bibliography

Ince-Askan H, Dolhain RJ. Pregnancy and rheumatoid arthritis. Best Pract Res Clin Rheumatol. 2015;29:580-96. [PMID: 26697768] doi:10.1016/j.berh.2015.07.001

Item 51   Answer: D

Educational Objective: Treat gouty cellulitis.

The most appropriate next step in management is treatment with prednisone. This patient has gouty cellulitis accompanying an attack of acute gouty arthritis of the ankle. This well-recognized manifestation is often misdiagnosed as bacterial cellulitis and treated (unsuccessfully) with antibiotics. Prednisone should resolve both the acute gouty arthritis and gouty cellulitis; a typical dose is 40 mg/d for 5 days.

NSAIDs such as indomethacin should be avoided in this patient who is anticoagulated with apixaban for atrial fibrillation.

Antibiotics such as intravenous clindamycin would be indicated for bacterial cellulitis, for which there is no evidence. There is not an expanding area of skin involvement, and two previous courses of antibiotics have not improved symptoms. Additionally, cellulitis would not explain the inflamed ankle joint. An infected joint with concomitant cellulitis is unlikely because of the protracted time course.

MRI of the lower leg would be appropriate to help define chronic osteomyelitis. This is unlikely, however, given the patient's lack of clear predisposing factors such as diabetes mellitus or an overlying skin ulcer, as well as normal plain radiographs after a month of symptoms.

Surgical debridement is the initial approach for necrotizing fasciitis. Necrotizing fasciitis, however, has a more fulminant course. It is unlikely in this afebrile, nontoxic-appearing patient with normal vital signs, whose symptoms have not significantly worsened during the past 4 weeks.

KEY POINT

- Prednisone is appropriate treatment for gouty cellulitis accompanying an attack of acute gouty arthritis.

Bibliography

Perez-Ruiz F, Castillo E, Chinchilla SP, Herrero-Beites AM. Clinical manifestations and diagnosis of gout. Rheum Dis Clin North Am. 2014;40:193-206. [PMID: 24703343] doi:10.1016/j.rdc.2014.01.003

Item 52   Answer: B

Educational Objective: Treat fibromyalgia.

The addition of pregabalin is the most appropriate treatment. This patient's current symptoms and history are consistent with her prior diagnosis of fibromyalgia. Patients with fibromyalgia typically benefit from validation of their symptoms by a physician because many patients have previously had their complaints disregarded by caregivers or family. In addition to psychological support and exercise, pharmacotherapy is a mainstay of fibromyalgia management. Three drugs are FDA approved for fibromyalgia: pregabalin, duloxetine, and milnacipran. Each provides an average benefit of approximately 30% reduction in pain. The latter two agents can also address coexisting mood disorder. This patient has already been appropriately started on duloxetine, and has had significant but insufficient pain improvement. Because patients with fibromyalgia often benefit from combination therapy, the addition of a new treatment, acting through a complementary mechanism, is indicated now for this patient. In contrast to the dual serotonin-norepinephrine reuptake inhibitor duloxetine, which enhances the suppression of pain signals, pregabalin inhibits glutamate release to directly reduce the passage of pain signals from the dorsal root ganglion. The combination is frequently of benefit.

Meloxicam is a long-acting NSAID that has better gastrointestinal tolerability than some other NSAIDs. However, NSAIDs have not shown reliable benefit for fibromyalgia pain.

Gabapentin shares its mechanism of action with pregabalin; although its pharmacokinetics are less reliable than pregabalin, and it is not FDA approved for this indication, its use in fibromyalgia is accepted; however, the discontinuation of duloxetine would be inadvisable.

Although dual serotonin-norepinephrine reuptake inhibitors are beneficial in fibromyalgia, selective serotonin reuptake inhibitors such as sertraline have not shown any benefit when used as single agents.

KEY POINT

- Combination pharmacologic therapy that takes advantage of complementary mechanisms of action may be helpful in some patients with fibromyalgia.

Bibliography

Gilron I, Chaparro LE, Tu D, Holden RR, Milev R, Towheed T, et al. Combination of pregabalin with duloxetine for fibromyalgia: a randomized controlled trial. Pain. 2016;157:1532-40. [PMID: 26982602] doi:10.1097/j.pain.0000000000000558

Item 53 Answer: D

Educational Objective: Treat interstitial lung disease associated with diffuse cutaneous systemic sclerosis.

Mycophenolate mofetil is the most appropriate treatment for this patient who has interstitial lung disease (ILD) associated with diffuse cutaneous systemic sclerosis. In systemic sclerosis (SSc), significant ILD occurs in 50% of patients with diffuse disease and in 35% of those with limited disease. The presence of anti–Scl-70 (DNA topoisomerase-1) antibodies increases the risk for ILD. Cyclophosphamide has been used to improve and/or stabilize lung involvement in SSc, but its utility is limited because it can only be taken for a limited time and the positive results are lost in the year after stopping cyclophosphamide. Recently, mycophenolate mofetil has been shown to be as effective as cyclophosphamide and is a medication that can be used for many years. Data indicate that mycophenolate mofetil can improve FVC in 75% of patients with SSc-ILD who are able to take this medication for 2 years. It can also

improve, similar to cyclophosphamide, the skin thickening associated with SSc in 71% of patients. This patient's FVC and D$_{LCO}$ are down compared with previous determinations, and the high-resolution CT scan of the chest shows findings consistent with nonspecific interstitial pneumonitis. Therefore, treatment with mycophenolate mofetil is appropriate.

In head-to-head comparisons, cyclophosphamide was as effective as mycophenolate mofetil in improving respiratory function and dyspnea, but mycophenolate mofetil was better tolerated than cyclophosphamide based on a longer time to patient withdrawal and was associated with a better safety profile, including lower incidence of leukopenia and thrombocytopenia.

High-dose glucocorticoids are frequently used in patients with SSc-ILD; however, there is no clear evidence of their benefit, and their use may convey an increased risk for scleroderma renal crisis and should be avoided.

Methotrexate does not have the data to support its use in SSc-ILD and because it can cause pulmonary fibrosis, it is not a good choice for this patient.

KEY POINT

- Mycophenolate mofetil is an appropriate treatment option for patients who have interstitial lung disease associated with systemic sclerosis.

Bibliography

Tashkin DP, Roth MD, Clements PJ, Furst DE, Khanna D, Kleerup EC, et al; Sclerodema Lung Study II Investigators. Mycophenolate mofetil versus oral cyclophosphamide in scleroderma-related interstitial lung disease (SLS II): a randomised controlled, double-blind, parallel group trial. Lancet Respir Med. 2016;4:708-19. [PMID: 27469583] doi:10.1016/S2213-2600(16)30152-7

Item 54 Answer: A

Educational Objective: Treat undifferentiated connective tissue disease with hydroxychloroquine.

The addition of hydroxychloroquine is the most appropriate treatment for this patient's arthritis symptoms. This patient has undifferentiated connective tissue disease (UCTD), a term used to describe an autoimmune disease that has clinical manifestations of other specific connective tissue diseases, but not enough positive features to satisfy diagnostic or classification criteria for any one disease. She has Raynaud phenomenon, inflammatory arthritis, and positive antinuclear antibodies, but does not have enough clinical findings to establish a more specific diagnosis. Over time, her condition may evolve into a specific connective tissue disease, most commonly systemic lupus erythematosus. Management of UCTD is the same as other connective tissue diseases and is based on the manifestations of the individual patient. This patient has not responded to a trial of an NSAID and has impaired activities of daily living; thus, she is a candidate for hydroxychloroquine.

Discontinuing naproxen and starting ibuprofen is not indicated because ibuprofen is not necessarily more effective than naproxen.

Obtaining radiography of the feet in a patient without symptoms or physical findings in the feet is unlikely to show any abnormality and thus will not provide any useful diagnostic information.

Repeating anti–double-stranded DNA antibody testing is not appropriate because the results are unlikely to have changed over a 1-month period. Repeat testing could be considered in the future if the patient's clinical condition changes.

Repeating antinuclear antibody testing will not provide further insight into the diagnosis, and the titer does not correlate with disease activity.

KEY POINT

- Treatment of undifferentiated connective tissue disease is the same as other connective tissue diseases and is based on the manifestations of the individual patient.

Bibliography

Mosca M, Tani C, Carli L, Bombardieri S. Undifferentiated CTD: a wide spectrum of autoimmune diseases. Best Pract Res Clin Rheumatol. 2012;26:73-7. [PMID: 22424194] doi:10.1016/j.berh.2012.01.005

Item 55   **Answer: D**

Educational Objective: **Recognize the most common side effect of a topical NSAID.**

The patient should be warned about localized skin rash as a possible side effect of topical NSAIDs recently prescribed for her knee osteoarthritis (OA). Topical NSAIDs such as diclofenac (available as a solution, spray, gel, or patch) provide similar pain relief as oral medications with fewer gastrointestinal effects. The American College of Rheumatology currently recommends topical NSAIDs rather than oral NSAIDs for patients aged 75 years or older because topical NSAIDs are considered to provide similar OA pain relief as oral medications, with greater gastrointestinal safety and tolerability. However, there are slightly more skin reactions (rash, itch, and burning) than placebo (rate ratio, 1.14 [95% CI, 0.51-2.55]). Topical diclofenac 1% gel may be less prone to produce local skin reactions compared with the solution, but it may be slightly less effective in reducing pain.

Simple analgesics are neither anti-inflammatory nor disease modifying but can help relieve pain in patients with arthritis. Topical analgesics (such as capsaicin and lidocaine) may be useful and can limit systemic drug exposure when only a single area is painful. Topical capsaicin is safe to use in the treatment of OA, but it can be associated with local irritation of the eyes and mucous membranes when drug residue is transferred from the fingers to these areas.

Intra-articular glucocorticoids can reduce OA knee pain within days to weeks. When a joint effusion is present, glucocorticoid injections can be particularly helpful after drainage of the excessive joint fluid. Local side effects include skin hypopigmentation, subcutaneous tissue atrophy, and joint infection.

KEY POINT

- Topical NSAIDs are recommended to treat osteoarthritis in patients aged 75 years or older because they provide similar pain relief as oral medications with greater gastrointestinal safety and tolerability, but with an increased incidence of skin irritation and rash.

Bibliography

Lin J, Zhang W, Jones A, Doherty M. Efficacy of topical non-steroidal anti-inflammatory drugs in the treatment of osteoarthritis: meta-analysis of randomised controlled trials. BMJ. 2004;329:324. [PMID: 15286056]

Item 56   **Answer: A**

Educational Objective: **Diagnose acute calcium pyrophosphate crystal arthritis.**

The most likely diagnosis is acute calcium pyrophosphate (CPP) crystal arthritis (pseudogout). Acute CPP crystal arthritis occurs episodically and is generally a condition that occurs in the elderly. The most frequently involved joints are knees and wrists. An acute attack is characterized by pain, warmth, tenderness, and swelling; signs of systemic inflammation may be present but are not universal. Attacks can last for weeks to months (in general, longer than gout attacks). Acute CPP crystal arthritis usually occurs in patients with osteoarthritis of involved joints, and plain radiographs may demonstrate chondrocalcinosis, seen as a thin radiopaque line of CPP deposition at chondral surfaces (most easily appreciated in the knees, pubic symphysis, and wrists). Ideally, acute CPP crystal arthritis is definitively diagnosed by identifying positively refringent rhomboid-shaped CPP crystals from joint fluid. However, there is rarely fluid to drain from a wrist, and even when fluid is obtainable, CPP crystals can be difficult to identify.

Gout appears less likely than acute CPP crystal arthritis given the joints involved and the lengthy nature of the attacks. Initially, gout usually affects the metatarsophalangeal joints, the mid foot, ankles, and knees, although in postmenopausal women the finger joints may be affected (especially those with pre-existing osteoarthritis). Even without treatment, most gout attacks resolve within 10 to 14 days. Additionally, the low serum urate level makes gout less likely.

Infectious arthritis is highly unlikely in this patient because symptoms began 2 weeks ago, she otherwise appears well, and her radiographs demonstrate no joint destruction (which would be expected 2 weeks into an untreated joint infection). Additionally, she had two prior similar episodes, and infectious arthritis is not self-limited or recurrent.

Palindromic rheumatism is an uncommon arthritis that is often a precursor to rheumatoid arthritis and is characterized by acute episodes of monoarthritis that last from 24 to 72 hours; attacks migrate between different appendicular joints, especially the metacarpophalangeal and proximal interphalangeal joints. The prolonged symptoms and joints in this case do not fit the pattern of palindromic rheumatism.

KEY POINT

- Acute calcium pyrophosphate crystal arthritis (pseudogout) is characterized by the sudden onset of pain, warmth, tenderness, and swelling of the affected joint, usually a knee or wrist; attacks are typically longer than those of gout.

Bibliography

Rosenthal AK, Ryan LM. Calcium Pyrophosphate Deposition Disease. N Engl J Med. 2016;374:2575-84. [PMID: 27355536] doi:10.1056/NEJMra1511117

Item 57   Answer: C

Educational Objective: Diagnose rheumatoid arthritis–related pleural effusion.

Rheumatoid pleuritis is the most likely cause of this patient's pleural effusion. Pleuritis is the most common rheumatoid arthritis (RA) pulmonary manifestation but is frequently asymptomatic; exudative pleural effusions may occur. According to the Light criteria, this pleural fluid is an exudate based upon an elevated pleural fluid lactate dehydrogenase (LDH) concentration greater than two thirds the upper limit of normal for serum LDH. In rheumatoid effusions, pleural leukocyte count is typically less than 5000/μL (5.0×10^9/L), pleural fluid glucose is less than 60 mg/dL (3.33 mmol/L), and pH is less than 7.3. This exudative pleural effusion is compatible with rheumatoid pleurisy, malignancy, and tuberculosis pleurisy.

Malignancy is a possible diagnosis accounting for this patient's pleural effusion. However, extremely low pleural fluid glucose concentrations are found only in rheumatoid pleurisy and empyema. Glucose concentration of approximately 30 to 60 mg/dL (1.7-3.3 mmol/L) is more typical of malignancy. In addition, pleural fluid lymphocytosis, particularly with lymphocyte counts representing 85% or more of the total nucleated cells, is not commonly associated with malignancies other than lymphoma. When in doubt, a chest CT with contrast should be performed in patients with pleural effusion of indeterminate cause.

The low leukocyte count and lymphocytic predominance is not compatible with an acute parapneumonic effusion.

Tumor necrosis factor α inhibitors such as etanercept increase the risk for tuberculosis. However, a previous negative tuberculin skin test and low pleural fluid adenosine deaminase measurement (<40 U/L) effectively rule out this diagnosis.

KEY POINT

- Pleuritis is the most common rheumatoid arthritis pulmonary manifestation but is frequently asymptomatic; exudative pleural effusions may occur.

Bibliography

Kelly C, Iqbal K, Iman-Gutierrez L, Evans P, Manchegowda K. Lung involvement in inflammatory rheumatic diseases. Best Pract Res Clin Rheumatol. 2016 Oct;30(5):870-888. doi: 10.1016/j.berh.2016.10.004. [PMID: 27964793]

Item 58   Answer: C

Educational Objective: Diagnose scleroderma renal crisis.

The most likely diagnosis is scleroderma renal crisis (SRC) in this patient with systemic sclerosis. Kidney involvement is common in systemic sclerosis. Up to 50% of patients have mild proteinuria, elevation in the plasma creatinine concentration, and/or hypertension, but most do not progress to chronic kidney disease. The most striking and life-threatening manifestation of kidney disease is SRC. SRC occurs in 10% to 15% of patients, and is more frequent in diffuse cutaneous systemic sclerosis (DcSSc) and in patients with anti-RNA polymerase III antibodies. SRC tends to occur early in the disease course; if untreated, it carries a mortality rate approaching 90%. The typical presentation is acute kidney injury and severe hypertension, mild proteinuria, urinalysis with few cells or casts, microangiopathic hemolytic anemia, and thrombocytopenia. Some patients develop pulmonary edema and hypertensive encephalopathy. Occasionally, patients remain normotensive despite kidney dysfunction. ACE inhibitors significantly improve kidney survival and decrease mortality among patients with SRC, regardless of the serum creatinine level.

Disseminated intravascular coagulation (DIC) is characterized by abnormal activation of coagulation, generation of thrombin, consumption of clotting factors, and peripheral destruction of platelets. DIC may result from various causes, including sepsis, obstetric emergencies, acute leukemias (especially acute promyelocytic leukemia), severe burns, venoms, and shock. It is not associated with a hypertensive emergency or urgency.

Hemolytic uremic syndrome (HUS) is caused by some strains of *Escherichia coli*, including the O157:H7 strain that produces Shiga-like toxin that targets the vascular endothelium of the glomerulus, causing cell death, breakdown of the endothelium, hemorrhage, and activation of platelets and inflammatory pathways resulting in intravascular thrombosis and hemolysis. It manifests as microangiopathic hemolytic anemia, thrombocytopenia, and acute kidney injury in the setting of dysentery. The absence of dysentery in this patient makes HUS an unlikely diagnosis.

Thrombotic thrombocytopenic purpura is characterized by abnormal activation of platelets and endothelial cells, deposition of fibrin in the microvasculature, and peripheral destruction of erythrocytes and platelets. The diagnosis is clinical and requires the presence of thrombocytopenia and microangiopathic hemolytic anemia in the absence of other causes of these findings such as SRC. In this patient with systemic sclerosis, the diagnosis of SRC is much more likely.

KEY POINT

- The typical presentation of scleroderma renal crisis is acute kidney injury and severe hypertension, mild proteinuria, urinalysis with few cells or casts, microangiopathic hemolytic anemia, and thrombocytopenia.

Answers and Critiques

Bibliography

Woodworth TG, Suliman YA, Furst DE, Clements P. Scleroderma renal crisis and renal involvement in systemic sclerosis. Nat Rev Nephrol. 2016;12:678-691. [PMID: 27641135] doi:10.1038/nrneph.2016.124

Item 59   **Answer: A**

Educational Objective: Diagnose Behçet syndrome.

The most likely diagnosis is Behçet syndrome, a systemic disease associated with inflammatory infiltration of multiple organs. The disease is characterized by recurrent painful oral and genital mucosal ulcerations, inflammatory eye disease (panuveitis, retinal vasculitis), and pathergy (an inflammatory response to skin prick with a sterile needle). Other clinical manifestations include venous thrombosis; central nervous system (CNS) manifestations such as brainstem lesions and aseptic meningitis, with the most common CNS symptoms being headache and diplopia; inflammatory arthritis (usually in the knees); skin lesions; and gastrointestinal inflammation/ulceration indistinguishable from inflammatory bowel disease. Behçet syndrome is most common in countries along the Silk Road and is more prevalent in men. The International Criteria for Behçet Disease are both sensitive and specific for the diagnosis and include the following weighted elements: genital aphthosis (2 points); ocular lesions (uveitis or retinal vasculitis) (2 points); oral aphthosis (1 point); skin lesions (pseudofolliculitis or erythema nodosum) (1 point); vascular lesions (superficial phlebitis, deep vein thrombosis, large vein thrombosis, arterial thrombosis, or aneurysm) (1 point); and pathergy (1 point). Three points are required to establish the diagnosis; this patient has 5 points.

Whereas Crohn disease can be associated with aphthous ulcers, uveitis, and peripheral arthritis, the lack of gastrointestinal symptoms make this an unlikely diagnosis.

Sarcoidosis can manifest as acute arthritis, bilateral hilar lymphadenopathy, and erythema nodosum, and a more chronic form of arthritis affects 1% to 4% of patients that may involve shoulders, hands, wrists, knees, and ankles. Uveitis is a common manifestation of sarcoidosis. Papular, nodular, and plaque-like skin lesions are common in sarcoidosis, but mucosal or genital ulcerations are not found.

Joint involvement occurs in 90% of patients with systemic lupus erythematosus (SLE), most commonly polyarthralgia, with frank arthritis involving both small and large peripheral joints found in 40% of patients. Bilateral knee inflammatory arthritis would be an unusual initial presentation for SLE. Oral ulcers can occur but are classically painless, and genital ulcers typically do not occur. Uveitis is one of the many ocular compilations of SLE but is relatively rare.

KEY POINT

- Behçet syndrome is characterized by recurrent painful oral and genital mucosal ulcerations, inflammatory eye disease, and pathergy.

Bibliography

International Team for the Revision of the International Criteria for Behçet's Disease (ITR-ICBD). The International Criteria for Behçet's Disease (ICBD): a collaborative study of 27 countries on the sensitivity and specificity of the new criteria. J Eur Acad Dermatol Venereol. 2014;28:338-47. [PMID: 23441863] doi:10.1111/jdv.12107

Item 60   **Answer: C**

Educational Objective: Treat chronic calcium pyrophosphate arthropathy.

Low-dose prednisone is the most appropriate treatment for this patient with chronic calcium pyrophosphate arthropathy, which may be present as two patterns: chronic calcium pyrophosphate (CPP) crystal inflammatory arthritis, and osteoarthritis with calcium pyrophosphate deposition (CPPD). Chronic CPP crystal inflammatory arthritis is a rare polyarthritis involving the wrists and metacarpophalangeal joints ("pseudo–rheumatoid arthritis"), with the absence of serologies associated with rheumatoid arthritis. The course may be marked by episodes of acute pseudogout, radiographic chondrocalcinosis, and lack of chronic inflammation on examination. Osteoarthritis with CPPD manifests as typical osteoarthritic findings involving joints not commonly associated with osteoarthritis (such as shoulders or metacarpophalangeal joints). Radiographic findings of osteoarthritis with CPPD (subchondral bone cysts, osteophytes, and subchondral sclerosis, consistent with osteoarthritis) often precede the onset of osteoarthritis. This patient presents with findings on examination and radiograph consistent with both patterns of chronic calcium pyrophosphate arthropathy. Treatment of chronic calcium pyrophosphate arthropathy can be difficult because there is a paucity of data. Options include low-dose glucocorticoids, low-dose colchicine, or NSAIDs to prevent inflammatory manifestations of the disease. For this patient, low-dose daily prednisone is appropriate.

Tumor necrosis factor (TNF)-α inhibitors have not been investigated as a treatment for chronic calcium pyrophosphate arthropathy, and beginning a TNF-α inhibitor such as adalimumab in not indicated. In this patient, the complete absence of response to one TNF-α inhibitor is another clue that rheumatoid arthritis was an incorrect diagnosis.

Allopurinol is a urate-lowering therapy, but calcium pyrophosphate deposition results from calcium pyrophosphate rather than uric acid deposition. The radiographic presence of chondrocalcinosis and osteoarthritic changes, as well as the absence of classic gouty erosions characterized by punched-out lesions with overhanging edges, argue against the diagnosis of chronic tophaceous gout. Finally, a low serum urate level and the absence of tophi also argue against the diagnosis of chronic tophaceous gout.

Methotrexate was recently found to be no better than placebo in a randomized trial for chronic calcium pyrophosphate arthropathy.

Although daily NSAID therapy can be a reasonable option, this patient is an elderly woman with hypertension and chronic kidney disease, making NSAIDs relatively contraindicated.

KEY POINT

- Treatment options for chronic calcium pyrophosphate arthropathy include low-dose glucocorticoids, low-dose colchicine, or NSAIDs to prevent inflammatory manifestations of the disease.

Bibliography

Rosenthal AK, Ryan LM. Calcium Pyrophosphate Deposition Disease. N Engl J Med. 2016;374:2575-84. [PMID: 27355536] doi:10.1056/NEJMra1511117

Item 61 **Answer: D**

Educational Objective: Treat drug-induced myopathy.

The most appropriate management is reduction of the prednisone dose in this patient with drug-induced myopathy caused by glucocorticoids. Glucocorticoid myopathy is a common consequence of prolonged treatment with high-dose glucocorticoids, as seen in this patient treated for polymyositis. Distinguishing between glucocorticoid-induced myopathy and active inflammatory myopathy is important, particularly in older patients for whom long-term glucocorticoid side effects can be particularly debilitating. The history is suggestive of glucocorticoid myopathy when a patient has been started on high-dose glucocorticoids within a few months, has cushingoid features, and has normal serum creatine kinase levels. No single feature is diagnostic on electromyogram (EMG) or muscle biopsy. Weakness can often be addressed by reducing the glucocorticoid dose and following the patient over the next 3 to 4 weeks to assess for gains in strength. Colchicine and hydroxychloroquine are also implicated as a cause of drug-induced myopathy. Statins are a frequent cause of myalgia and/or asymptomatic serum creatine kinase elevations and, rarely, statin use can result in an immune-mediated necrotizing myopathy associated with antibodies to the enzyme HMG-CoA reductase.

An EMG could potentially reveal findings of low amplitude motor unit potentials or be normal in glucocorticoid myopathy. However, the initial clinical improvement and reduction in the muscle enzymes with reduction in glucocorticoid dose most strongly suggest drug-induced myopathy, and an EMG in this situation is unlikely to provide helpful results.

In glucocorticoid-induced myopathy, nonspecific atrophy of type IIb fibers without necrosis or inflammation can be seen that would help substantiate the diagnosis. However, muscle biopsy is an invasive procedure that is not indicated in a patient in whom initial clinical improvement and normalization of muscle enzyme levels has occurred, suggesting the diagnosis of glucocorticoid-induced myopathy.

Immunosuppressive therapy with azathioprine is used for glucocorticoid-resistant disease or glucocorticoid sparing.

Reducing the azathioprine dose is not likely to be of diagnostic or therapeutic benefit because proximal muscle weakness is not an adverse effect of azathioprine.

KEY POINT

- Glucocorticoid myopathy should be suspected in a patient with recent initiation of high-dose glucocorticoids, cushingoid features, initial clinical improvement, and reduction in serum creatine kinase levels who has an increase in weakness with reduction in the glucocorticoid dose; treatment is appropriate dose reduction or discontinuation if possible.

Bibliography

Fasano S, Alves SC, Isenberg DA. Current pharmacological treatment of idiopathic inflammatory myopathies. Expert Rev Clin Pharmacol. 2016:1-12. [PMID: 26708717]

Item 62 **Answer: E**

Educational Objective: Diagnose Takayasu arteritis.

The most likely diagnosis is Takayasu arteritis, a rare granulomatous large-vessel vasculitis affecting the aorta and its major branches and pulmonary arteries. This disease predominantly affects females typically less than age 30 years and of Asian ancestry. Aneurysms and stenoses of large arteries cause symptoms of claudication in the extremities, discrepancies in blood pressure between the arms, and reduced pulses. Involvement of the aorta can lead to aortic insufficiency and heart failure. This rare complication is a leading cause of morbidity and mortality in patients with Takayasu arteritis. This patient has upper extremity claudication, reduced radial pulse, evidence of inflammation (elevated erythrocyte sedimentation rate, anemia) and new-onset aortic insufficiency with dilated aortic root, all consistent with the diagnosis of Takayasu arteritis.

Giant cell arteritis (GCA) is a large-vessel granulomatous vasculitis that can also affect the great vessels of the chest, leading to a similar presentation, but is unlikely given this patient's young age; GCA affects individuals over age 50 years.

IgA vasculitis is a small-vessel vasculitis mediated by immune complexes predominantly containing IgA. It does not involve the large vessels and almost always causes a rash, not seen in this patient.

Kawasaki disease is a medium-vessel vasculitis that begins in childhood, manifesting with a rash and other mucocutaneous findings. It can affect coronary vessels, leading to cardiac complications such as heart failure. This patient developed initial symptoms as an adult, and has no rash, making Kawasaki disease an unlikely diagnosis.

Polyarteritis nodosa (PAN) is a medium-vessel vasculitis that can affect multiple organ systems. Cardiac involvement as well as large-vessel involvement is not a typical manifestation of PAN, making this diagnosis unlikely.

Answers and Critiques

KEY POINT

- Takayasu arteritis is a rare chronic granulomatous vasculitis seen in young Asian women that mainly affects the aorta and its major branches as well as the coronary and pulmonary arteries, resulting in claudication, cardiac ischemia, aortic or mitral regurgitation, aortic dissection, and renal artery stenosis.

Bibliography

de Souza AW, de Carvalho JF. Diagnostic and classification criteria of Takayasu arteritis. J Autoimmun. 2014;48-49:79-83. [PMID: 24461381] doi:10.1016/j.jaut.2014.01.012

Item 63   Answer: A

Educational Objective: Initiate folic acid in a patient with rheumatoid arthritis who is starting methotrexate.

In addition to methotrexate, folic acid, 1 mg/d, should be initiated in this patient with rheumatoid arthritis (RA). RA is characterized by a chronic inflammatory polyarthritis affecting large and small joints with a predilection for the small joints of the hands and feet. Patients with RA typically report joint pain and inflammatory symptoms, including swelling and morning stiffness often lasting several hours. Joint swelling (softness or bogginess of the affected joint) is palpable on joint examination. Glucocorticoids, such as prednisone, act rapidly to control inflammation and joint symptoms, and can be useful until slower-acting disease-modifying antirheumatic drugs (DMARDs) achieve full effect. DMARD treatment typically begins with weekly administration of methotrexate, which is the anchor drug in RA and is used in both monotherapy and combination therapy. Daily folic acid supplementation with 1 mg (or weekly folinic acid supplementation) has been found to reduce the mucosal, hematologic, hepatic, and gastrointestinal side effects of methotrexate. Folic acid supplementation also reduces discontinuation of methotrexate for any reason. Methotrexate blocks the cellular utilization of folic acid, and folate depletion is considered to be the cause of most of the side effects associated with methotrexate therapy. Supplementation with folic acid reduces the incidence of side effects without any loss of methotrexate efficacy in treating RA. Folic acid can be taken on the same day as methotrexate because folic acid and methotrexate enter the cell via different pathways. Folinic acid is the reduced form of folate and is typically reserved for patients who have not had a satisfactory response to folic acid. Folinic acid is considerably more expensive than folic acid, and proper timing and administration of folinic acid is complex.

Niacin, thiamine, and vitamin C have no known utility in treating RA or preventing methotrexate side effects.

KEY POINT

- Folic acid supplementation should be initiated in patients beginning therapy with methotrexate to reduce the risk of side effects and discontinuation of methotrexate.

Bibliography

Shea B, Swinden MV, Ghogomu ET, Ortiz Z, Katchamart W, Rader T, et al. Folic acid and folinic acid for reducing side effects in patients receiving methotrexate for rheumatoid arthritis. J Rheumatol. 2014;41:1049-60. [PMID: 24737913] doi:10.3899/jrheum.130738

Item 64   Answer: E

Educational Objective: Diagnose Löfgren syndrome.

No further testing is necessary. This patient has a triad of bihilar adenopathy, arthritis, and erythema nodosum, consistent with Löfgren syndrome, a common rheumatologic manifestation of sarcoidosis. Diagnostic specificity for sarcoidosis is 95% when all three parts of the triad are present, thus making further testing unnecessary. The most common joints involved are ankles, followed by knees and wrists. Löfgren syndrome has a good prognosis with disease remission within 2 to 16 weeks.

Biopsy of a hilar lymph node demonstrating noncaseating granulomas consistent with the diagnosis of sarcoidosis is unnecessary in this patient who clinically has Löfgren syndrome.

Biopsy of a shin lesion will demonstrate septal panniculitis without primary vasculitis that is consistent with erythema nodosum. The diagnosis of erythema nodosum is usually clinical, but biopsy may be helpful in patients with atypical presentations, such as lesions located in areas other than the anterior shins. In this case, biopsy will not add any further useful information.

Rheumatoid arthritis (RA) is a systemic autoimmune disorder that typically presents as a symmetric inflammatory polyarthritis. Characteristically affected joints include the proximal interphalangeal and metacarpophalangeal joints of the hands and feet and the wrists, but other joints can also be involved. Rheumatoid factor is ordered as part of the evaluation of RA but is unnecessary in a patient with acute arthritis, erythema nodosum, and hilar lymphadenopathy.

Synovial fluid analysis is likely to demonstrate inflammation but is not specific for sarcoidosis versus other rheumatologic diseases. Joint infection is unlikely in this patient with multiple swollen joints, rather than a single joint, and the presence of other findings specific for Löfgren syndrome.

KEY POINT

- The presence of acute arthritis, bilateral hilar lymphadenopathy, and erythema nodosum is 95% specific for Löfgren syndrome.

Bibliography

O'Regan A, Berman JS. Sarcoidosis. Ann Intern Med. 2012;156:ITC5-1, ITC5-2, ITC5-3, ITC5-4, ITC5-5, ITC5-6, ITC5-7, ITC5-8, ITC5-9, ITC5-10, ITC5-11, ITC5-12, ITC5-13, ITC5-14, ITC5-15; quiz ITC5-16. [PMID: 22547486] doi:10.7326/0003-4819-156-9-201205010-01005

Item 65   Answer: D

Educational Objective: Diagnose IgA vasculitis.

Skin biopsy with immunofluorescence is appropriate in this patient with purpura, abdominal pain, and arthralgia, which is the classic triad for IgA vasculitis (Henoch-Schönlein purpura).

CONT.

IgA vasculitis is the most common childhood vasculitis (incidence, 20/100,000) and tends to appear after upper respiratory infections. IgA vasculitis is rarer among adults. IgA vasculitis is an IgA immune complex–mediated small-vessel vasculitis that almost always affects the skin but frequently affects the bowel, leading to pain, bleeding, and occasionally intussusception; less commonly, it affects the kidneys and rarely causes pulmonary hemorrhage. Biopsy of the most accessible affected organ, in this case the skin, will establish the diagnosis by demonstrating leukocytoclastic vasculitis with predominance of IgA deposits on immunofluorescence. Furthermore, skin biopsy is easily obtainable and does not expose the patient to radiation or contrast agents or the risks of kidney biopsy. Kidney biopsy is reserved for patients in whom the diagnosis is uncertain or if there is clinical evidence of severe kidney involvement. Biopsy findings are characterized by IgA deposition in the mesangium on immunofluorescence microscopy that is identical to that in IgA nephropathy.

Mesenteric angiography may demonstrate reduced blood flow and possibly irregularities in small vessels consistent with vasculitis, but it will not establish the specific diagnosis of IgA-mediated vasculitis. With the exception of angiography, radiologic testing is not specific for vasculitis; the features of IgA vasculitis in the bowel such as edema from inflammation or poor blood supply may occur in other conditions such as infectious enterocolitis, inflammatory bowel disease, or ischemic bowel disease.

The diagnosis of IgA vasculitis is based on the clinical picture in both children and adults. Laboratory studies are nonspecific but confirm systemic inflammation. IgA levels are sometimes elevated in IgA vasculitis but are not sensitive or specific enough to establish the diagnosis.

KEY POINT

- The classic triad for IgA vasculitis (Henoch-Schönlein purpura) is purpura, abdominal pain, and arthralgia; diagnosis is established with biopsy of the affected organ.

Bibliography

Audemard-Verger A, Pillebout E, Guillevin L, Thervet E, Terrier B. IgA vasculitis (Henoch-Shönlein purpura) in adults: Diagnostic and therapeutic aspects. Autoimmun Rev. 2015;14:579-85. [PMID: 25688001] doi:10.1016/j.autrev.2015.02.003

Item 66   Answer: D

Educational Objective: Screen for the HLA-B*5801 allele in a patient at high risk for allopurinol hypersensitivity.

HLA-B*5801 allele testing is the most appropriate next step in management. This patient with gout is at high risk for allopurinol sensitivity. His risk factors include diuretic use, ethnicity (Thai descent), and chronic kidney disease. Patients of Thai, Han Chinese, and Korean descent have a higher likelihood of having the HLA-B*5801 allele, which confers a high risk for allopurinol sensitivity. Allopurinol hypersensitivity

is characterized by DRESS (drug reaction, eosinophilia, and systemic symptoms) syndrome and can result in kidney failure and death; allopurinol should be discontinued at the first sign of a rash. The presence of the HLA-B*5801 allele is a contraindication to prescribing allopurinol; therefore, this patient should be screened before beginning urate-lowering therapy.

The absence of the HLA-B*5801 allele does not guarantee protection against allopurinol hypersensitivity. Febuxostat is a nonpurine, noncompetitive xanthine oxidase inhibitor, which is a viable alternative to allopurinol. It can be used in patients with mild to moderate chronic kidney disease and is safe to try after an adverse reaction or failure with allopurinol. Febuxostat is approximately 10 times more expensive than generic allopurinol.

Probenecid should be avoided in patients with chronic kidney disease, as the drug requires intact kidney function.

There is no suggestion of an antinuclear antibody (ANA)–related disease such as systemic lupus erythematosus, and testing for ANA should not be performed in patients with low pretest probability of disease. The presence of ANA does not correlate with the risk for drug hypersensitivity. Therefore, there is no indication for ANA testing.

KEY POINT

- Risk factors for allopurinol sensitivity include diuretic use, chronic kidney disease, and the presence of the HLA-B*5801 allele in certain Asian ethnic groups.

Bibliography

Saokaew S, Tassaneeyakul W, Maenthaisong R, Chaiyakunapruk N. Cost-effectiveness analysis of HLA-B*5801 testing in preventing allopurinol-induced SJS/TEN in Thai population. PLoS One. 2014;9:e94294. [PMID: 24732692] doi:10.1371/journal.pone.0094294

Item 67   Answer: C

Educational Objective: Diagnose spondyloarthritis in a patient with enthesitis.

Spondyloarthritis is the most likely diagnosis in this patient with enthesitis. Spondyloarthritis refers to a group of disorders that share an overlapping set of features, including inflammation of the axial skeleton, tendons, and entheses (insertion of tendon to bone); tendon and enthesis calcification; an association with HLA-B27; and mucocutaneous, gastrointestinal, and ocular inflammation. The four disorders of spondyloarthritis are ankylosing spondylitis, psoriatic arthritis, inflammatory bowel disease–associated arthritis, and reactive arthritis. The enthesis is a complex structure at the site of insertion of a tendon or ligament onto the bone. Inflammation of the enthesis (enthesitis) is highly suggestive of spondyloarthritis. When enthesitis is particularly severe, the inflammation may extend along the associated tendon and local ligaments, resulting in dactylitis ("sausage digits"). This patient has dactylitis, with diffuse inflammatory swelling of multiple digits, making spondyloarthritis the likely cause of this patient's presentation.

Infectious arthritis typically presents with pain, swelling, warmth, and erythema of a single joint, accompanied by fever and constitutional symptoms, and is not associated with enthesitis/dactylitis.

Rheumatoid arthritis is characterized by a chronic inflammatory polyarthritis affecting large and small joints with a predilection for the small joints of the hands and feet and is not associated with enthesitis/dactylitis.

System lupus erythematosus (SLE) should be considered in any patient who presents with unexplained multisystem disease. The most common early SLE manifestations include constitutional symptoms (fever, weight loss, or severe fatigue), arthralgia/arthritis, and skin disease. Joint involvement occurs in 90% of patients with SLE, with inflammatory polyarthralgia the most common presentation. SLE is unlikely due to the lack of rash or other clinical features; furthermore, it is not associated with enthesitis/dactylitis.

KEY POINT

- Enthesitis is highly suggestive of spondyloarthritis; when particularly severe, the inflammation may extend along the associated tendon and local ligaments, resulting in dactylitis ("sausage digits").

Bibliography

Ehrenfeld M. Spondyloarthropathies. Best Pract Res Clin Rheumatol. 2012;26:135-45. [PMID: 22424199] doi:10.1016/j.berh.2012.01.002

Item 68   Answer: D

Educational Objective: Diagnose tuberculous vertebral osteomyelitis.

The most likely diagnosis is tuberculous vertebral osteomyelitis (Pott's disease), the most common form of skeletal tuberculosis. Skeletal tuberculosis accounts for 10% to 35% of cases of extrapulmonary tuberculosis. Spinal involvement usually results from the hematogenous spread of *Mycobacterium tuberculosis* into the cancellous bone tissue of the vertebral bodies, from a primary pulmonary focus or extrapulmonary foci such as the lymph nodes. Predisposing factors for skeletal tuberculosis include previous tuberculosis infection, malnutrition, alcoholism, diabetes mellitus, and HIV infection. Delays in diagnosis are common because the onset of symptoms is insidious, and disease progression is slow. The duration of symptoms prior to diagnosis may range from weeks to years. The lower thoracic spine is the most frequently involved segment; common symptoms are back pain, fever, weight loss, and neurologic abnormalities. Paraplegia is the most devastating complication. Diagnosis is suggested by typical clinical presentation, along with evidence of past exposure to tuberculosis or concomitant visceral tuberculosis, and findings on neuroimaging modalities. Bone tissue or abscess samples from needle or surgical biopsy stained for acid-fast bacilli and/or positive cultures are most helpful in diagnosis.

Herniated intervertebral disk usually occurs in the lower lumbar spine (at L4-5 or L5-S1 levels) and typically causes pain and sometimes sensory symptoms radiating down the leg(s). This patient's constitutional symptoms of chills, weight loss, and low-grade fever, as well as image findings of erosion in the vertebral body and paravertebral swelling, are not consistent with herniated intervertebral disk.

Multiple myeloma is the most common primary malignant neoplasm of the skeletal system, and the vertebral column is a commonly affected site. The classic radiographic appearance includes multiple, small, well-circumscribed, lytic, punched-out, round lesions that can be found in the skull, pelvis, and spine on skeletal survey, not erosive changes as seen in this patient.

Osteoporosis with vertebral compression fracture may cause severe back pain and the thoracolumbar area is a common site, but patients do not typically experience neurologic or constitutional symptoms. Erosive changes with surrounding fusiform paravertebral swelling suggest another diagnosis.

KEY POINT

- In tuberculous vertebral osteomyelitis, the lower thoracic spine is the most frequently involved segment; common symptoms are back pain, fever, weight loss, and neurologic abnormalities.

Bibliography

Garg RK, Somvanshi DS. Spinal tuberculosis: a review. J Spinal Cord Med. 2011;34:440-54. [PMID: 22118251] doi:10.1179/2045772311Y.0000000023

Item 69   Answer: A

Educational Objective: Diagnose fibromyalgia in a man in the absence of discrete tender points.

The most likely diagnosis is fibromyalgia. The characteristic features of fibromyalgia are widespread chronic pain, fatigue, and sleep disorders, which are frequently accompanied by impaired cognitive function, mood disorders, and symptoms such as headache, gastrointestinal symptoms, and paresthesia. Although this patient initially appears to have specific joint symptoms, he is actually experiencing widespread (including nonarticular) pain. This widespread pain, together with poor/nonrestorative sleep, fatigue, and cognitive dysfunction (in this case, difficulty concentrating), is consistent with fibromyalgia. The absence of tender points is not relevant; men with fibromyalgia frequently do not experience tender points. Other features experienced by patients (bowel symptoms, anxiety/depression, low-grade fever, low-titer/borderline antinuclear antibodies) are not diagnostic of fibromyalgia but are consistent with its presence.

The clinical manifestations of hypothyroidism include fatigue, cold intolerance, constipation, weight gain, impaired concentration, dry skin, edema, depression, mood changes, muscle cramps, and myalgia. A normal thyroid-stimulating hormone level excludes hypothyroidism.

This patient's physical examination demonstrates full range of motion of the joints without crepitus, making osteoarthritis less likely. Additionally, osteoarthritis cannot explain his diffuse body pain, difficulty sleeping, chronic fatigue, bowel symptoms, headache, and difficulty concentrating.

Rheumatoid arthritis (RA) is characterized by pain and swelling in multiple (>3) small joints of the hands and/or feet, along with morning stiffness lasting at least 1 hour. Initial symptoms often worsen gradually over weeks to months. RA frequently interferes with activities of daily living, including occupational and recreational activities. Constitutional symptoms such as increased fatigue and malaise are common. Depression and myalgia may occur and, less often, fever, anorexia, and weight loss. Physical examination reveals tenderness and swelling of the joints, sometimes with warmth and erythema; symmetric joint involvement is common. This patient lacks the synovitis characteristic of RA.

KEY POINT

- The characteristic features of fibromyalgia are widespread chronic pain, fatigue, and sleep disorders, which are frequently accompanied by impaired cognitive function, mood disorders, and symptoms such as headache, gastrointestinal symptoms, and paresthesia.

Bibliography

Clauw DJ. Fibromyalgia: a clinical review. JAMA. 2014;311:1547-55. [PMID: 24737367] doi:10.1001/jama.2014.3266

Item 70   Answer: E

Educational Objective: Treat class V (membranous) lupus nephritis.

Mycophenolate mofetil is the most appropriate treatment of this patient's kidney disease. Classification of lupus nephritis is based on findings by light microscopy, electron microscopy, and immunofluorescence. This patient with recently diagnosed systemic lupus erythematosus (SLE) now presents with proteinuria likely due to lupus nephritis (likely class V, membranous). Guidelines recommend aggressive therapy with immunosuppressives for significant kidney involvement. A number of immunosuppressive therapies are beneficial in the treatment of SLE nephritis, including mycophenolate mofetil, cyclophosphamide, azathioprine, and rituximab. In the treatment of isolated class V lupus nephritis, especially without kidney dysfunction, mycophenolate mofetil is the most appropriate initial immunosuppressive therapy based on the guideline recommendations. Importantly, mycophenolate mofetil is teratogenic and has been associated with fetal harm and death; it must be stopped 3 months before a planned pregnancy.

Adalimumab has not been shown to be effective in lupus nephritis and may potentially worsen the disease based on animal data.

Belimumab may be considered in patients with continued SLE activity after standard therapy has been tried and found to be ineffective. Its role in the treatment of lupus nephritis continues to evolve but is currently not well defined. Its use in this patient should not be considered before having tried standard therapy.

Cyclophosphamide may be considered in this patient and used appropriately in patients with lupus nephritis but is not an appropriate first choice due to a higher rate of side effects compared with mycophenolate mofetil, as well as its effect on reducing fertility and premature menopause. Cyclophosphamide is typically reserved for severe active nephritis to induce remission, followed by mycophenolate mofetil or possibly azathioprine as maintenance therapy.

Methotrexate is not effective in lupus nephritis and may be associated with toxicity in a patient with kidney disease.

KEY POINT

- Mycophenolate mofetil is the most appropriate initial immunosuppressive therapy in the treatment of isolated class V lupus nephritis, especially without kidney dysfunction.

Bibliography

Hahn BH, McMahon MA, Wilkinson A, Wallace WD, Daikh DI, Fitzgerald JD, et al; American College of Rheumatology. American College of Rheumatology guidelines for screening, treatment, and management of lupus nephritis. Arthritis Care Res (Hoboken). 2012;64:797-808. [PMID: 22556106] doi:10.1002/acr.21664

Item 71   Answer: C

Educational Objective: Treat psoriatic arthritis.

The most appropriate medication to add to this patient's treatment regimen is a tumor necrosis factor (TNF)-α inhibitor such as infliximab. In patients with psoriatic arthritis who have uncontrolled disease while taking methotrexate at a dose of 25 mg weekly, the addition of a TNF-α inhibitor is indicated. Randomized controlled trials have established the efficacy of the combination of methotrexate and TNF-α inhibitors for reducing symptoms, restoring function, and limiting joint damage. Other biologics shown to be effective include ustekinumab and secukinumab.

Abatacept is a biologic disease-modifying agent that targets the T-cell costimulation pathway and is used in the treatment of rheumatoid arthritis. A single randomized controlled trial has shown that abatacept could be efficacious in psoriatic arthritis. However, in a patient with psoriatic arthritis in whom a TNF-α inhibitor has not been used, abatacept is not the appropriate next choice in management due to limited experience in these patients.

Hydroxychloroquine is a long-acting anti-inflammatory medication that interferes with the innate immune system inflammatory response and is used to treat rheumatoid arthritis, systemic lupus erythematosus, and dermatomyositis. It has been reported to be associated with an increased incidence of severe cutaneous reactions in psoriasis and is not the best choice.

Rituximab is a monoclonal antibody that targets CD20+ B cells used in the treatment of rheumatoid arthritis, vasculitis, and various malignancies. It has not been used in the treatment of psoriatic arthritis.

- In recalcitrant psoriatic arthritis, the combination of methotrexate and a tumor necrosis factor α inhibitor has shown efficacy in managing joint symptoms and slowing the progression of radiographic damage, including joint space narrowing and erosions.

Bibliography

Elyoussfi S, Thomas BJ, Ciurtin C. Tailored treatment options for patients with psoriatic arthritis and psoriasis: review of established and new biologic and small molecule therapies. Rheumatol Int. 2016;36:603-12. [PMID: 26892034] doi:10.1007/s00296-016-3436-0

Item 72   Answer: A

Educational Objective: Treat ankylosing spondylitis with NSAIDs.

The most appropriate treatment is an NSAID such as diclofenac for this patient with ankylosing spondylitis, a chronic inflammatory disease affecting the axial skeleton (including sacroiliac joints), entheses, and peripheral joints. It has a strong familial predilection, the strongest association with HLA-B27 among the forms of spondyloarthritis, and a male predominance. This man's history is suggestive of ankylosing spondylitis, with symptoms of inflammatory back pain, the presence of HLA-B27, a family history of ankylosing spondylitis, and a change in his exercise routine. He is early in the course of his disease and has not developed plain radiographic or laboratory abnormalities. Continuous full-dose NSAIDs are first-line therapy and can help relieve pain and stiffness. Studies of continuous full-dose NSAIDs demonstrate symptomatic relief as well as reduced sacroiliac and spine inflammation as seen on MRI in some patients. In a young man with no medical comorbidities, they are associated with a low incidence of side effects. Patients with ankylosing spondylitis are more likely to respond to NSAIDs and do so more rapidly and completely than patients with chronic low back pain from other causes.

Results from most randomized controlled trials of methotrexate use in ankylosing spondylitis have shown no benefit, and it is therefore not appropriate in this patient.

A considerable amount of more recent data suggests that tumor necrosis factor (TNF)-α inhibitors can be particularly helpful in the management of symptoms of ankylosing spondylitis. However, NSAIDs remain first-line therapy. There is variability in the expression of disease, and some patients can be managed with complete symptom relief without immunosuppression. The efficacy of TNF-α inhibitors for symptom relief needs to be weighed against their cost, potential side effects, and the fact that these agents have not been definitively established to be disease modifying.

Sulfasalazine has historically been used in the treatment of ankylosing spondylitis, but its use as second-line therapy has declined as more effective agents, such as TNF-α inhibitors, have emerged. This patient's primary site of involvement is the spine, and many experts now relegate the use of sulfasalazine for treatment of the peripheral arthritis associated with ankylosing spondylitis and only if NSAIDs

are ineffective and a TNF-α inhibitor is not available or affordable.

- Continuous full-dose NSAIDs are first-line therapy for ankylosing spondylitis.

Bibliography

Taurog JD, Chhabra A, Colbert RA. Ankylosing Spondylitis and Axial Spondyloarthritis. N Engl J Med. 2016;374:2563-74. [PMID: 27355535] doi:10.1056/NEJMra1406182

Item 73   Answer: D

Educational Objective: Treat knee osteoarthritis with physical therapy and exercise.

Physical therapy and a graduated leg muscle strengthening exercise program are appropriate for this patient with knee osteoarthritis. For patients with osteoarthritis, an individualized management plan includes education on osteoarthritis and joint protection, an exercise regimen, weight loss, proper footwear, and assistive devices as appropriate. Physical activity includes graduated aerobic exercise and strength training, with attention paid to bolstering strengthening periarticular structures and minimizing injury. The patient's main symptom is stiffness, not pain, and he prefers nonpharmacologic therapy at this time, which is most appropriate from a management perspective as well. Muscle weakness is common in knee osteoarthritis, possibly related to disuse, and muscle strengthening has been associated with reduced pain and improved function. All treatment guidelines agree that a muscle strengthening exercise program should be part of the patient's management plan.

Because the patient has a history of peptic ulcer disease, ibuprofen is not advisable. He also chooses not to take medication for his knee symptoms, and it is unclear whether ibuprofen would help his main symptom of stiffness.

Intra-articular glucocorticoids are useful agents in knee osteoarthritis, particularly as second-line therapies. Similar to ibuprofen, it is unclear whether this treatment would help the patient with his stiffness.

A knee MRI is not indicated in a patient without knee buckling or locking or signs of instability, all of which may indicate an unstable meniscal tear that needs surgical management. Incidental meniscal tears are common MRI findings in the middle-aged population, and especially in patients with knee osteoarthritis. Studies have shown that patients with knee osteoarthritis and meniscal tears experience similar long-term improvements in pain and function with physical therapy compared with arthroscopic surgery, and that arthroscopic surgery may even pose higher harms.

- Treatment guidelines recommend that a muscle strengthening exercise program should be part of the management plan for knee osteoarthritis.

Bibliography

McAlindon TE, Bannuru RR, Sullivan MC, Arden NK, Berenbaum F, Bierma-Zeinstra SM, et al. OARSI guidelines for the non-surgical management of knee osteoarthritis. Osteoarthritis Cartilage. 2014;22:363-88. [PMID: 24462672] doi:10.1016/j.joca.2014.01.003

Item 74   Answer: A

Educational Objective: Diagnose acute cutaneous lupus erythematosus.

This patient has acute cutaneous lupus erythematosus (ACLE) and most likely has systemic lupus erythematosus (SLE). The cutaneous manifestations of SLE are essential to recognize because skin findings are key diagnostic criteria. Because the subtypes of SLE are important to distinguish, the dermatologic examination is crucial. The malar (butterfly) rash of ACLE consists of bright erythematous patches over both cheeks and the nasal bridge, almost always sparing the nasolabial folds (in contrast to the more violaceous facial erythema of dermatomyositis, which often involves that crease). The malar rash of ACLE can occur simultaneously with other findings of SLE or may precede other symptoms of SLE by months or years. The rash can last a variable length of time from hours to weeks and typically recurs or worsens with sun exposure. Essentially all patients with ACLE have or will develop SLE; therefore, all patients should receive a thorough evaluation for systemic involvement.

Erysipelas is a superficial cellulitis involving the lymphatics that often presents as a violaceous-red, edematous, well-demarcated plaque on the face or lower extremities secondary to group A streptococci. Patients are extremely uncomfortable and often have systemic symptoms such as fever and malaise. When on the face, the presentation of erysipelas is not symmetrically distributed as it is with ACLE.

Rosacea often has inflammatory papules, small pustules, and telangiectasias, and tends to involve the nasolabial folds. These manifestations are rare to absent in SLE.

Seborrheic dermatitis is often characterized by a greasy scale and tends to involve the nasolabial folds, eyebrows, and scalp. None of these manifestations is present in this patient.

A less widely known subtype of cutaneous lupus is subacute cutaneous lupus erythematosus. The typical clinical eruption consists of circular or polycyclic scaly erythematous patches and papulosquamous plaques over the forearms, chest, or especially the upper back, in a V-shaped configuration. This pattern in not present in this patient.

KEY POINT

- The malar (butterfly) rash of acute cutaneous lupus erythematosus (ACLE) consists of bright erythematous patches over both cheeks and the nasal bridge, almost always sparing the nasolabial folds; essentially all patients with ACLE have or will develop systemic lupus erythematosus.

Bibliography

Okon LG, Werth VP. Cutaneous lupus erythematosus: diagnosis and treatment. Best Pract Res Clin Rheumatol. 2013;27:391-404. [PMID: 24238695] doi:10.1016/j.berh.2013.07.008

Item 75   Answer: B

Educational Objective: Diagnose C1-C2 subluxation in a patient with rheumatoid arthritis.

The most appropriate diagnostic test to perform next is radiography of the cervical spine with flexion/extension views. Patients with long-standing (generally 10 years or more) rheumatoid arthritis (RA) are at risk of developing C1-C2 subluxation. Inflammation from RA can lead to attenuation of the transverse ligament that normally limits the posterior motion of the odontoid process of the C2 vertebrae. Instability around the odontoid can impinge upon posterior structures, including the spinal cord and vertebral arteries. Common symptoms include a sensation of the head falling off, drop attacks, and painless paresthesia of the hands and feet; rarely, sudden death can occur. Initial imaging should be radiography of the cervical spine with flexion/extension views; if results are abnormal, MRI should then be performed. Consideration of surgery is necessary for patients with significant subluxation, especially if symptomatic. Patients with long-standing RA undergoing general anesthesia for any kind of surgery should have cervical spine radiography with flexion/extension views to assess for atlantoaxial subluxation, which can lead to neurologic compromise when the neck is extended during intubation.

Electromyography is the primary test used to diagnose lower motor neuron conditions such as focal neuropathies, polyneuropathies, motor neuron diseases, and myopathy. Nerve conduction studies are used to assess peripheral nerve system function and can classify peripheral nerve conduction abnormalities due to axonal degeneration, demyelination, and conduction block. In most clinical situations involving peripheral nerve or muscle disease, nerve conduction studies and electromyography are performed and interpreted at the same time. Electrodiagnostic studies are not helpful in a myelopathy as seen with C1-C2 subluxation.

The neurologic symptoms associated with vitamin B_{12} deficiency typically include paresthesia and ataxia, more often in the lower extremities. This patient has intermittent symptoms and no evidence of a peripheral neuropathy on examination. A normal complete blood count makes vitamin B_{12} deficiency less likely, although neurologic complications may occur without hematologic manifestations of deficiency.

Hypothyroidism can cause distal peripheral neuropathy (which is often painful) and carpal tunnel syndrome. The lack of painful paresthesias and a normal neurologic examination make hypothyroidism neuropathy an unlikely diagnosis.

KEY POINT

- Patients with long-standing rheumatoid arthritis are at risk for developing C1-C2 subluxation; symptoms include a sensation of the head falling off, drop attacks, and painless paresthesia of the hands and feet.

Bibliography

Del Grande M, Del Grande F, Carrino J, Bingham CO 3rd, Louie GH. Cervical spine involvement early in the course of rheumatoid arthritis. Semin Arthritis Rheum. 2014;43:738-44. [PMID: 24444595] doi:10.1016/j.semarthrit.2013.12.001

Answers and Critiques

Item 76   Answer: B

Educational Objective: Diagnose neuropsychiatric systemic lupus erythematosus.

Neuropsychiatric systemic lupus erythematosus (NPSLE) is the most likely diagnosis in this patient with systemic lupus erythematosus (SLE). NPSLE prevalence is high in patients with SLE (75%) and may involve central and/or peripheral nervous systems, with the most common manifestations being headache, mild cognitive dysfunction, and mood disorder. Acute presentations, including seizures and psychosis, happen infrequently (<5%) but require aggressive symptomatic as well as disease-specific treatment. This patient has no sensory or motor deficits and presents with confusion, along with a nonfocal neurologic examination. She also shows signs of active SLE disease, including clinical evidence (fatigue, rash, arthritis) and laboratory findings (low complements and a high erythrocyte sedimentation rate). She has elevated protein in the cerebral spinal fluid (CSF), and radiologic studies show diffuse white matter changes. These findings suggest that NPSLE is the likely cause for the mental status changes/psychosis and aseptic meningitis.

This patient does not have acute bacterial meningitis because she lacks fever (seen in >75% of patients) and neck stiffness, and she has a normal cell count and glucose on CSF.

This patient's clinical presentation is not suggestive of seizures: she is alert and awake without involuntary movements, is following commands, and has no findings suggestive of ongoing seizure/status epilepticus.

Steroid-induced psychosis is seen in patients taking high doses of glucocorticoids (usually >1 mg/kg/d) and is very unusual at doses less than 20 mg/d. This patient's dose is only 5 mg/d, making steroid-induced psychosis unlikely.

KEY POINT

- Neuropsychiatric systemic lupus erythematosus prevalence is high in patients with systemic lupus erythematosus, with the most common manifestations being headache, mild cognitive dysfunction, and mood disorder; severe acute presentations, including seizures and psychosis, occur infrequently.

Bibliography
Popescu A, Kao AH. Neuropsychiatric systemic lupus erythematosus. Curr Neuropharmacol. 2011;9:449-57. [PMID: 22379459] doi:10.2174/157015911796557984

Item 77   Answer: B

Educational Objective: Predict long-term prognosis of Kawasaki disease.

A history of coronary artery aneurysm is the most important disease complication determining the patient's need for extensive evaluation and his long-term prognosis. Kawasaki disease (KD) is a medium-vessel vasculitis that affects children and is very rare in adults. KD presents as fever, rash, cervical lymphadenopathy, prominent nonexudative conjunctivitis, and oral mucosal and lip changes. Coronary vessel vasculitis, aneurysm formation, and other cardiac complications (such as heart failure, pericarditis, and arrhythmias) may develop. Up to 25% of untreated patients develop coronary artery aneurysms as long-term sequelae of KD; intravenous immunoglobulin (IVIG) treatment reduces the incidence of aneurysms, but 10% to 20% of patients do not respond. Estimates indicate that 4% to 8% of patients treated with IVIG will develop aneurysms. Thrombosis or stenosis of these aneurysms can lead to ischemia and myocardial infarction. It is important to identify and follow patients at risk for long-term cardiac complications of KD, because they may require preventive therapy with aspirin or other antithrombotic medications. With the exception of the complications related to the coronary arteries, most patients with KD completely recover from multisystem acute inflammation. Patients without abnormalities need no specific cardiology surveillance, but those with persistent coronary aneurysm may require periodic electrocardiography, echocardiography, and/or coronary artery imaging as part of a long-term surveillance program.

Recommendations about the nature and frequency of continued surveillance of patients recovering from KD, as well as physical activity restrictions, are provided by the American Heart Association and are based upon the coronary artery status of the patient. In the absence of coronary aneurysm, the available data suggest that the risk for coronary artery disease is low. For example, a large cohort study showed that among patients with KD, 5% had persistent coronary aneurysm, and long-term adverse cardiovascular events occurred in 8% with persistent coronary aneurysm versus 0% without persistent aneurysm. However, the nature and frequency of long-term surveillance are still unclear. An ongoing cohort study of Japanese children with a history of KD growing into adulthood will better inform the medical community on the best long-term surveillance and management plan.

A past history of bundle branch block, myocarditis, or pericarditis does not appear to be associated with the same risk for long-term cardiovascular events as does the presence of coronary aneurysm.

KEY POINT

- Persistent coronary artery aneurysm conveys the greatest risk for long-term cardiovascular events in survivors of childhood Kawasaki disease.

Bibliography
McCrindle BW, Rowley AH, Newburger JW, et al. Diagnosis, Treatment, and Long-Term Management of Kawasaki Disease: A Scientific Statement for Health Professionals From the American Heart Association. Circulation. 2017;135:e927-e999. [PMID: 28356445] doi:10.1161/CIR.0000000000000484

Item 78   Answer: C

Educational Objective: Prevent osteoarthritis with weight loss.

Recommending weight loss in order to lower the likelihood that she will develop osteoarthritis (OA) is the most appropriate choice. Obesity is the strongest modifiable risk factor for OA incidence. Multiple studies have shown that higher BMI categories have proportionally higher risk of developing radiographic and symptomatic knee OA. A recent randomized clinical trial showed that a reduction of ≥5 kg or 5% of body weight over a 30-month period reduces the risk for the onset of radiographic knee OA in middle-aged overweight and obese women. Another recent study of obese and overweight patients found that subjects who lost weight over 48 months showed significantly lower knee cartilage degeneration, as assessed with MRI, compared with those whose weight was stable.

Chondroitin sulfate supplementation has not been studied to lower the risk for developing incident OA. There are promising but inconclusive data on whether chondroitin sulfate has a salutary effect on the progression of structural changes in established knee OA.

Limited studies have examined the association of vitamin D with incident OA, and available data thus far have not shown that low vitamin D confers a greater risk of incident OA. There is no evidence that vitamin D supplementation reduces the incidence of OA.

Suggesting that running will increase her risk of knee OA is not appropriate. Although not completely conclusive, the medical literature generally supports the idea that running does not contribute to the degeneration of articular cartilage in joints that are neuroanatomically normal. Some studies using advanced MRI techniques showed that moderate exercise in subjects at high risk for OA may be associated with favorable joint composition changes, which could have chondroprotective effects on the knee. Additionally, some studies suggest that quadriceps muscle weakness may be a risk for knee OA incidence. Nonetheless, there is a clear association with knee OA and antecedent knee injury, such as meniscal or cruciate ligament tears, so while stopping running may not be a beneficial recommendation, taking precaution to avoid injury would be prudent.

KEY POINT

- Obesity is the strongest modifiable risk factor for osteoarthritis incidence; weight loss can lower the risk for developing the disease.

Bibliography

Roos EM, Arden NK. Strategies for the prevention of knee osteoarthritis. Nat Rev Rheumatol. 2016;12:92-101. [PMID: 26439406] doi:10.1038/nrrheum.2015.135

Item 79   Answer: A

Educational Objective: Treat scleroderma renal crisis.

The most appropriate treatment for this patient with scleroderma renal crisis is the ACE inhibitor captopril. This patient has features of systemic sclerosis (SSc), including a history of Raynaud phenomenon, gastroesophageal reflux disease, and skin changes typical of this disease. She also has features that occur in patients with scleroderma renal crisis, including

hypertensive emergency, headache, microangiopathic hemolytic anemia (schistocytes on the peripheral blood smear), thrombocytopenia, elevated serum creatinine levels, and proteinuria. Approximately 75% of cases of scleroderma renal crisis occur in the first 4 years of SSc disease onset. Scleroderma renal crisis can be seen in both limited and diffuse forms of SSc but more often in those with rapidly progressive diffuse disease. Anti-RNA polymerase III antibodies serve as a marker for increased risk for scleroderma renal crisis as well as extensive skin disease. The use of ACE inhibitors has dropped the 1-year mortality of scleroderma renal crisis from 76% to 15%. The mechanism of action of ACE inhibitors is believed to be mitigation of the effect of interstitial fibrosis and vascular dysfunction in the glomerular arterial bed. Treatment with an ACE inhibitor (typically captopril) should be initiated promptly in SSc patients with even mild hypertension or otherwise unexplained elevations in serum creatinine levels or acute kidney injury. Angiotensin receptor blockers (ARBs) are an alternative for patients who cannot take ACE inhibitors, although ARBs are less effective for managing scleroderma renal crisis.

Cyclophosphamide is an immunosuppressive agent and not effective in scleroderma renal crisis.

Glucocorticoids, such as methylprednisolone, are implicated as potential risk factors for the development of scleroderma renal crisis and are not indicated for this patient.

In patients with hypertensive emergency, blood pressure must be lowered quickly with short-acting intravenous antihypertensive infusions to limit end-organ damage. Intravenous nitroprusside is often a first choice for patients with hypertensive emergencies. It can be titrated quickly to achieve blood pressure control. However, it does nothing to address the underlying physiological cause of scleroderma renal crisis and is inferior to ACE inhibitors on reducing mortality.

KEY POINT

- Features of scleroderma renal crisis include hypertensive emergency, headache, microangiopathic hemolytic anemia, thrombocytopenia, elevated serum creatinine levels, and proteinuria; treatment involves ACE inhibitors, typically captopril.

Bibliography

Woodworth TG, Suliman YA, Furst DE, Clements P. Scleroderma renal crisis and renal involvement in systemic sclerosis. Nat Rev Nephrol. 2016;12:678-691. [PMID: 27641135] doi:10.1038/nrneph.2016.124

Item 80   Answer: C

Educational Objective: Treat early rheumatoid arthritis with methotrexate.

The most appropriate treatment at this time is methotrexate. This patient has early rheumatoid arthritis (RA) with moderate disease activity measured by the clinical disease activity index (CDAI). Methotrexate is an anchor drug in RA and is the preferred initial monotherapy, as it both controls symptoms and prevents joint damage. Clinical trials have demonstrated that 30% to 50% of patients treated with methotrexate monotherapy will show no disease progression as measured by hand and foot radiographs. Close dose titration (up to as high as 25 mg per week) based on her CDAI score is necessary, as is monitoring for the development of joint damage by radiography or ultrasonography. Ultrasonography is capable of identifying erosions earlier than radiography and can identify continued inflammation even in asymptomatic patients with no detectable synovitis on examination. If methotrexate alone does not lead to remission, a second disease-modifying treatment should be added.

Prednisone may improve symptoms and is disease modifying in conjunction with methotrexate, but long-term side effects (such as diabetes mellitus and osteoporosis) limit its usefulness as primary therapy in RA. Prednisone is primarily used as short-term therapy for disease flares and for temporary symptom control while waiting for long-term medications to become effective. Prednisone should be used at the lowest effective dose for the shortest period possible.

NSAIDs convey anti-inflammatory, analgesic, and antipyretic effects. As such, ibuprofen may address pain and swelling but is not considered disease modifying and will not slow the progression of disease. The major role for NSAIDs in the treatment of RA is for temporary symptom control while waiting for the effect of disease-modifying treatments such as methotrexate to be realized.

Although first-line therapy for lupus nephritis and potentially useful in systemic sclerosis, mycophenolate mofetil does not have a clearly defined role in the treatment of RA. A clinical trial of mycophenolate mofetil in RA showed no benefit compared with placebo.

KEY POINT

- In rheumatoid arthritis, methotrexate is an anchor drug and is the preferred initial monotherapy.

Bibliography

Singh JA, Saag KG, Bridges SL Jr, Akl EA, Bannuru RR, Sullivan MC, et al. 2015 American College of Rheumatology guideline for the treatment of rheumatoid arthritis. Arthritis Rheumatol. 2016;68:1-26. [PMID: 26545940] doi:10.1002/art.39480

Item 81   Answer: C

Educational Objective: Diagnose glucocorticoid-induced osteonecrosis.

Plain radiography of the left hip is the most appropriate initial test for this patient with subacute hip pain. She has lupus nephritis that requires treatment with glucocorticoids. Both glucocorticoid treatment and systemic lupus erythematosus are risk factors for osteonecrosis, which causes death of an area of bone due to compromised blood supply. Other common risk factors include prior fracture or radiation exposure, excessive alcohol use, and sickle cell anemia. Osteonecrosis typically affects the ends of long bones, including the femoral head, humeral head, and distal femur. The involved

area of bone collapses, often leading to rapidly progressive osteoarthritis. Patients with hip osteonecrosis present with groin pain (that is, true hip pain) occasionally radiating to the buttock, which worsens with ambulation; osteoarthritis can present in the same way, but would not be expected in a 34-year-old patient. Physical findings include reduced range of motion of the hip, altered gait, and pain with weight bearing. Plain radiography is the initial radiographic study of choice, although MRI is the gold standard for diagnosis and may be required if plain radiography is not diagnostic. Early radiographic findings include bone density changes, sclerosis, and, eventually, cyst formation. Subchondral radiolucency producing the "crescent sign" indicates subchondral collapse. End-stage disease is characterized by collapse of the femoral head, joint-space narrowing, and degenerative changes.

Dual-energy x-ray absorptiometry is useful to assess bone density in patients on chronic glucocorticoid therapy. Although it may establish the presence of osteoporosis, it cannot determine the cause of pain and has little role in the evaluation of acute symptoms such as hip pain.

MRI is the best method for detecting early bone edema caused by osteonecrosis when plain radiographs are normal. MRI is preferred for diagnostic use in patients with nondiagnostic plain radiographs. However, for end-stage disease, MRI is more expensive than plain radiography, and it may be unnecessary if plain radiography is diagnostic.

Ultrasonography can be used to evaluate for trochanteric bursitis as the cause of lateral hip pain but would not be useful to check for osteonecrosis.

KEY POINT

- Plain radiography is the initial radiographic study of choice for osteonecrosis, and MRI is the modality of choice for sensitive evaluation of early disease when plain radiographs are normal.

Bibliography

Weinstein RS. Glucocorticoid-induced osteonecrosis. Endocrine. 2012; 41:183-90. [PMID: 22169965] doi:10.1007/s12020-011-9580-0

Item 82   Answer: A

Educational Objective: Diagnose infectious arthritis.

Arthrocentesis followed by intravenous antibiotics is the appropriate next step in management of this immunocompromised patient with suspected infectious arthritis. This patient is immunosuppressed due to both his underlying rheumatoid arthritis (RA) and his medications. Additionally, other than the left knee, it appears that his arthritis is well controlled, raising concern for a cause other than a flare of his RA, including infectious arthritis. The hallmarks of a joint infection are warmth, erythema, pain, and swelling. The typical bacterial infectious arthritis develops over days. Joint infections are commonly limited to a single joint; the knee is the most common site, but the hip, wrist, and ankle are also commonly affected. Fever and rigors may occur but are not universally present (60% of patients); absence of fever

CONT.

therefore does not exclude an infected joint. When infectious arthritis is suspected, the synovial fluid must be aspirated and assessed for leukocyte count, Gram stain, culture, and crystal analysis. Joint aspiration should be performed before initiating antibiotics whenever possible. Infectious arthritis must be expeditiously recognized and treated to prevent joint damage; therefore, intravenous antibiotics should be initiated right after arthrocentesis if the suspicion for infectious arthritis is high, as in this case. A synovial fluid leukocyte count of >50,000/µL (50 × 10^9/L), and especially ≥100,000/µL (100 × 10^9/L), strongly suggests an infectious process.

Colchicine is a useful medication for inflammatory arthritis caused by crystals composed of monosodium urate or calcium pyrophosphate. The lack of response to naproxen suggests that crystal-associated arthritis is an unlikely diagnosis. More importantly, infection must be ruled out with arthrocentesis before colchicine therapy is initiated.

Starting prednisone for a presumed RA flare would not be appropriate until infectious arthritis was ruled out by performing arthrocentesis and analyzing synovial fluid for leukocyte count and cultures. The elevated leukocyte count and erythrocyte sedimentation rate cannot differentiate whether the underlying cause of the patient's arthritis is infection or RA flare.

Adding sulfasalazine to the patient's medication regimen would only be appropriate if his RA was not well controlled (swelling, pain, and tenderness in multiple joints). Single joint involvement is highly suspicious of another diagnosis, particularly infection.

KEY POINT

- Arthrocentesis followed by intravenous antibiotics is appropriate for patients with suspected infectious arthritis.

Bibliography
Wang DA, Tambyah PA. Septic arthritis in immunocompetent and immunosuppressed hosts. Best Pract Res Clin Rheumatol. 2015;29:275-89. [PMID: 26362744] doi:10.1016/j.berh.2015.05.008

Item 83   Answer: E

Educational Objective: Diagnose hepatitis C virus–related cryoglobulinemic vasculitis.

Hepatitis C antibody testing is the most appropriate test to perform next in this patient who likely has cryoglobulinemic vasculitis. This patient has a small-vessel vasculitis documented on skin biopsy, along with Raynaud symptoms, arthralgia, sensory neuropathy, and abnormal urinalysis that may represent glomerulonephritis. The presence of cryoglobulins in this setting suggests cryoglobulinemic vasculitis; positive rheumatoid factor and low C4 are characteristic. Ninety percent of cases of mixed cryoglobulinemia are associated with hepatitis C virus infection; this infection may go unrecognized for many years before the development of vasculitis. It is important to assess for hepatitis C virus infection in an individual with cryoglobulinemia; treatment of the hepatitis

C virus infection will also treat the cryoglobulinemia and the vasculitis.

In the absence of sclerodactyly, dilated capillary loops of fingernail beds, or digital pitting, the patient has no clinical features aside from Raynaud phenomenon to support a diagnosis of systemic sclerosis; therefore, anticentromere antibody testing is not indicated.

Similarly, the patient has no joint swelling on physical examination, making a diagnosis of rheumatoid arthritis much less likely; therefore, anti–cyclic citrullinated peptide antibody testing is not needed.

Anti–Jo-1 antibodies are found in patients with antisynthetase syndrome, which causes myositis and interstitial lung disease. This patient lacks these clinical features, as well as inflammatory arthritis and mechanic's hands (hyperkeratotic fissuring of the palmar and lateral surfaces of the fingers) that are often part of the syndrome. Therefore, he should not be tested for these antibodies.

Anti–U1-ribonucleoprotein antibodies is associated with systemic lupus erythematosus and mixed connective tissue disease, an overlap disease containing features of myositis, systemic sclerosis and lupus; however, the patient has negative antinuclear antibodies and aside from Raynaud phenomenon and joint pain has no other clinical features suggestive of these conditions.

KEY POINT

- Ninety percent of cases of mixed cryoglobulinemia are associated with hepatitis C virus infection; therefore, assessing for hepatitis C virus infection in an individual with cryoglobulinemia is indicated.

Bibliography
Cacoub P, Comarmond C, Domont F, Savey L, Saadoun D. Cryoglobulinemia vasculitis. Am J Med. 2015;128:950-5. [PMID: 25837517] doi:10.1016/j.amjmed.2015.02.017

Item 84   Answer: B

Educational Objective: Diagnose psoriatic arthritis.

The most likely diagnosis is psoriatic arthritis. Characteristic features of psoriatic arthritis include psoriasis, enthesitis, dactylitis ("sausage digits"), tenosynovitis, arthritis of the distal interphalangeal joints, asymmetric oligoarthritis, and spondylitis. This patient has an asymmetric, oligoarticular arthritis involving the small joints of the hands (particularly the distal joints) and feet, a history of dactylitis, negative autoantibodies, and new bone formation and pencil-in-cup deformities on radiographs, all of which are compatible with the diagnosis of psoriatic arthritis. Patients with a characteristic pattern of psoriatic joint involvement (especially distal interphalangeal arthritis and/or dactylitis), but without apparent psoriasis, should undergo a thorough examination for occult psoriatic skin changes (for example, scalp, umbilicus, gluteal cleft, genitals) and careful nail examination. Although the characteristic skin rash is absent, the patient did have psoriatic nail changes characterized by onycholysis, pitting, and trachyonychia (roughened surface).

Gout can occur as a monoarticular or oligoarticular inflammatory arthritis, most typically starting in the first metatarsophalangeal joint but, subsequently, involving joints in the upper and lower extremities. An increasingly polyarticular pattern, however, is not likely to be seen in a patient without kidney disease, without hyperuricemia, and without medication exposure that might be expected to increase the serum urate level.

Reactive arthritis is an inflammatory arthritis that occurs in the setting of a defined antecedent infection, usually of the genitourinary or gastrointestinal tract. These cases often present as an asymmetric oligoarthritis. Up to 50% of cases resolve by 6 months, but 20% of patients progress to chronic disease. This patient has arthritis lasting almost a decade in the setting of psoriasis and should not be attributed to reactive arthritis.

Rheumatoid arthritis is characterized by a symmetric polyarticular inflammatory arthritis involving the proximal interphalangeal and metacarpophalangeal joints in the hands and the analogous joints in the feet, and commonly affecting the wrists and ankles. Radiographic findings include periarticular osteopenia and marginal (near the edges of the joint) erosions. This patient does not have physical, radiographic, or laboratory findings (negative rheumatoid factor and anti–cyclic citrullinated peptide antibodies) to support this diagnosis.

KEY POINT

- Characteristic features of psoriatic arthritis include psoriasis, enthesitis, dactylitis, tenosynovitis, arthritis of the distal interphalangeal joints, asymmetric oligoarthritis, and spondylitis.

Bibliography

Raychaudhuri SP, Wilken R, Sukhov AC, Raychaudhuri SK, Maverakis E. Management of psoriatic arthritis: Early diagnosis, monitoring of disease severity and cutting edge therapies. J Autoimmun. 2017;76:21-37. [PMID: 27836567] doi:10.1016/j.jaut.2016.10.009

Item 85   Answer: C

Educational Objective: Evaluate kidney disease in systemic lupus erythematosus.

Kidney biopsy should be performed to assess this patient's kidney disease. Lupus nephritis occurs in up to 70% of patients with systemic lupus erythematosus (SLE); the presence of anti–double-stranded DNA antibodies is a marker for risk. This patient's symptoms and laboratory findings, including constitutional symptoms, inflammatory polyarthritis, a malar (butterfly) rash, positive autoantibodies (antinuclear, anti-Smith, and anti–double-stranded DNA antibodies), hypocomplementemia, and proteinuria, are suggestive of SLE. She likely has the nephrotic syndrome due to lupus nephritis, and further evaluation is needed. Kidney disease is frequent in SLE and can be seen in 10% to 30% of patients at initial presentation. There are six different pathologic classes of kidney involvement in SLE with

significant prognostic and therapeutic implications. Kidney biopsy is the diagnostic test of choice to assess and categorize the kidney disease and should be performed in most cases. Indications for kidney biopsy are as follows: increasing serum creatinine without explanation, proteinuria >1000 mg/24 h, proteinuria >500 mg/24 h with hematuria, and proteinuria >500 mg/24 h with cellular casts.

Testing for antiphospholipid antibodies is appropriate to complete this patient's evaluation but will not help to further assess her kidney disease.

CT of the abdomen and pelvis may reveal masses or retroperitoneal obstruction but is unlikely to be helpful in diagnosing the cause of the nephrotic syndrome. Renal vein thrombosis can present with proteinuria but cannot account for this patient's rash, polyarthritis, or hypocomplementemia.

Renal arteriography should be performed in patients with medium-vessel vasculitis such as polyarteritis nodosa. This patient has SLE, and the vasculitis in SLE is small-vessel immune complex–mediated, in which arteriogram is usually normal and would unnecessarily expose the patient to nephrotoxic dye.

Serum and urine protein electrophoresis can assess a myeloproliferative disorder, which is not suspected in this patient with rash, polyarthritis, and the nephrotic syndrome.

KEY POINT

- Kidney biopsy is the diagnostic test of choice to assess and categorize kidney disease in patients with systemic lupus erythematosus and is usually essential to make therapeutic decisions.

Bibliography

Almaani S, Meara A, Rovin BH. Update on lupus nephritis. Clin J Am Soc Nephrol. 2016. [PMID: 27821390]

Item 86   Answer: C

Educational Objective: Manage neuropathic side effects of leflunomide.

The most appropriate next step in management is to stop leflunomide. Leflunomide inhibits lymphocyte activation by blocking the pyrimidine synthesis pathway. It is approved to treat rheumatoid arthritis (RA), in which its efficacy is comparable to methotrexate. Common toxicities include gastrointestinal upset, diarrhea, aminotransferase elevations, cytopenias, infection, and teratogenesis. An uncommon side effect is peripheral neuropathy, which is usually axonal and may include sensory, motor, or mixed findings. The neuropathy can be severe but is usually self-limited if the drug is discontinued, highlighting the importance of early recognition. Low-dose methotrexate in combination with leflunomide is an infrequently employed, but proven, strategy for treating refractory RA.

Beginning gabapentin as a treatment for peripheral neuropathy would be an appropriate adjunctive therapy to stopping leflunomide, but the definitive treatment is to stop the offending agent.

High-dose glucocorticoids would be appropriate in the setting of rheumatoid vasculitis. Although peripheral neuropathy may be present in this rare complication of RA, rheumatoid vasculitis invariably occurs in the setting of poorly controlled disease. In addition, other manifestations of vasculitis would typically be present, including cutaneous findings (ulcers) and ocular disease (scleritis, episcleritis, uveitis). This patient has well-controlled RA and has no associated systemic or cutaneous findings of vasculitis, making the diagnosis extremely unlikely and the need for increasing the prednisone unnecessary.

Methotrexate inhibits folic acid metabolism and increases extracellular adenosine levels. It is the recommended initial disease-modifying antirheumatic drug for most patients with RA. Methotrexate is administered weekly along with daily folic acid supplementation, which limits toxicity without affecting efficacy. Potential toxicities include hepatitis and bone marrow suppression (leukopenia, anemia). Patients with liver disease should not receive methotrexate, and limiting alcohol intake is strongly advised. Methotrexate does not cause peripheral neuropathy and should not be discontinued.

KEY POINT

- An uncommon side effect of leflunomide is peripheral neuropathy, and definitive treatment is discontinuation of the medication.

Bibliography

Richards BL, Spies J, McGill N, Richards GW, Vaile J, Bleasel JF, et al. Effect of leflunomide on the peripheral nerves in rheumatoid arthritis. Intern Med J. 2007;37:101-7. [PMID: 17229252]

Item 87   Answer: C

Educational Objective: Treat tophaceous gout with appropriate urate-lowering therapy.

Increasing allopurinol to 500 mg/d is the most appropriate next step in management for this patient with symptomatic tophaceous gout. Although she has stage 3 chronic kidney disease (with an estimated glomerular filtration rate <60 mL/min/1.73 m^2), she is tolerating allopurinol, 400 mg/d, without issue and does not take a diuretic, so she is not at high risk for allopurinol hypersensitivity. Allopurinol can be titrated to a maximum of 800 mg/d in 100-mg increments.

It is important to note that two recently published guidelines differ regarding the role of pharmacologic urate-lowering therapy in patients with gout. The 2016 American College of Physicians guideline (http://annals.org/aim/article/2578528/management-acute-recurrent-gout-clinical-practice-guideline-from-american-college) notes a lack of evidence supporting a specific target level for urate lowering; this guideline stresses discussing the risks and benefits of urate-lowering therapy with patients and suggests a "treat to avoid symptoms" approach without specifically considering the serum urate levels. The 2016 European League Against Rheumatism (EULAR) recommendations support a "treat-to-target" approach (consistent with the 2012 American College of Rheumatology gout guidelines), reducing the serum urate level to less than 6.0 mg/dL (0.35 mmol/L) in patients without tophi and less than 5.0 mg/dL (0.30 mmol/L) in patients with tophi. Based on both the ACP and EULAR guidelines, this patient meets criteria for more aggressive therapy.

Adding probenecid might be reasonable in some cases but is contraindicated in this patient because of her estimated glomerular filtration rate of less than 60 mL/min/1.73 m^2, tophi, and recurrent nephrolithiasis.

Pegloticase is a costly drug that should be considered only when other options have been exhausted.

Increasing colchicine to twice daily for prophylaxis of acute attacks offers no clear benefit over once daily dosing. More importantly, this would not affect the serum urate level or cause resorption of the tophi.

KEY POINT

- For patients with inadequately treated tophaceous gout who tolerate allopurinol, the dose can be titrated to a maximum of 800 mg/d in 100-mg increments to alleviate symptoms.

Bibliography

Qaseem A, Harris RP, Forciea MA; Clinical Guidelines Committee of the American College of Physicians. Management of Acute and Recurrent Gout: A Clinical Practice Guideline From the American College of Physicians. Ann Intern Med. 2017;166:58-68. [PMID: 27802508] doi:10.7326/M16-0570

Item 88   Answer: C

Educational Objective: Identify pulmonary arterial hypertension as a leading cause of mortality in mixed connective tissue disease.

Pulmonary arterial hypertension (PAH) and interstitial lung disease are the two conditions most commonly associated with premature mortality in patients like this with mixed connective tissue disease (MCTD). MCTD is rare (1:1,000,000). Age at onset is between 30 and 50 years, with a 9:1 female predominance. Most patients have no known risk factors. MCTD is an overlap syndrome that includes features of systemic lupus erythematosus (SLE), systemic sclerosis, and/or polymyositis in the presence of anti-U1-ribonucleoprotein (RNP) antibodies. More than 50% of patients with MCTD have hand edema and synovitis at disease onset. About one third develop myositis, and nearly half develop decreased esophageal motility and fibrosing alveolitis. PAH occurs in 20%, with fatigue often the initial symptom. PAH (and interstitial lung disease) is associated with poor prognosis and is a major cause of mortality in patients with MCTD. The course of MCTD is variable; the likelihood of developing PAH, interstitial lung disease, and/or cardiovascular disease increases with disease duration. Regular follow-up and monitoring for these conditions is warranted. Patients with MCTD should undergo high-resolution CT of the chest, echocardiography, and pulmonary function testing.

Central nervous system (CNS) disease is common in MCTD, with trigeminal neuralgia occurring in up to 25% of patients. CNS vasculitis is extremely rare, and CNS disease is not typically a cause of mortality in patients with MCTD.

Pericarditis is likely the most common cardiac manifestation of MCTD and while contributing to excess morbidity, it does not result in premature death. As with other chronic inflammatory diseases, premature atherosclerosis is common in patients with MCTD and can contribute to both morbidity and early mortality.

Kidney disease is found in approximately 25% of patients with MCTD and most often presents as a membranous nephropathy that typically does not lead to premature death. Glomerulonephritis is rarely observed. Renovascular hypertension as seen in systemic sclerosis is a rare cause of mortality.

KEY POINT

- In patients with mixed connective tissue disease, pulmonary arterial hypertension and interstitial lung disease are associated with premature mortality; therefore, regular follow-up and monitoring for these conditions is warranted.

Bibliography

Hajas A, Szodoray P, Nakken B, Gaal J, Zöld E, Laczik R, et al. Clinical course, prognosis, and causes of death in mixed connective tissue disease. J Rheumatol. 2013;40:1134-42. [PMID: 23637328] doi:10.3899/jrheum.121272

Item 89   Answer: C

Educational Objective: Treat osteoarthritis with intra-articular glucocorticoids.

Intra-articular glucocorticoid injection is an appropriate treatment option for this patient with knee osteoarthritis (OA) not adequately controlled with acetaminophen or an exercise program. Given the localized nature of her symptoms, and her more specific desire for short-term relief while she travels, she could benefit from targeted treatment. Despite a lack of high quality of evidence, trials comparing intra-articular glucocorticoids and placebo generally show that the treatment is safe and may significantly improve pain and function for patients in the short term. Furthermore, U.S. and international OA guidelines support the use of intra-articular glucocorticoids for knee OA. A recent 2-year study has called the efficacy and long-term safety of intra-articular glucocorticoid injections into question, with possible negative effects on cartilage thickness, an outcome with unclear clinical meaning. Arthrocentesis and joint injections are safe procedures in patients receiving therapeutic doses of anticoagulation therapy, and are rarely associated with significant bleeding.

Alendronate is an osteoporosis medication that inhibits bone resorption via actions on osteoclasts or on osteoclast precursors. Risedronate, another bisphosphonate, has been studied in osteoarthritis, but results have not been favorable for OA symptom modification. Risedronate did reduce a marker of cartilage degradation; nevertheless, it is not a currently recommended OA treatment.

For patients with symptomatic knee OA, the American Academy of Orthopaedic Surgeons recommends against the use of arthroscopy with debridement. This recommendation is based on evidence from randomized trials and systematic reviews that fail to show benefit for knee pain with or without radiographic knee OA.

Pregabalin, which binds to the $\alpha2$-δ subunit of voltage-gated calcium channels within the central nervous system and inhibits excitatory neurotransmitter release, is not a recognized treatment for OA. It is currently FDA approved for fibromyalgia, neuropathic pain, postherpetic neuralgia, and partial-onset seizures. Because it can cause euphoria, pregabalin is categorized as a schedule V controlled substance.

Tramadol is a centrally acting synthetic opioid analgesic that also weakly inhibits the reuptake of norepinephrine and serotonin. Tramadol may rarely be warranted to control pain in patients with OA who have not responded to other agents or are poor candidates for other interventions to treat painful joints, such as surgery. Compared with placebo, tramadol results in a statistically significant but relatively small improvement of OA-related knee pain. Significant side effects sufficient to warrant drug discontinuation include nausea, vomiting, and constipation.

KEY POINT

- Intra-articular glucocorticoid injection is a treatment option for patients with localized osteoarthritis.

Bibliography

Jüni P, Hari R, Rutjes AW, Fischer R, Silletta MG, Reichenbach S, et al. Intra-articular corticosteroid for knee osteoarthritis. Cochrane Database Syst Rev. 2015:CD005328. [PMID: 26490760] doi:10.1002/14651858.CD005328.pub3

Item 90   Answer: C

Educational Objective: Treat refractory systemic lupus erythematosus with belimumab.

Belimumab is the most appropriate therapeutic option to consider in this patient with a history of systemic lupus erythematosus (SLE) who continues to have active disease manifestations primarily affecting the skin and joints while she is on appropriate standard immunosuppressive therapy, including glucocorticoids. She has not been able to tolerate other immunosuppressive agents commonly used to treat active disease manifestations. Therefore, an alternative approach or escalation of the therapy is appropriate for this patient. Belimumab is FDA approved as an addition to standard therapy in patients who have SLE with mild to moderately active disease. Belimumab is designed to inhibit B-lymphocyte stimulator (BLyS) protein. BLyS plays a key role in the selection, maturation, and survival of B cells, and it has a significant role in the pathogenesis of SLE. The addition of belimumab to standard therapy reduces disease activity levels and delays flares in patients with serologically active SLE or prior glucocorticoid use. Its use is also associated with improved quality of life in appropriately selected patients. Belimumab has been found to be most effective in patients with mucocutaneous and joint manifestations; its role in other disease manifestations continues to be studied and evolve.

Abatacept is a T-cell costimulatory inhibitor that has been tried in SLE but not found to be effective.

Adalimumab is a tumor necrosis factor (TNF)-α inhibitor effective in the treatment of rheumatoid arthritis and spondyloarthritis. Blocking TNF in patients with SLE has not been effective and may potentially worsen the disease.

The interleukin (IL)-17 inhibitor secukinumab is an approved therapy for psoriatic arthritis and ankylosing spondylitis. The role of IL-17 and its blockade in SLE is under investigation but is currently not well elucidated in SLE. Secukinumab has not been studied in SLE and is not an appropriate therapy.

KEY POINT

- Belimumab is FDA approved as an addition to standard therapy in patients who have systemic lupus erythematosus with persistent mild to moderately active disease.

Bibliography

Garcia A, De Sanctis JB. A review of clinical trials of belimumab in the management of systemic lupus erythematosus. Curr Pharm Des. 2016;22:6306-6312. [PMID: 27587201] doi:10.2174/138161282266616083110 3254

Item 91   Answer: C

Educational Objective: Diagnose diffuse idiopathic skeletal hyperostosis.

Diffuse idiopathic skeletal hyperostosis (DISH) is the most likely diagnosis. DISH is a noninflammatory condition involving ossification of spinal ligaments and entheses. DISH can be asymptomatic or present in various ways, including as pain and stiffness in the spine, with the thoracic spine being most often involved. Although features such as ligamentous ossification are shared with ankylosing spondylitis, the sacroiliac joints are not involved in DISH. The most characteristic radiographic change of DISH is confluent ossification of at least four contiguous vertebral levels, usually on the right side of the spine. The left-sided sparing is possibly related to mechanical pressure from the aorta, and its pulsations, as a barrier toward production of bony hyperostosis on the left side.

Ankylosing spondylitis is characterized by bilateral sacroiliac joint abnormalities on spinal radiographs. Other spinal sections may also be involved, but sacroiliac joint involvement is cardinal for diagnosis. Inflammatory back pain is the most common symptom and is usually comprised of four of five of the following features: onset of back discomfort before the age of 40 years; insidious onset; improvement with exercise; no improvement with rest; and pain at night (with improvement upon arising).

Calcium pyrophosphate deposition may affect the axial spine but more often affects the peripheral skeleton. It is often asymptomatic, is not known to have a predilection for a particular segment of the spine, and appears as punctate

and linear radiodensities of calcification within the cartilage on radiographs. It does not result in ossification of spinal ligaments and entheses.

Psoriatic arthritis can affect the spine, with inflammatory back pain symptoms similar to those listed with ankylosing spondylitis. Differences between psoriatic arthritis and DISH include that sacroiliac joints may be asymmetrically involved in psoriatic arthritis but are not involved in DISH, and the spondylitis is random and not necessarily continuous in psoriatic arthritis, whereas a defining characteristic of DISH is involvement of four or more vertebral bodies. DISH syndesmophytes (ligamentous ossification) are located on the anterior and lateral margins of vertebrae, but they tend to be nonmarginal in psoriatic arthritis.

KEY POINT

- Diffuse idiopathic skeletal hyperostosis is a noninflammatory condition that involves ossification of spinal ligaments and entheses and usually presents as back pain and stiffness; characteristic radiographic changes include confluent ossification of at least four contiguous vertebral levels, usually on the right side of the spine.

Bibliography

Mader R, Verlaan JJ, Buskila D. Diffuse idiopathic skeletal hyperostosis: clinical features and pathogenic mechanisms. Nat Rev Rheumatol. 2013;9:741-50. [PMID: 24189840] doi:10.1038/nrrheum.2013.165

Item 92   Answer: C

Educational Objective: Diagnose colchicine and clarithromycin drug interaction.

Discontinuation of colchicine and clarithromycin is the most appropriate next step in management. The coadministration of colchicine and clarithromycin can result in potentially fatal colchicine toxicity that manifests as rhabdomyolysis, acute kidney injury, and pancytopenia. Colchicine is metabolized in the liver by the CYP3A4 cytochrome and should be avoided in patients taking CYP3A4 inhibitors such as clarithromycin and fluconazole. Coadministration with clarithromycin is particularly concerning, because there have been several case reports of fatal outcomes with the combination (even when taken for a short time). Once the patient recovers, however, colchicine may be reinitiated (as it is the combination of the two drugs that led to the current scenario).

High-dose glucocorticoid therapy would be indicated in the event of immune-mediated hemolytic anemia and leukopenia (Evans syndrome). Colchicine toxicity, however, is not immune mediated and would not respond to glucocorticoids.

Plasma exchange would be appropriate for thrombotic thrombocytopenic purpura (TTP). Although TTP can cause thrombocytopenia and acute kidney injury, the lack of schistocytes on blood smear argues against microangiopathic hemolytic anemia, and other features of TTP such as fever and mental status changes are also absent. Plasma exchange is not effective for colchicine toxicity.

CONT.

There is no need to discontinue febuxostat; this drug can be continued in patients with chronic kidney disease and would not cause the clinical picture described.

KEY POINT

• Coadministration of colchicine and CYP3A4 inhibitors (such as clarithromycin and fluconazole) should be avoided because potentially fatal colchicine toxicity with kidney failure, rhabdomyolysis, and bone marrow suppression may occur.

Bibliography

Hung IF, Wu AK, Cheng VC, Tang BS, To KW, Yeung CK, et al. Fatal interaction between clarithromycin and colchicine in patients with renal insufficiency: a retrospective study. Clin Infect Dis. 2005;41:291-300. [PMID: 16007523]

Item 93   Answer: D

Educational Objective: Diagnose subacute cutaneous lupus erythematosus.

This patient has subacute cutaneous lupus erythematosus (SCLE) and likely has systemic lupus erythematosus (SLE). She has a new rash on the torso with annular and patchy papular areas. This rash is most likely SCLE, a photosensitive rash occurring especially on the arms, neck, upper trunk, and face. The rash can be annular with central clearing or papulosquamous with patchy erythematous plaques and papules. In some patients, the rash may have both of the characteristics, as seen in this patient. SCLE often has a fine scale that may leave postinflammatory hypo- or hyperpigmentation. SCLE is associated with anti-Ro/SSA antibodies, with a prevalence of 75%. About 50% of patients with SCLE also have SLE. These patients more typically have mild systemic symptoms, most commonly arthritis and myalgias; patients with lupus vasculitis, central nervous system lupus, and nephritis are found in less than 10% of patients with SCLE. Psoriasis can present with similar lesions but are usually photoresponsive (improve with sun exposure), unlike this patient.

Essentially 100% of patients with acute cutaneous lupus erythematosus (ACLE) have SLE. ACLE may present in multiple forms, with the most commonly recognized being a characteristic localized malar (butterfly) eruption. Less commonly it can appear as a generalized eruption, which typically appears as an erythematous maculopapular eruption of sun-exposed skin such as the extensor surfaces of the arms and hands.

Patients with dermatomyositis frequently have areas of poikiloderma with ill-defined patchy erythema and "salt-and-pepper" dyspigmentation accompanied by telangiectasias on the chest or upper back. There may be slightly violaceous erythema over the "V" of the neck, chest, and the upper back (the "Shawl sign") or on the lateral hips (the "holster sign").

Discoid lupus erythematosus (DLE) occurs in 20% of patients with SLE but more commonly occurs as an isolated, nonsystemic finding; patients with isolated DLE usually do not go on to develop SLE. DLE usually affects the scalp and

face and presents as hypo- and/or hyperpigmented, possibly erythematous, patches or thin plaques that may be variably atrophic or hyperkeratotic.

KEY POINT

• Subacute cutaneous lupus erythematosus (SCLE) can present as annular with central clearing or papulosquamous with patchy erythematous plaques and papules, and both forms can be seen in the same patient; about 50% of patients with SCLE also have systemic lupus erythematosus.

Bibliography

Okon LG, Werth VP. Cutaneous lupus erythematosus: diagnosis and treatment. Best Pract Res Clin Rheumatol. 2013;27:391-404. [PMID: 24238695] doi:10.1016/j.berh.2013.07.008

Item 94   Answer: D

Educational Objective: Diagnose ankylosing spondylitis.

The most appropriate test to perform next is plain radiography of the sacroiliac joints. This patient has features of inflammatory back pain (onset before age 45 years, duration >3 months, insidious onset, morning stiffness >30 minutes, improvement with exercise, no improvement with rest, awaking from pain with improvement on arising, alternating buttock pain), as well as antecedent history of anterior uveitis. He should therefore be evaluated for ankylosing spondylitis. The American College of Radiology appropriateness criteria recommend radiography of the sacroiliac joints and spine as the initial evaluation of patients with inflammatory sacroiliac or back symptoms for evidence of sacroiliitis, including erosions, evidence of sclerosis, and widening, narrowing, or partial ankylosis of the sacroiliac joints. The presence of such findings would confirm the diagnosis of ankylosing spondylitis.

A bone scan lacks specificity for the changes of sacroiliitis and is not of value in the diagnosis of ankylosing spondylitis.

CT of the sacroiliac joints is not considered an appropriate initial diagnostic test for ankylosing spondylitis. It exposes the patient to unnecessary amounts of radiation.

MRI is also unnecessary in most cases of suspected ankylosing spondylitis because the diagnosis can often be confirmed with less costly radiography. Although MRI is more sensitive than radiography or CT in detecting sacroiliitis, it is less specific and can result in a high yield of false-positive test results. MRI may be useful to detect inflammation in patients with high clinical suspicion but normal or equivocal radiographs.

KEY POINT

• Plain radiography of the sacroiliac joints should be obtained in patients with suspected ankylosing spondylitis to evaluate for evidence of sacroiliitis, including erosions, sclerosis, and widening, narrowing, or partial ankylosis of the sacroiliac joints.

Bibliography

Taurog JD, Chhabra A, Colbert RA. Ankylosing spondylitis and axial spondyloarthritis. N Engl J Med. 2016;374:2563-74. [PMID: 27355535] doi:10.1056/NEJMra1406182

Item 95   Answer: C

Educational Objective: Prevent gout attacks during the initiation of urate-lowering therapy.

Discontinuing colchicine and beginning an NSAID such as meloxicam is the most appropriate next step to decrease the frequency of this patient's gout attacks. He has experienced several acute gout attacks since beginning allopurinol 2 months ago. It is common to experience "mobilization attacks" at the initiation of urate-lowering therapy, which occur when urate body stores shift from joints and soft tissues to the vasculature. Hence, all patients beginning urate-lowering therapy should also receive a prophylactic agent to prevent against mobilization flares for 6 to 12 months, without which the average patient will experience several acute attacks. Colchicine is the primary prophylactic agent employed (once or twice daily) for this role, but low-dose glucocorticoids and low-dose NSAIDs are also effective. Choice of therapy should be tailored to the individual's comorbid conditions. This patient is currently taking colchicine, which is most likely causing the diarrhea. In this case, discontinuation of colchicine and initiating a low-dose NSAID such as meloxicam is the most appropriate choice. All NSAIDs are considered equivalent for this purpose.

Adding prednisone would be a reasonable option for prophylaxis but is not ideal for this patient with insulin-dependent type 2 diabetes mellitus, because even low-dose glucocorticoids may result in hyperglycemia and increase insulin requirements.

Adding the uricosuric agent probenecid or increasing the allopurinol would not afford protection against mobilization flares because they are both urate-lowering agents, not prophylactic agents. Intensifying urate-lowering therapy would be a reasonable choice if the recurrent attacks are thought to represent a failure of urate-lowering therapy, rather than mobilization attacks, as is suspected with this patient.

Increasing colchicine would be a reasonable option, were it not for the diarrhea that began with the institution of colchicine 2 months ago. Diarrhea is one of the most common side effects of colchicine, and increasing the dose would worsen gastrointestinal toxicity.

KEY POINT

- All patients with gout beginning urate-lowering therapy should also receive a prophylactic agent such as colchicine, low-dose glucocorticoids, or low-dose NSAIDs to prevent mobilization flares; the choice of prophylactic drug is determined by patient comorbidities.

Bibliography

Latourte A, Bardin T, Richette P. Prophylaxis for acute gout flares after initiation of urate-lowering therapy. Rheumatology (Oxford). 2014;53:1920-6. [PMID: 24758886] doi:10.1093/rheumatology/keu157

Item 96   Answer: B

Educational Objective: Diagnose hip osteonecrosis related to systemic lupus erythematosus.

MRI of the hip is the most appropriate test to perform next in this patient with systemic lupus erythematosus (SLE) and a past exposure to high-dose glucocorticoids, who now presents with unexplained groin pain. She is at high risk for developing osteonecrosis affecting the hip/femur. Osteonecrosis is a serious complication of SLE that most commonly affects the hips but can also involve other large joints and should be suspected when there is otherwise unexplained pain and/or reduced range of motion. Chronic prednisone doses (>20 mg/d), severe/active SLE, and vasculitis are all associated with increased risk. Hip radiography can detect advanced disease, but MRI is the modality of choice for sensitive evaluation of early disease. Small lesions can improve and resolve spontaneously, but larger lesions usually lead to bony collapse and structural sequelae. MRI should be performed in this patient with normal pelvic and hip radiographs.

The American College of Radiology (ACR) approach to imaging for suspected osteonecrosis recommends CT only for patients who cannot undergo MRI. CT is somewhat more sensitive than plain radiography in the diagnosis of osteonecrosis but not nearly as sensitive as MRI.

Radionuclide bone scan will detect increased bone turnover at the junction, osteonecrosis, and reactive bone resulting in an image of increased tracer uptake surrounding a cold area (doughnut sign). However, radionuclide bone scan is significantly less sensitive and less specific than MRI in the detection of early osteonecrosis lesions and is not usually recommended as a first-line diagnostic test.

If MRI cannot be performed in patients with suspected early osteonecrosis, a reasonable alternative is bone scan with single photon emission CT (SPECT). This imaging modality is more sensitive than radiography, but the ACR Appropriateness Criteria for Osteonecrosis of the Hip designated SPECT as a second-line test to MRI for the detection of early lesions.

KEY POINT

- Osteonecrosis is a complication of systemic lupus erythematosus most commonly affecting the hips and should be suspected when there is otherwise unexplained pain and/or reduced range of motion; MRI is the modality of choice for evaluation of early disease.

Bibliography

Gontero RP, Bedoya ME, Benavente E, Roverano SG, Paira SO. Osteonecrosis in systemic lupus erythematosus. Reumatol Clin. 2015;11:151-5. [PMID: 25441491] doi:10.1016/j.reuma.2014.05.005

153

Index

A **NAME AND ADDRESS (Please complete.)**

Last Name   First Name   Middle Initial

Address

Address cont.

City   State   ZIP Code

Country

Email address

ACP®
American College of Physicians
Leading Internal Medicine, Improving Lives

Medical Knowledge Self-Assessment Program® 18

B **Order Number**
(Use the 10-digit Order Number on your MKSAP materials packing slip.)

C **ACP ID Number**
(Refer to packing slip in your MKSAP materials for your 8-digit ACP ID Number.)

TO EARN *CME Credits and/or MOC Points* YOU MUST:

1. Answer all questions.
2. Score a minimum of 50% correct.

- -

TO EARN *FREE* INSTANTANEOUS *CME Credits and/or MOC Points* ONLINE:

1. Answer all of your questions.
2. Go to **mksap.acponline.org** and enter your ACP Online username and password to access an online answer sheet.
3. Enter your answers.
4. You can also enter your answers directly at **mksap.acponline.org** without first using this answer sheet.

To Submit Your Answer Sheet by Mail or FAX for a $20 Administrative Fee per Answer Sheet:

1. Answer all of your questions and calculate your score.
2. Complete boxes A-H.
3. Complete payment information.
4. Send the answer sheet and payment information to ACP, using the FAX number/address listed below.

D **Required Submission Information if Applying for MOC**

Birth Month and Day
M M   D D

ABIM Candidate Number

COMPLETE FORM BELOW ONLY IF YOU SUBMIT BY MAIL OR FAX

Last Name   First Name   MI

Payment Information. Must remit in US funds, drawn on a US bank.
The processing fee for each paper answer sheet is $20.

☐ Check, made payable to ACP, enclosed

Charge to   ☐ **VISA**   ☐ **MasterCard**   ☐ **AMERICAN EXPRESS**   ☐ **DISCOVER**

Card Number _____

Expiration Date _____ / _____
                 MM   YY

Security code (3 or 4 digit #s) _____

Signature _____

Fax to: 215-351-2799

Mail to:
Member and Customer Service
American College of Physicians
190 N. Independence Mall West
Philadelphia, PA 19106-1572

E TEST TYPE

TEST TYPE	Maximum Number of CME Credits
○ Cardiovascular Medicine	30
○ Dermatology	16
○ Gastroenterology and Hepatology	22
○ Hematology and Oncology	33
○ Neurology	22
○ Rheumatology	22
○ Endocrinology and Metabolism	19
○ General Internal Medicine	36
○ Infectious Disease	25
○ Nephrology	25
○ Pulmonary and Critical Care Medicine	25

F CREDITS OR POINTS CLAIMED ON SECTION
1 hour = 1 credit or 1 point

Enter the number of credits earned on the test to the nearest quarter hour. Physicians should claim only the credit commensurate with the extent of their participation in the activity.

G
Enter your score here.

Instructions for calculating your own score are found in front of the self-assessment test in each book. You must receive a minimum score of 50% correct.

_____ %

Credit Submission Date:_____

H

☐ I want to submit for CME credits

☐ I want to submit for CME credits and MOC points.

1 Ⓐ Ⓑ Ⓒ Ⓓ Ⓔ
2 Ⓐ Ⓑ Ⓒ Ⓓ Ⓔ
3 Ⓐ Ⓑ Ⓒ Ⓓ Ⓔ
4 Ⓐ Ⓑ Ⓒ Ⓓ Ⓔ
5 Ⓐ Ⓑ Ⓒ Ⓓ Ⓔ
6 Ⓐ Ⓑ Ⓒ Ⓓ Ⓔ
7 Ⓐ Ⓑ Ⓒ Ⓓ Ⓔ
8 Ⓐ Ⓑ Ⓒ Ⓓ Ⓔ
9 Ⓐ Ⓑ Ⓒ Ⓓ Ⓔ
10 Ⓐ Ⓑ Ⓒ Ⓓ Ⓔ
11 Ⓐ Ⓑ Ⓒ Ⓓ Ⓔ
12 Ⓐ Ⓑ Ⓒ Ⓓ Ⓔ
13 Ⓐ Ⓑ Ⓒ Ⓓ Ⓔ
14 Ⓐ Ⓑ Ⓒ Ⓓ Ⓔ
15 Ⓐ Ⓑ Ⓒ Ⓓ Ⓔ
16 Ⓐ Ⓑ Ⓒ Ⓓ Ⓔ
17 Ⓐ Ⓑ Ⓒ Ⓓ Ⓔ
18 Ⓐ Ⓑ Ⓒ Ⓓ Ⓔ
19 Ⓐ Ⓑ Ⓒ Ⓓ Ⓔ
20 Ⓐ Ⓑ Ⓒ Ⓓ Ⓔ
21 Ⓐ Ⓑ Ⓒ Ⓓ Ⓔ
22 Ⓐ Ⓑ Ⓒ Ⓓ Ⓔ
23 Ⓐ Ⓑ Ⓒ Ⓓ Ⓔ
24 Ⓐ Ⓑ Ⓒ Ⓓ Ⓔ
25 Ⓐ Ⓑ Ⓒ Ⓓ Ⓔ
26 Ⓐ Ⓑ Ⓒ Ⓓ Ⓔ
27 Ⓐ Ⓑ Ⓒ Ⓓ Ⓔ
28 Ⓐ Ⓑ Ⓒ Ⓓ Ⓔ
29 Ⓐ Ⓑ Ⓒ Ⓓ Ⓔ
30 Ⓐ Ⓑ Ⓒ Ⓓ Ⓔ
31 Ⓐ Ⓑ Ⓒ Ⓓ Ⓔ
32 Ⓐ Ⓑ Ⓒ Ⓓ Ⓔ
33 Ⓐ Ⓑ Ⓒ Ⓓ Ⓔ
34 Ⓐ Ⓑ Ⓒ Ⓓ Ⓔ
35 Ⓐ Ⓑ Ⓒ Ⓓ Ⓔ
36 Ⓐ Ⓑ Ⓒ Ⓓ Ⓔ
37 Ⓐ Ⓑ Ⓒ Ⓓ Ⓔ
38 Ⓐ Ⓑ Ⓒ Ⓓ Ⓔ
39 Ⓐ Ⓑ Ⓒ Ⓓ Ⓔ
40 Ⓐ Ⓑ Ⓒ Ⓓ Ⓔ
41 Ⓐ Ⓑ Ⓒ Ⓓ Ⓔ
42 Ⓐ Ⓑ Ⓒ Ⓓ Ⓔ
43 Ⓐ Ⓑ Ⓒ Ⓓ Ⓔ
44 Ⓐ Ⓑ Ⓒ Ⓓ Ⓔ
45 Ⓐ Ⓑ Ⓒ Ⓓ Ⓔ

46 Ⓐ Ⓑ Ⓒ Ⓓ Ⓔ
47 Ⓐ Ⓑ Ⓒ Ⓓ Ⓔ
48 Ⓐ Ⓑ Ⓒ Ⓓ Ⓔ
49 Ⓐ Ⓑ Ⓒ Ⓓ Ⓔ
50 Ⓐ Ⓑ Ⓒ Ⓓ Ⓔ
51 Ⓐ Ⓑ Ⓒ Ⓓ Ⓔ
52 Ⓐ Ⓑ Ⓒ Ⓓ Ⓔ
53 Ⓐ Ⓑ Ⓒ Ⓓ Ⓔ
54 Ⓐ Ⓑ Ⓒ Ⓓ Ⓔ
55 Ⓐ Ⓑ Ⓒ Ⓓ Ⓔ
56 Ⓐ Ⓑ Ⓒ Ⓓ Ⓔ
57 Ⓐ Ⓑ Ⓒ Ⓓ Ⓔ
58 Ⓐ Ⓑ Ⓒ Ⓓ Ⓔ
59 Ⓐ Ⓑ Ⓒ Ⓓ Ⓔ
60 Ⓐ Ⓑ Ⓒ Ⓓ Ⓔ
61 Ⓐ Ⓑ Ⓒ Ⓓ Ⓔ
62 Ⓐ Ⓑ Ⓒ Ⓓ Ⓔ
63 Ⓐ Ⓑ Ⓒ Ⓓ Ⓔ
64 Ⓐ Ⓑ Ⓒ Ⓓ Ⓔ
65 Ⓐ Ⓑ Ⓒ Ⓓ Ⓔ
66 Ⓐ Ⓑ Ⓒ Ⓓ Ⓔ
67 Ⓐ Ⓑ Ⓒ Ⓓ Ⓔ
68 Ⓐ Ⓑ Ⓒ Ⓓ Ⓔ
69 Ⓐ Ⓑ Ⓒ Ⓓ Ⓔ
70 Ⓐ Ⓑ Ⓒ Ⓓ Ⓔ
71 Ⓐ Ⓑ Ⓒ Ⓓ Ⓔ
72 Ⓐ Ⓑ Ⓒ Ⓓ Ⓔ
73 Ⓐ Ⓑ Ⓒ Ⓓ Ⓔ
74 Ⓐ Ⓑ Ⓒ Ⓓ Ⓔ
75 Ⓐ Ⓑ Ⓒ Ⓓ Ⓔ
76 Ⓐ Ⓑ Ⓒ Ⓓ Ⓔ
77 Ⓐ Ⓑ Ⓒ Ⓓ Ⓔ
78 Ⓐ Ⓑ Ⓒ Ⓓ Ⓔ
79 Ⓐ Ⓑ Ⓒ Ⓓ Ⓔ
80 Ⓐ Ⓑ Ⓒ Ⓓ Ⓔ
81 Ⓐ Ⓑ Ⓒ Ⓓ Ⓔ
82 Ⓐ Ⓑ Ⓒ Ⓓ Ⓔ
83 Ⓐ Ⓑ Ⓒ Ⓓ Ⓔ
84 Ⓐ Ⓑ Ⓒ Ⓓ Ⓔ
85 Ⓐ Ⓑ Ⓒ Ⓓ Ⓔ
86 Ⓐ Ⓑ Ⓒ Ⓓ Ⓔ
87 Ⓐ Ⓑ Ⓒ Ⓓ Ⓔ
88 Ⓐ Ⓑ Ⓒ Ⓓ Ⓔ
89 Ⓐ Ⓑ Ⓒ Ⓓ Ⓔ
90 Ⓐ Ⓑ Ⓒ Ⓓ Ⓔ

91 Ⓐ Ⓑ Ⓒ Ⓓ Ⓔ
92 Ⓐ Ⓑ Ⓒ Ⓓ Ⓔ
93 Ⓐ Ⓑ Ⓒ Ⓓ Ⓔ
94 Ⓐ Ⓑ Ⓒ Ⓓ Ⓔ
95 Ⓐ Ⓑ Ⓒ Ⓓ Ⓔ
96 Ⓐ Ⓑ Ⓒ Ⓓ Ⓔ
97 Ⓐ Ⓑ Ⓒ Ⓓ Ⓔ
98 Ⓐ Ⓑ Ⓒ Ⓓ Ⓔ
99 Ⓐ Ⓑ Ⓒ Ⓓ Ⓔ
100 Ⓐ Ⓑ Ⓒ Ⓓ Ⓔ
101 Ⓐ Ⓑ Ⓒ Ⓓ Ⓔ
102 Ⓐ Ⓑ Ⓒ Ⓓ Ⓔ
103 Ⓐ Ⓑ Ⓒ Ⓓ Ⓔ
104 Ⓐ Ⓑ Ⓒ Ⓓ Ⓔ
105 Ⓐ Ⓑ Ⓒ Ⓓ Ⓔ
106 Ⓐ Ⓑ Ⓒ Ⓓ Ⓔ
107 Ⓐ Ⓑ Ⓒ Ⓓ Ⓔ
108 Ⓐ Ⓑ Ⓒ Ⓓ Ⓔ
109 Ⓐ Ⓑ Ⓒ Ⓓ Ⓔ
110 Ⓐ Ⓑ Ⓒ Ⓓ Ⓔ
111 Ⓐ Ⓑ Ⓒ Ⓓ Ⓔ
112 Ⓐ Ⓑ Ⓒ Ⓓ Ⓔ
113 Ⓐ Ⓑ Ⓒ Ⓓ Ⓔ
114 Ⓐ Ⓑ Ⓒ Ⓓ Ⓔ
115 Ⓐ Ⓑ Ⓒ Ⓓ Ⓔ
116 Ⓐ Ⓑ Ⓒ Ⓓ Ⓔ
117 Ⓐ Ⓑ Ⓒ Ⓓ Ⓔ
118 Ⓐ Ⓑ Ⓒ Ⓓ Ⓔ
119 Ⓐ Ⓑ Ⓒ Ⓓ Ⓔ
120 Ⓐ Ⓑ Ⓒ Ⓓ Ⓔ
121 Ⓐ Ⓑ Ⓒ Ⓓ Ⓔ
122 Ⓐ Ⓑ Ⓒ Ⓓ Ⓔ
123 Ⓐ Ⓑ Ⓒ Ⓓ Ⓔ
124 Ⓐ Ⓑ Ⓒ Ⓓ Ⓔ
125 Ⓐ Ⓑ Ⓒ Ⓓ Ⓔ
126 Ⓐ Ⓑ Ⓒ Ⓓ Ⓔ
127 Ⓐ Ⓑ Ⓒ Ⓓ Ⓔ
128 Ⓐ Ⓑ Ⓒ Ⓓ Ⓔ
129 Ⓐ Ⓑ Ⓒ Ⓓ Ⓔ
130 Ⓐ Ⓑ Ⓒ Ⓓ Ⓔ
131 Ⓐ Ⓑ Ⓒ Ⓓ Ⓔ
132 Ⓐ Ⓑ Ⓒ Ⓓ Ⓔ
133 Ⓐ Ⓑ Ⓒ Ⓓ Ⓔ
134 Ⓐ Ⓑ Ⓒ Ⓓ Ⓔ
135 Ⓐ Ⓑ Ⓒ Ⓓ Ⓔ

136 Ⓐ Ⓑ Ⓒ Ⓓ Ⓔ
137 Ⓐ Ⓑ Ⓒ Ⓓ Ⓔ
138 Ⓐ Ⓑ Ⓒ Ⓓ Ⓔ
139 Ⓐ Ⓑ Ⓒ Ⓓ Ⓔ
140 Ⓐ Ⓑ Ⓒ Ⓓ Ⓔ
141 Ⓐ Ⓑ Ⓒ Ⓓ Ⓔ
142 Ⓐ Ⓑ Ⓒ Ⓓ Ⓔ
143 Ⓐ Ⓑ Ⓒ Ⓓ Ⓔ
144 Ⓐ Ⓑ Ⓒ Ⓓ Ⓔ
145 Ⓐ Ⓑ Ⓒ Ⓓ Ⓔ
146 Ⓐ Ⓑ Ⓒ Ⓓ Ⓔ
147 Ⓐ Ⓑ Ⓒ Ⓓ Ⓔ
148 Ⓐ Ⓑ Ⓒ Ⓓ Ⓔ
149 Ⓐ Ⓑ Ⓒ Ⓓ Ⓔ
150 Ⓐ Ⓑ Ⓒ Ⓓ Ⓔ
151 Ⓐ Ⓑ Ⓒ Ⓓ Ⓔ
152 Ⓐ Ⓑ Ⓒ Ⓓ Ⓔ
153 Ⓐ Ⓑ Ⓒ Ⓓ Ⓔ
154 Ⓐ Ⓑ Ⓒ Ⓓ Ⓔ
155 Ⓐ Ⓑ Ⓒ Ⓓ Ⓔ
156 Ⓐ Ⓑ Ⓒ Ⓓ Ⓔ
157 Ⓐ Ⓑ Ⓒ Ⓓ Ⓔ
158 Ⓐ Ⓑ Ⓒ Ⓓ Ⓔ
159 Ⓐ Ⓑ Ⓒ Ⓓ Ⓔ
160 Ⓐ Ⓑ Ⓒ Ⓓ Ⓔ
161 Ⓐ Ⓑ Ⓒ Ⓓ Ⓔ
162 Ⓐ Ⓑ Ⓒ Ⓓ Ⓔ
163 Ⓐ Ⓑ Ⓒ Ⓓ Ⓔ
164 Ⓐ Ⓑ Ⓒ Ⓓ Ⓔ
165 Ⓐ Ⓑ Ⓒ Ⓓ Ⓔ
166 Ⓐ Ⓑ Ⓒ Ⓓ Ⓔ
167 Ⓐ Ⓑ Ⓒ Ⓓ Ⓔ
168 Ⓐ Ⓑ Ⓒ Ⓓ Ⓔ
169 Ⓐ Ⓑ Ⓒ Ⓓ Ⓔ
170 Ⓐ Ⓑ Ⓒ Ⓓ Ⓔ
171 Ⓐ Ⓑ Ⓒ Ⓓ Ⓔ
172 Ⓐ Ⓑ Ⓒ Ⓓ Ⓔ
173 Ⓐ Ⓑ Ⓒ Ⓓ Ⓔ
174 Ⓐ Ⓑ Ⓒ Ⓓ Ⓔ
175 Ⓐ Ⓑ Ⓒ Ⓓ Ⓔ
176 Ⓐ Ⓑ Ⓒ Ⓓ Ⓔ
177 Ⓐ Ⓑ Ⓒ Ⓓ Ⓔ
178 Ⓐ Ⓑ Ⓒ Ⓓ Ⓔ
179 Ⓐ Ⓑ Ⓒ Ⓓ Ⓔ
180 Ⓐ Ⓑ Ⓒ Ⓓ Ⓔ